Emotional Intelligence: An International Handbook

Emotional Intelligence
An International Handbook

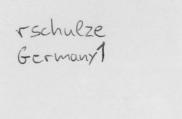

Edited by

Ralf Schulze
Richard D. Roberts

HOGREFE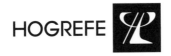

Library of Congress Cataloging-in-Publication Data
is available via the Library of Congress Marc Database under the
LC Control Number 2004114391

Library and Archives Canada Cataloguing in Publication

Emotional intelligence : an international handbook / Ralf Schulze, Richard D. Roberts (eds.).

Includes bibliographical references.
ISBN 0-88937-283-7

1. Emotional intelligence. I. Schulze, Ralf II. Roberts, Richard D.

BF576.E674 2004   152.4   C2004-906074-0

© 2005 by Hogrefe & Huber Publishers

PUBLISHING OFFICES
USA: Hogrefe & Huber Publishers, 875 Massachusetts Avenue, 7th Floor,
                Cambridge, MA 02139
                Phone (866) 823-4726, Fax (617) 354-6875; E-mail info@hhpub.com
EUROPE: Hogrefe & Huber Publishers, Rohnsweg 25, 37085 Göttingen, Germany
                Phone +49 551 49609-0, Fax +49 551 49609-88, E-mail hh@hhpub.com

SALES & DISTRIBUTION
USA: Hogrefe & Huber Publishers, Customer Services Department,
                30 Amberwood Parkway, Ashland, OH 44805
                Phone (800) 228-3749, Fax (419) 281-6883, E-mail custserv@hhpub.com
EUROPE: Hogrefe & Huber Publishers, Rohnsweg 25, 37085 Göttingen, Germany
                Phone +49 551 49609-0, Fax +49 551 49609-88, E-mail hh@hhpub.com

CORPORATE OFFICE
Hogrefe & Huber Publishers, Inc., 218 Main Street, Suite 485, Kirkland WA 98033

OTHER OFFICES
CANADA: Hogrefe & Huber Publishers, 1543 Bayview Avenue, Toronto, Ontario M4G 3B5
SWITZERLAND: Hogrefe & Huber Publishers, Länggass-Strasse 76, CH-3000 Bern 9

Hogrefe & Huber Publishers
Incorporated and registered in the State of Washington, USA, and in Göttingen, Lower Saxony,
Germany

Printed and bound in Germany
ISBN 0-88937-283-7

Foreword

The field of emotional intelligence (EI) has moved forward in dramatic ways since Jack Mayer and I published our first article on EI in 1990. In just a brief decade and a half, our state of knowledge has matured to the extent that an international handbook is now possible. And if we look back further, to the seminal and influential articles on social intelligence (even the ones doubting its existence), practical intelligence, and intrapersonal intelligence, we have clearly come further still. But now is not the time for complacency in EI research. Although we may have traveled a good ways down the road from those earlier days, it is only in recent years that there is an emerging consensus in the EI literature on definitions, best methods of measurement, and expectations for what EI should predict.

Perhaps what is most helpful about this handbook is that it very quickly does what many books and articles do not do: It clearly differentiates the genuinely scientific approach to EI from popularizations. In doing so, the chapters herein hold EI to the highest standard. Not only must EI have heuristic value, but it cannot be merely old wine in new bottles or an interesting idea impossible to operationalize. We have argued for some time that the most useful approach to EI is one that considers it a set of interrelated skills. In that sense, we define emotional intelligence as involving both the capacity to reason about emotions and to use emotions in order to assist reasoning. We believe EI includes abilities to identify emotions accurately in oneself and in other people, understand emotions and emotional language, manage emotions in oneself and in other people, and use emotions to facilitate cognitive activities and motivate adaptive behavior. These skills are ones that can be measured and that are not easily incorporated into definitions (and measures) of existing constructs such as social competence or personality.

The chapters in this handbook also place ideas about EI into the context of general theories and research pertaining to intelligence, emotion, and personality. This is more important than it might sound at first. One of the difficulties with popular ideas about EI is that characteristics of humans that are adaptive and desirable but have little to do with intelligence or emotion are sometimes classified as EI. These have included task persistence, zeal, optimism, good character, morality, and the like. It is important to consider what EI is but also what it is not. The most useful measures of EI should show only modest correlations with general intelligence and should be largely unassociated with standard measures of personality such as those mapping on to the "Big Five".

Couching EI—especially as measured—within conventional ideas about intelligence more generally, such as its overlap with social intelligence and whether EI is best thought of as fluid, crystallized, or both, is also characteristic of many of the chapters in this handbook, and these perspectives are quite helpful. In other writing, we have tried to argue that EI meets the traditional standards—more or less—for what it means for some construct to be an intelligence. At first we asked this question in order to be provocative. But over time, it has turned into a more serious line of inquiry that is very much assisted by the kind of discussion that can be found here. As one of the author teams suggests, the interpretation of research results is greatly benefited by definitional and theoretical coherence in this area. Relating EI to other similar-sounding kinds of intelligence also motivates greater clarity in describing what is unique to EI.

A part of this handbook is devoted to issues of measurement. And these are welcome discussions. Although we have preferred ability-based measures to self-report inventories, there is no gold-standard yet in this field, and all measurement approaches pose serious challenges. Self-report measures may be prone to self-aggrandizement and other reporting biases and may have little discriminant validity with respect to typical personality measures. Ability measures present the dilemma of how we define a "correct" or, at least, a better or more adaptive answer? Reference to consensual norms or the responses of experts are two approaches, but they also represent interesting conceptual questions: What if the masses tend to be misguided in this area? Who, exactly, should be considered an expert? Measurement issues are not going to be easily resolved, but like the editors of this volume, I agree that future approaches need to emphasize the assessment of emotion-related abilities in ongoing, fluid situations and not just draw upon crystallized emotional knowledge.

Perhaps some of the most exciting work—but also where clever ideas far outstrip available data—is in the application of EI to education, work, psychopathology, and physical health. Appropriate speculation about the potential utility of EI, as both theory and as a set of measurable constructs, is featured in the final set of chapters here. The possibilities seem limitless, and the imaginative uses of EI already observed in the field are encouraging.

One area still needing considerably more attention—and the lack of research in this area is especially obvious in an international handbook—concerns culture. Is EI a culture-bound construct? Certainly display rules for emotional expression are culturally specific (just compare how people behave at funerals in different parts of the world). But are the underlying skills involved in identifying, understanding, managing, and using emotion also different across cultures? We think, in general, that they are not, but we really do not know for sure. And how might knowledge of cultural differences (e.g., in which cultures is giving honest feedback to your boss about his terrible idea an adaptive behavior and in which is it maladaptive?) be incorporated in theories and measures of EI? These are questions still needing to be addressed.

Reading these chapters is very satisfying and not just because so many of the contributors are friends whose thoughts about emotional intelligence I have always respected. These are thoughtful commentaries that steer the field in the right direction. They guide us clearly with respect to what we need to do next. And they make it salient that globalization has contributed to great scientific strides forward in understanding EI.

PETER SALOVEY

YALE UNIVERSITY
NEW HAVEN, CT, USA

Preface

Emotional intelligence (EI) is a relatively recent addition to the set of psychological constructs that are the subject of scientific investigation. Although it can be argued that the roots of EI may be traced back to the start of the last century, the bulk of books, research, and peer-review publications exploring EI have appeared within the last 15 years. At the time of writing this preface, a literature search in the PsycINFO database indicated 700 or so publications using the term *emotional intelligence*, with only three publications appearing before 1990. However, EI has enjoyed a much more chequered history than these figures might, on first blush, suggest. Even though it is not easy to tell exactly how many of these publications are more a critique of the concept, rather than a constructive research effort, the ratio of critical commentary to empirical research appears remarkably high by available scientific standards.

The use of the term EI by mass media is even more recent. The speed with which the term *emotional intelligence* has been adopted and its accompanying enthusiasm by the general public is certainly remarkable. Arguably, not since Freud, has a psychological term had a comparable history of welcomed reception by laypeople, nor as wide-ranging influence on popular culture (witnessed by the fact that, among other things, books, toys, films, and even robots employ it as an advertising jingle). However, the number, strength, and veracity of supposedly scientifically founded claims associated with EI also appears unprecedented. For example, EI has variously been portrayed as the psychological factor *most* relevant for success in almost any field of application (i.e., in the home, workplace, and school). Claims of this sort simply lack scientific support, certainly on balance of available evidence.

As a result of this short (yet colorful) history, the concept of EI is associated with a relatively large literature, much controversy, and a remarkable tension between scientific and popular accounts. The editors of this book opine that this situation calls for focused, systematic research to clarify the issues, as well as more open dialogue between theoretical and applied researchers, on the one hand, and practitioners, on the other. We also feel that the field of EI is in need of diverse scientific approaches, rigorously examining the theoretical underpinnings of EI from multi-disciplinarian perspectives including intelligence research, the psychology of emotions, personality psychology, social psychology, psychometrics, and artificial intelligence. Practical implications for educational, organizational, and clinical contexts need also to be considered. To accomplish such an ambitious set of goals, while maintaining heterogeneity of perspectives and coping with the growing research demand, international research collaboration seems essential. It was the editors' intention, through invitations to each of the current contributors, to assemble a group of experts that would give this volume a truly international flavor.

A disclaimer appears in order before we provide a look ahead to the topics covered in the book. The editors consider themselves neither high priests nor gravediggers devoted to either elevating or burying the concept of EI. As paradoxical as it might seem, we try to be as dispassionate as possible about this emotion-laden concept and the discussion surrounding it. Theories, measurement approaches, and applications of EI deserve balanced scientific discourse in order to advance psychological research and applications, as well as to provide scientific background for informed discussions in the public forum. We hope that this edited volume contributes to this goal by providing scholarly presentations as described in the following paragraphs.

This edited book brings together experts from around the world to present their perspectives on the scientific status of EI. In five parts of the book, theories of EI, assessment approaches, and research on the antecedents and consequences in occupational, educational, and clinical settings are presented. In these contributions, empirical evidence supporting or contradicting common assumptions about the nature of EI, and its relationships with other psychological constructs, are highlighted. The book thereby offers a critical appraisal of the scientific status of EI.

Part I introduces basic ideas, concepts, and frames of reference for theories, measures, and applications of EI. The editors of the book and two distinguished scholars, Gerald Matthews and Moshe Zeidner, provide a brief introduction to these basic concepts. This chapter provides background from intelligence, individual differences, measurement, and emotions research, which allow non-experts, in particular, to follow arguments put forth over the duration of the volume.

In Part II, a range of theoretical approaches are presented, their strength and weaknesses are highlighted, and conclusions on the status of EI theories are drawn. Aljoscha Neubauer and Harald Freudenthaler (Chapter 2) begin this section by providing a review of the most prominent models of EI. This chapter represents an indispensable resource for those readers who have not been introduced to current models and controversies in the field. In the next chapter by David Schultz, Carroll Izard, and Jo Ann Abe, a different perspective is taken. The focus of this chapter lies on the connections between emotion systems and EI, and the latter's development, in particular. This chapter enables the reader to view the field from a different theoretical angle by highlighting the connection between EI and emotions research. Perhaps to the surprise of the uninitiated reader, most models of EI are more heavily influenced by intelligence, rather than emotions, research. Hence, Chapter 3 can be regarded as an addition and complement to most other chapters, which are geared towards individual differences approaches. Chapter 4 by Joseph Ciarrochi and Claire Godsell introduces a new theory for human suffering, upon which a framework of EI is based. As for the previous chapter dealing with emotions systems, the authors broaden the set of theoretical perspectives by describing an approach to EI from yet another research tradition.

Historically, the field of EI has important conceptual predecessors in intelligence research that are closely connected to theoretical components of EI. Social intelligence (SI) appears among the most important of these forerunners. Sue-Mee Kang, Jeanne Day, and Naomi Meara (Chapter 5) elaborate on relationships between EI and SI. The overlap between these two concepts is stressed both on a theoretical and empirical level. Kang, Day, and Meara highlight many reasons why these areas should be considered in close connection and point to future areas of research that deserve more detailed attention. The last chapter of Part II, by Elizabeth Austin and Donald Saklofske, discusses communalities and differences between EI, SI, and practical intelligence (PI). They bring these three concepts together, delineate conceptual and empirical differences, and present data to support the widely disputed assertion that EI is incrementally valid for certain criteria. The authors of Chapter 6 facilitate the comprehension of subtle differences between theoretical approaches to these intelligences, by providing both a schema and set of criteria to comparatively evaluate these concepts.

The chapters in Part III of the book are devoted to measurement of EI. Chapter 7, by Oliver Wilhelm, provides an overview of measurement models of EI, especially those approaches that conceptualize EI as an ability, rather than a personality, trait. Basic models are explicated throughout this chapter as the reader is simultaneously guided through many of the conceptual assumptions underlying available assessment procedures. A critical issue for EI measurement is thereafter discussed in Chapter 8 by Peter Legree, Joseph Psotka, Trueman Tremble, and Dennis Bourne. The authors present an elaborate rationale for one of the most widely used procedures to score test-takers responses on EI ability tests, namely consensus scoring. Since scoring examinee's test responses remains a vexing issue for objective forms of EI assessment, this chapter is remarkably important. It not only provides a rationale justifying the assignment of scores using a consensual approach but also provides data supporting the basic premises that these contributors put forth.

In Chapter 9, Juan Carlos Pérez, K. V. (Dino) Petrides, and Adrian Furnham give a concise overview of trait EI and provide a comprehensive list and classification of measures of this concept. They present the state-of-the-art approach to trait EI assessment, which designates the conceptual approach to EI as a personality characteristic. Part III concludes with a chapter by Susanne Weis and Heinz-Martin Süß. They report a facetted approach to the measurement of SI, with supporting empirical data for their hypothesized model. A feature of this chapter is the connection drawn, especially at the measurement level, between the areas of SI and EI research. It therefore provides an excellent synthesis of the communalities and differences highlighted in earlier chapters focusing on theory.

Part IV is devoted to applications of EI. In the first contribution to this section, Thomas Goetz, Anne Frenzel, Reinhard Pekrun, and Nathan Hall (Chapter 11) discuss the theoretical background, and application opportunities, of EI in the educational context. A theoretical model is put forward that positions EI in the context of learning and achievement. The authors highlight the significance of EI in this applied domain while drawing important research implications. In Chapter 12, Rebecca Abraham gives an overview of another domain where EI is widely applied: the workplace. The reader is introduced to basic tenets and findings from this field, where leadership, performance feedback, and organizational commitment are covered.

In Chapter 13, James Parker shows why EI is relevant for clinical applications and provides references to empirical research in support of his claims. One concept of central importance, discussed throughout this chapter, is alexithymia: a deficit in perceiving, understanding, and communicating emotional experiences. The concluding chapter to Part IV, by Elisabeth Engelberg and Lennart Sjöberg, links EI and interpersonal skills. In reviewing pertinent literature, it brings to the reader's attention the fact that EI is highly relevant for social interaction and personal relationships, as well as showing, through empirical data, how EI can be linked to such applied issues as faking in high-stakes testing.

Each of the various approaches, findings, and conclusions made by these contributors are integrated in the fifth, and final, part of the book. In Chapter 15, the editors team up again with Moshe Zeidner and Gerald Matthews to synthesize the results and conclusions of the various chapters and analyze what we have learned and what we may have missed from the preceding commentaries. Unresolved issues in scientific research, which might be the subject of future research efforts, are highlighted, with a view to providing an account of both the current and projected scientific status of EI.

We are much obliged to the chapter authors for their invaluable scientific contributions and their cooperation in making this book possible. We hope that these interesting and thought provoking ideas, concepts, and empirical applications of EI will prove to be insightful and advance the readers understanding and knowledge of this elusive construct and the many controversies surrounding it. We are also grateful to the following "heroic" (least in our eyes) persons who helped typeset this book with LATEX, provided valuable critical input, engaged in fruitful discussions, and/or otherwise kept our emotions from over-ruling our intelligence (and vice-versa): Niklas Ahn, Cristina Aicher, Blixa Bargeld, Lionel Benevides, King Buzzo, Alexander Freund, John Garcia, Michael Gira, Heiko Großmann, Julia Haubrich, Al Jourgensen, Nadine Kespe, Sabine Ludwig, Carolyn MacCann, Omar A. Rodriguez-Lopez, Matthew D. Roberts, Roudy Trouvé, Crazy Horse Weber, and Cedric Bixler Zavala.

RALF SCHULZE
RICHARD D. ROBERTS
MARCH 2005, PRINCETON, MÜNSTER, & SYDNEY

Contributors

ABE, JO ANN A. Psychology Department, Southern Connecticut State University, 501 Crescent Street, New Haven, CT 06515, USA;
EMail: abej1@southernct.edu

ABRAHAM, REBECCA Nova Southeastern University, Farquhar Center for Undergraduate Studies, 3301 College Avenue, Fort Lauderdale, FL 33314, USA;
EMail: abraham@polaris.acast.nova.edu

AUSTIN, ELIZABETH School of Philosophy, Psychology and Language Sciences, University of Edinburgh, 7 George Square, Edinburgh EH8 9JZ, UK;
EMail: elizabeth.austin@ed.ac.uk

BOURNE, DENNIS American Psychological Association–OEMA, 750 First Street, NE, Washington, DC 20002, USA;
EMail: dbourne@apa.org

CIARROCHI, JOSEPH Department of Psychology, University of Wollongong, Wollongong, New South Wales, Australia, 2522;
EMail: joec@uow.edu.au

DAY, JEANNE Department of Psychology, University of Notre Dame, 118 Haggar Hall, Notre Dame, IN 46556, USA;
EMail: jday@nd.edu

ENGELBERG, ELISABETH Center for Economic Psychology, Stockholm School of Economics, P.O. Box 6501, SE-113 83 Stockholm, Sweden;
EMail: Elisabeth.Engelberg@hhs.se

FRENZEL, ANNE C. Institute of Educational Psychology, University of Munich, Leopoldstrasse 13, D-80802 Munich, Germany;
EMail: zirngibl@edupsy.uni-muenchen.de

FREUDENTHALER, HERIBERT Institut für Psychologie, Abteilung Differentielle Psychologie, Karl-Franzens-Universität Graz, Universitätsplatz 2, A-8010 Graz, Austria;
EMail: freudent@email.kfunigraz.ac.at

FURNHAM, ADRIAN Dept of Psychology, University College London , 26 Bedford Way, London WC1H 0 AP, UK;
EMail: a.furnham@ucl.ac.uk

GODSELL, CLAIRE   Department of Psychology, University of Wollongong, Wollongong, New South Wales, Australia, 2522;
EMail: clg07@uow.edu.au

GOETZ, THOMAS   Institute of Educational Psychology, University of Munich, Leopoldstrasse 13, D-80802 Munich, Germany;
EMail: goetz@edupsy.uni-muenchen.de

HALL, NATHAN   Department of Psychology, University of Manitoba, Winnipeg, Manitoba R3T 2N2, Canada;
EMail: umhallnc@cc.UManitoba.CA

IZARD, CARROLL E.   Department of Psychology, University of Delaware, 200 Academy St 104, Newark, DE 19716-2577, USA;
EMail: izard@udel.edu

KANG, SUN-MEE   Department of Psychology, California State University, 18111 Nordhoff Street, Northridge, CA 91330-8255, USA;
EMail: skang@csun.edu

LEGREE, PETE   U.S. Army Research Institute, SARU (ATTN: TAPC-ARI-RS), 5001 Eisenhower Avenue, Alexandria, VA 22333 USA;
EMail: legree@ari.army.mil

MATTHEWS, GERALD   Department of Psychology, University of Cincinnati, PO BOX 210376, Cincinnati, OH 45221-0376, USA
EMail: matthegd@email.uc.edu

MEARA, NAOMI   Department of Psychology, University of Notre Dame, 118 Haggar Hall, Notre Dame, IN 46556, USA
EMail: Meara.1@nd.edu

NEUBAUER, ALJOSCHA C.   Institut für Psychologie, Abteilung Differentielle Psychologie, Karl-Franzens-Universität Graz, Universitätsplatz 2, A-8010 Graz, Austria;
EMail: aljoscha.neubauer@uni-graz.at

PARKER, JAMES   Department of Psychology, Otonabee College, Trent University, Peterborough, Ontario, K9J 7B8, Canada;
EMail: jparker@trentu.ca

PEKRUN, REINHARD   Institute of Educational Psychology, University of Munich, Leopoldstrasse 13, D-80802 Munich, Germany;
EMail: pekrun@edupsy.uni-muenchen.de

PÉREZ, JUAN CARLOS   Faculty of Education, UNED, Senda del Rey, 7 28040 Madrid, Spain;
EMail: jcperez@bec.uned.es

PETRIDES, K. V.   Institute of Education, University of London, 25 Woburn Square, London WC1H 0AA, UK;
EMail: k.petrides@ioe.ac.uk

PSOTKA, JOSEPH   U.S. Army Research Institute, SARU (ATTN: TAPC-ARI-RS), 5001 Eisenhower Avenue, Alexandria, VA 22333-5600, USA; EMail: psotka@ari.army.mil

SAKLOFSKE, DONALD   Educational Psychology and Special, Education, College of Education, University of Saskatchewan, Canada; EMail: don.saklofske@usask.ca

SCHULTZ, DAVID A.   Department of Psychology, University of Maryland – Baltimore County, 1000 Hilltop Circle, MP 330, Baltimore, MD 21250, USA; EMail: dschultz@umbc.edu

SJÖBERG, LENNART   Center for Economic Psychology, Stockholm School of Economics, P.O. Box 6501, SE-113 83 Stockholm, Sweden; EMail: le.sjberg@telia.com

SÜSS, HEINZ-MARTIN   Institut für Psychologie, Otto-von-Guericke-Universität, Postfach 4120, D-39016 Magdeburg, Germany; EMail: heinz-martin.suess@gse-w.uni-magdeburg.de

TREMBLE, TRUEMAN   U.S. Army Research Institute, SARU (ATTN: TAPC-ARI-RS), 5001 Eisenhower Avenue, Alexandria, VA 22333-5600, USA; EMail: tremble@ari.army.mil

WEIS, SUSANNE   Institut für Psychologie, Otto-von-Guericke-Universität, Postfach 4120, D-39016 Magdeburg, Germany; EMail: sweis@rumms.uni-mannheim.de

WILHELM, OLIVER   Institut für Psychologie, Humboldt-Universität Berlin, Rudower Chaussee 18, D-12489 Berlin, Germany; EMail: oliver.wilhelm@rz.hu-berlin.de

ZEIDNER, MOSHE   University of Haifa, School of Education, Mt. Carmel, 31999, Israel; EMail: Zeidner@research.haifa.ac.il

Contents

Part I

Introduction

1

Theory, Measurement, and Applications of Emotional Intelligence: Frames of Reference

Ralf Schulze
Educational Testing Service, USA
Westfälische Wilhelms-Universität Münster, Germany

Richard D. Roberts
Educational Testing Service, USA
University of Sydney, Australia

Moshe Zeidner
University of Haifa, Israel

Gerald Matthews
University of Cincinnati, USA

Summary

This chapter provides an introduction to theory, measurement, and applications of psychological constructs, with special reference to that set of concepts standing at the interface of emotional intelligence (EI) research. In particular, we provide the reader with a brief overview of the fields of intelligence, emotions, and personality research. We also discuss the importance of measurement in individual differences psychology and a subset of the methods that are often utilized by researchers working in this sub-discipline. Finally, we suggest the potential importance of EI in applied fields. Throughout these passages, we aim to establish the frames of reference for subsequent chapters in order to facilitate the reader's understanding of the many issues raised by contributors to this edited volume.

1.1   INTRODUCTION

Traditional approaches to cognitive assessment generally require the solution to an abstract problem (e.g., rotating an object in three-dimensional space) or some factual item that is important to the dominant culture (e.g., knowing the meaning of words), for which responses are scored as either right or wrong. Thus assessed, cognitive ability provides the single best psychological predictor of many real-life criteria. For example, meta-analyses have suggested that cognitive measures predict job and academic performance better than any other measured concept of psychological, sociological, or demographic significance (see, e.g., Schmidt & Hunter, 1998). However, while noteworthy, these relationships are actually constrained by rather modest limits. For example, even when cognitive tests are combined with other, well-established, psychological measures (e.g., personality, biographical data) and statistical corrections are made for a range of artifacts, validity coefficients for the prediction of real-life criteria seldom exceed .60 (e.g., Jensen, 1998; Matthews, Zeidner, & Roberts, 2002; Neisser et al., 1996). Moreover, cognitive constructs have often been criticized for being culturally and/or ethnically insensitive, ecologically questionable, and largely contrived. Findings from meta-analyses, along with attendant criticisms of cognitive tests, have spurred researchers to explore new psychological domains that might collectively raise the level of prediction while simultaneously addressing critical concerns.

In the current book, a range of specialists will argue that emotional intelligence (EI), along with two closely related constructs (i.e., social and practical intelligence) represent important psychological phenomena that have so far been given limited consideration by scientists working within this tradition. Broadly conceived, EI, which is discussed more often in the book than the other two constructs, represents a form of ability that processes and benefits from the emotional system (Matthews et al., 2002; Matthews, Roberts, & Zeidner, 2004; Mayer, Salovey, & Caruso, 2000). Of note, it may comprise an entire family of constructs that may be juxtaposed to concepts that derive from traditional approaches to the measurement of academic intelligence. In turn, each EI construct may add incremental validity (over and above cognitive abilities, as typically measured) to the prediction of real-life outcome variables, including physical health, academic performance, perceived quality of life, and psychological well-being.

In this opening chapter, we provide an overview of intelligence models, emotions theories, and a construct that has come to be closely related to EI because of the proliferation of self-report measures used to assess it: personality. We also explore various methods and techniques frequently used by scientists working in these fields. In the penultimate section we touch briefly on applied issues, before closing with some comments on how this chapter is to be viewed in the context of the entire volume.

1.2   HUMAN INTELLECTUAL ABILITIES

Scientific understanding of human abilities has gained much from the research of Carroll (1993), who summarized and integrated over 400 studies conducted within the factor analytic tradition (Roberts, Markham, Zeidner, & Matthews, 2005). Carroll's reanalysis of each data set led him to a model having three levels (or strata). On Stratum I lay primary mental abilities. On Stratum II are a variety of broad cognitive abilities also identified by Cattell, Horn, and associates in their theory of fluid and crystallized intelligence (e.g., Horn & Noll, 1994). Finally, on the third-stratum is a general intelligence factor. The importance of Carroll's concepts extends to educational interventions, public policy on testing, and sociological issues (see, e.g., Spearitt, 1996). It is also likely to guide theory and research in individual differences for some time (Roberts et al., 2005).

The uniqueness of Carroll's (1993) model is that virtually all models of cognitive abilities may be subsumed under its broad umbrella. In the passages that follow, we introduce each of these models, which contributors to this volume will variously refer to. Before leaving Carroll, it is perhaps appropriate to note that he did make suggestive comments of direct relevance to issues raised by contributors to this book (i.e., emotional, social, and practical intelligence). In particular, Carroll (1993) notes that there is evidence for a domain of behavioral knowledge, which is relatively independent from Stratum II constructs, certainly in some data sets. He also suggests that this domain requires more careful and systematic exploration than had been accomplished up to the time of his writing.

1.2.1   Structural Models of Intelligence

In the following subsections, we present a selection of prominent structural models of intelligence. They are all very closely related to a statistical technique called *factor analysis* that will not be explained in this chapter. For a deeper understanding of structural models of intelligence—and factor analysis, which many theories of EI draw upon—the reader is referred to Schulze (2005).

Psychometric g.   Perhaps the most famous theory of intelligence is that offered by Spearman (e.g., 1923) who proposed that there are two factors underlying mental test performance: a general factor (g) and specific factors (s). Specific factors are unique to performance on any cognitive test, whereas the general factor permeates performance on all intellectual tasks. As a consequence, Spearman postulated that g alone is of psychological significance. Individual differences in g are the result of differences in the magnitude of mental energy invested in any given task. It is worth noting that a strict g account of human intelligence would render the concept of EI quite problematic; by definition, EI requires the presence of at least one other intelligence (e.g., something we might call rational intelligence) for the qualifier (i.e., emotional) to have currency (Matthews et al., 2002). This notion is clearly inconsistent with a single-factor intelligence model.

Primary mental abilities.   In a significant departure from Spearman, Thurstone (e.g., 1938) proposed, and later provided supportive evidence for, primary mental abilities (PMAs), which collectively comprise intelligence. While originally finding thirteen such factors, Thurstone eventually settled on nine that he was both able to consistently validate and assign psychological labels. The PMAs so derived include: verbal comprehension, verbal fluency, number facility, spatial visualization, memory, inductive reasoning, deductive reasoning, practical problem reasoning, and perceptual speed. These factors are not ordered in any particular way and are thus of equal importance in detailing the structure of intelligent behavior (for this reason, Thurstone's model is sometimes called an *oligarchic theory*).

Structure-of-intellect model.   While the number of factors in Thurstone's theory is large, Guilford (e.g., 1967, 1988) took a more extreme view in positing that some 180 factors comprise intelligence. Accordingly, for Guilford, every mental task involves three aspects (also called *facets*): operation, content, and product. There are six kinds of operations in this model, five types of content, and six varieties of products. The *structure of intellect* has been symbolized as a rectangular prism composed of 180 ($6 \times 5 \times 6$) smaller prisms. Each dimension of this prism corresponds to one of the three ingredients (i.e., operation, content, and product) with each of the 180 possible combinations of these three categories forming even smaller rectangular prisms. An early appeal of this model was its ability to incorporate both creativity and social intelligence (what Guilford calls behavioral cognition [see, e.g., O'Sullivan & Guilford, 1975]) into its structure—psychological dimensions that few models of intelligence include. For this reason, the reader may note that several of the chapter authors refer to the structure-of-intellect model in their commentaries.

Gf-Gc theory.   Various critics bring into question each of the preceding theories highlighted above; for example, the number of PMAs has shown to exceed nine, though equally the data attest that there are considerably less than 180. Moreover, PMAs tend to cluster together, suggesting a hierarchical arrangement of factors. For this reason, contemporary focus has been given to hierarchical models of intelligence. In the most prominent of these—the theory of fluid (Gf) and crystallized (Gc) ability—there is considered to be enough structure among established PMAs to define several distinct types of intelligence. Empirical evidence, from several lines of inquiry, supports the distinctions between factors of this theory (e.g., Cattell, 1971; Horn & Noll, 1994; Roberts et al., 2005). Data have shown that these broad factors: (1) involve different underlying cognitive processes; (2) share different predictive validities; (3) are differentially sensitive to intervention; and (4) appear to be subject to different sets of learning and genetic influences.

The most compelling evidence for the distinctions between these constructs comes from factor analytic and developmental research. The main distinguishing feature between Gf and Gc is the amount of formal education and acculturation that is present either in the content of, or operations required during, tests used to measure these abilities. It is well established that Gf depends to a much smaller extent on formal education experiences than does Gc. Moreover, while Gc remains constant or improves slightly over the course of an individual's life span, Gf generally declines as a function of age. Besides Gf and Gc, evidence suggests the existence of broad visualization (Gv), broad auditory function (Ga), short-term acquisition and retrieval (SAR), tertiary storage and retrieval (TSR), and broad speediness (Gs). In isolation, each construct represents a broad organization of ability that involves mental processes, for which each factor is purported to have a neurophysiological counterpart.

1.2.2   Systems Theories of Intelligence

Two contemporary theorists—Gardner (1993) and Sternberg (1985)—have proposed intelligence models that attempt to be fairly encompassing in dealing with both the internal and external world of the human being. Because such theories view intelligence as a complex system, they are often referred to as *system models*, a point of departure used to demarcate them from the structural models covered above. Such systems models, in expanding the subject matter of intelligence research, include concepts that structural models would not necessarily view as intelligence. Perhaps because of their breadth, EI researchers often embrace systems theory accounts of intelligence more strongly than they do structural theories. For example, one will find no mention in Goleman (1995) of structural models of human cognitive abilities, although he cites Gardner's theory to support scientific evidence for EI quite frequently.

Multiple intelligences.   Gardner's (1993) theory of "multiple intelligences" derives from consideration of criteria, such as domains where extraordinary degrees of talent/giftedness are exemplified, deficits in brain-damaged individuals have been isolated, or there appears an evolutionary history and plausibility. In all, Gardner posits seven independent types of intelligence. These include: linguistic intelligence, spatial intelligence, logical-mathematical intelligence, musical intelligence, bodily-kinesthetic intelligence, intrapersonal intelligence, and interpersonal intelligence. The final two intelligences cover the individual's attempts to understand both their own and other people's behaviors, motives, and/or emotions. Clearly, both of these constructs are relevant to EI.

Triarchic theory.   Sternberg (1985) has also emphasized a departure from traditional conceptualizations, defining intelligence as "purposive adaptation to, and selection and shaping of, real-world environments relevant to one's life" (p. 45). By recourse to various analogies, Sternberg shows that academic intelligence, as assessed by psychometric tests, is imperfectly related to the ability to function intelligently in everyday life. On this basis, he goes "beyond IQ" to emphasize different aspects of intellectual functioning, prominent of which is practical intelligence (PI), a concept that contributors to this volume actually discuss in some detail. According to Sternberg, PI is especially dependent on acquired tacit knowledge, which is procedural rather than declarative, informal rather than formal, and generally learnt without explicit instruction. In short, tacit knowledge is reflected in knowing what to do in a given situation, and getting on and doing it. It occurs without ever necessarily being taught what to do, how to do it, or being able to articulate why you are doing it.

Practical, social, and emotional intelligence share a focus on acquired knowledge (declarative and procedural), flexible cognitive-retrieval mechanisms, and problem solving that does not lend itself to one correct solution. Recently, Hedlund and Sternberg (2000) argued that the main distinguishing feature between each concept lies in the content of the knowledge, and the types of problems, emphasized. Thus, "unlike many approaches to understanding social and emotional intelligence, the tacit-knowledge approach ... limits the definition of practical intelligence to cognitive ability (such as knowledge acquisition) rather than encompassing an array of individual differences variables" (Hedlund & Sternberg, 2000, p. 157). Elsewhere, we have suggested three categories of tacit knowledge that directly impinge upon EI: managing self, managing others, and managing tasks (Matthews et al., 2002).

Concluding thoughts on intelligence theories.   This brief foray into theories of intelligence suggests that the concept of EI has a richer history than many of its principal advocates often imply. Our commentary also suggests that paramount to the development of EI models should be how constructs comprising it align with intelligence models (whether they be structural or systems approaches). This issue raises many questions; for example, is EI really a new form of ability or can it be subsumed under one or more already existing constructs? Presently we know very little of how EI relates to broad cognitive abilities, or how EI relates to practical and social intelligence. Because these are important scientific issues, in several chapters that follow, contributors take up these issues in considerable detail.

1.3   EMOTIONS THEORY

In this section, we give the reader some background on consensus and controversies surrounding the study of emotions that contributors to this book will often draw upon, albeit sometimes implicitly. Our aim is to equip the reader with sufficient information to critically evaluate the status of EI models, measures, and applications discussed throughout the book for its correspondence with features outlined in the account of emotions theory that follows. Notably, this topic is often given a relatively minor role in accounts of EI, though underlying many of the approaches discussed in the current volume are issues highlighted throughout this section.

In particular, we will come to find that there are a range of EI theories. One reason for this state-of-affairs appears to be the fact that psychological theories of emotions result in several, incompatible approaches. Emotions have been related to a set of largely independent (i.e., modular) brain systems; to a central executive control system residing in the frontal cortex; to dimensions of sub-jective experience measured by questionnaires; and to information-processing routines for self-regulation. Indeed, from a scientific standpoint, the subjective nature of emotions constitutes a complex problem, which specialists are forced to grapple with. Although there are physical counterparts to emotions (e.g., facial expressions), they are primarily defined by labels attached to conscious awareness (e.g., feelings of sorrow). Psychological science has a materialist basis; hence it is enigmatic why any material object, including the brain, has the property of awareness (Matthews et al., 2002). The broad answer to this problem has been to construe emotions as corresponding to some underlying process or system, which can be described in materialist terms. Thus con-ceived, emotions might represent a type of learning, specific brain systems, properties of information-processing mechanisms, and so forth.

Researchers also differ in their conceptions of the correspondences between emotions and physical reality. A disconnect between theorists concerns the centrality of subjective experience. Biological theorists are inclined to down-play subjective emotion (see, e.g., Damasio, 1999; Panksepp, 1998). For them, emotion is (1) fundamentally a state of specific neural systems, (2) activated by motivationally significant stimuli, and (3) a construct difficult to observe. The activity of the system is expressed through various responses including auto-nomic nervous system activity, behaviors, and subjective feelings, which are conceptually distinct from emotions (Damasio, 1999). Conversely, emotions may be seen as a subset of conscious experience. This approach is identified with the operationalization of emotions through self-report measures. There is a large literature on the measurement of emotions and feeling states, which uses standard psychometric techniques to identify and validate dimensions of feeling (see Matthews et al., 2002).

Another disjuncture among emotions theories concerns how emotions inter-relate with cognition and motivation. Emotions are typically associated both with evaluations of personal significance and with motivations to act. For ex-ample, fear correlates with evaluations of personal threat and with the incli-nation to escape the feared object. Traditionally, emotion (subsumable under the superordinate category of *affect*), motivation (also referred to as *conation*), and cognition make up a three-fold classification used in many areas of psy-chology. Emotion thus represents a distinct system, separate from motivation and cognition, though interacting with them. Given separate domains, there are various conceptions of the inter-relationships between them. One view is that emotions are chained to motivations and cognitions (Plutchik, 1980);[1]

---

[1]It is interesting to note that most prominent social psychological theories of attitude–behavior relationships—for example, the theory of reasoned action and theory of planned behavior (see Schulze & Wittmann, 2003)—contain exactly such links as one of their cornerstones.

another is that emotions "combine motivational, cognitive, adaptational, and physiological processes into a single complex state that involves several levels of analysis" (Lazarus, 1991, p. 6). Viewed from this perspective, the feasibility of studying EI comes to depend on the way that a researcher assumes affect, conation, and cognition are linked.

Yet another disconnect among theories of emotions refers to the extent to which feeling states are free-floating in some specific interaction with the external environment. A distinction is often made between emotions and moods (e.g., Ortony, Clore, & Collins, 1988). An emotion is transient, tied to a particular stimulus (or event), and appears quite complex and differentiated because it reflects an individual's cognition of an event. Moods, by contrast, are more free-floating, need not refer to any particular object, and may persist longer than emotions. Moods also appear more easily reduced to a small set of basic dimensions. Much emotions theory explicitly suggests that emotions are grounded in specific interactions with the environment, a proposition that jars with the actual content of emotions measures, which often assess general feelings, rather than feelings about some event.

1.3.1   Issues in Conceptualizing Emotions

Singular or multiple?   Emotion may be defined as a high-level mental property (e.g., Lazarus, 1991) or as an attribute of physiological functioning (Damasio, 1999). Emotions may also be identified with parts of conscious experience, with latent systems whose state may be unconscious, or with psychophysiological systems of causal relevance. Currently, there is little that is definitive in the empirical evidence to decide which definition is the most efficacious. Generally, it is useful to apply a three-level cognitive science framework (Pylyshyn, 1999). Depending on the research context, it appears useful to see emotion as (1) a property of brain systems, (2) information-processing, or, (3) abstracted personal meanings that do not map onto neural or cognitive architectures in any simple way (Matthews et al., 2002).

It appears useful to distinguish two families of emotions theory. The first type of theory starts with a conceptual analysis of emotion, distinguishing emotions from other aspects of mental life and attempting to delineate defining features of general and specific emotions. Different instances of theory differ in fundamental issues relating to definition, consciousness, and causality. The common theme, however, is that emotion is a construct, which may be distinguished from the subjective feelings that are one of several manifest expressions of emotions. This approach may be grounded in terms of models from cognitive psychology (Lazarus, 1991) and neuroscience (Panksepp, 1998) or in philosophical-conceptual terms (Ben Ze'ev, 2000). The implications of the model may be explored empirically through studies of various types of response, including self-report, overt behavior, and physiology.

The second type of theory starts with an operationalization of affect, for example, through a questionnaire that measures the intensity of feelings (e.g., happiness). Research then moves to explain the causes and consequences of the constructs indexed by the questionnaire. Mood research is usually of this kind. For example, Thayer (e.g., 1996) has identified energy and tension as two fundamental aspects of mood, and explored their antecedents and psychological consequences in empirical studies. However, there is reason to suspect that more specific emotions can be grounded in the same operational approach and some authors have developed self-report emotions measures (see, e.g., Izard, Libero, Putnam, & Haynes, 1993). Whereas the first approach addresses emotion primarily as a universal psychological quality, the second is especially concerned with individual differences: why people are more or less emotional than one another and the behavioral consequences of this individual variation.

Central or peripheral?   Another key conceptual issue in the study of emotions is the extent that emotions are based in physical reality. If emotions reflect the workings of a material system, it is important to identify the system (or systems) concerned. Historically, debates surrounding the source of emotions have addressed whether emotions are centrally or peripherally generated (i.e., whether emotions are a direct reflection of some brain system, or whether emotions are constructed from cues provided by peripheral signals; e.g., sweaty palms). The centralist view gains credence from evidence that emotions are influenced by damage to certain brain areas and by drugs such as cocaine, heroin, and ecstasy that affect neurochemistry. Support for the peripheralist position comes from studies showing that, within limits, the way humans experience bodily activity seems to feed into emotional experience (e.g., Parkinson, 1996).

Centralist thinking can be traced to Darwin's view that emotions are concomitants of physiological reactions (e.g., crying when sad evolved from the response of the eye to a foreign object). Darwin's studies of emotions aimed to show that responses were innate, appearing reflexively to trigger stimuli of evolutionary significance. Contemporary studies emphasize specific brain systems believed to have evolved to handle stimuli that are motivationally significant. These include evolutionarily relatively primitive systems, such as the amygdala, and areas in the frontal lobes of the cerebral cortex, whose development is an especially human characteristic. Evidence for the role of these systems in emotion comes from studies of experimentally-induced brain lesions in animals, and accidental damage in humans (e.g., Damasio, 1999). Links between the various neurotransmitters of the brain and emotions are also important (Panksepp, 1998). The general position is that various brain systems analyze incoming stimuli for reward, punishment, and other motivational implications, and concurrently produce both emotions and physiological change.

The peripheralist perspective, although acknowledging biology, emphasizes a more psychological basis for emotions. Its progenitor, William James, saw emotion as a form of perception based on awareness of signals from peripheral bodily organs, such as the heart and skin. Common sense suggests that if we encounter a snake, this event causes a state of fear, and so we run away. James turned common sense around by proposing that the threatening event elicits pre-organized bodily reactions. These include physiological responses such as accelerated heart rate, shallow breathing, and the like, and behaviors, such as flight. Awareness of these responses is emotion: running away precedes fear. While peripheralism fell out of favor in the first part of the twentieth century, the principal legacy of this tradition remains focused interest in the role of feedback from physiological systems in producing emotions (e.g., Damasio, 1999). Moreover, James' work, by referring to individual's personal idiosyncrasies, memories, and associations as shaping emotions, introduced psychology into emotions research.

Cognitive theories.   The cognitive revolution, which commenced in the early 1960s, led to a fundamental reexamination of almost every domain of psychological enquiry. The idea that mental processes can be compared to symbolic computer programs allowed theorists to detach emotions from biological substrate. Studies conducted under this framework found that both subjective distress and autonomic nervous system responses (e.g., skin conductance) depended on the orientation given to the individual and their strategy for dealing with distressing material (e.g., Lazarus & Alfert, 1964). The cognitive approach was also bolstered by clinical studies suggesting that emotional disorders derived from maladaptive cognitions (e.g., Beck, 1967). These theorists pointed to the role of faulty knowledge and styles of interpreting events as the underlying source of cognitions.

Cognitive theories can be expressed in both centralist and peripheralist terms. They are centralist to the extent that information-processing directly outputs emotional states. For example, Simon (1967) suggests that emotions reflect interruptions to ongoing behavior; it has also been argued that appraisal processes generate emotions. Evaluating an event as a threat (consciously or unconsciously) may necessarily produce anxiety, and anxiety may require a prior threat appraisal. As with biological centralism, this concept of emotions suggests that there exists a concomitant, central (cognitive) process. However, there is not necessarily any simple one-to-one mapping between specific cognitions and emotions. Averill (1980), for example, makes an important distinction between pre-reflective and reflective experience. Pre-reflective awareness is the raw stuff of experience, generated, presumably, by unconscious analysis of events, and common to animals and humans. Reflective experience refers to the subsequent, meaning-based reconceptualization of experience. Extending this line of reasoning, transactional theories (e.g., Lazarus, 1991) see emotions as an index of some abstracted personal meaning. Specific information-processing routines, such as a threat appraisal, may feed into the personal meaning, but do not rigidly determine it. Instead, the emotion reflects a construction of meaning based on the various cues provided by analysis of the eliciting event.

Functions of emotions.   Following on from the legacy left by Darwin, evolutionary psychology views emotions as resulting from natural selection, operating around the Pleistocene epoch, when our species separated from its lower primate precursors. Hence, we might expect that emotions will sometimes conflict with adaptation to modern cultures and technology. In many countries, spiders are non-existent (or trivial) sources of threat, so phobic responses to house spiders will simply be disruptive, however adaptive they might have been in earlier environments. Other adaptive challenges such as handling conflict with other people and seeking a mate may not have changed so much, with emotions playing the same roles as in prehistory.

If emotions are adaptive, then that specific emotion has, through natural selection and/or learning, the function of promoting some desired outcome. However, it is also clear that emotions may have a range of consequences, some unintended. We might distinguish direct and indirect consequences of emotions. A direct consequence would reflect the adaptive purpose of the emotion, such as, in the case of fear, a mobilization for flight (a biological preparedness), or readiness to compete in a high stakes examination (a culturally-influenced acquired personal meaning). An indirect consequence would be an outcome unrelated to adaptive function, such as the distraction that may result from anxiety, or the health problems that may follow from chronic stress.

1.3.2   Issues in Measuring Emotions

Dimensions of emotions.   Normal scientific practice implies a good operationalization of emotions, that is, reliable and valid scales that represent a focus for research linking emotions scales to causes and consequences. In fact, dimensional approaches to emotions have been surprisingly controversial, reflecting a rift between conceptually-driven and data-driven theories. For example, Lazarus (1991) argues that providing dimensions to emotions obscures the distinctive relational themes to which each emotion relates. According to this view, emotions are seen as discrete states, rather than points in a multidimensional continuum, although the strength of the emotion may vary continuously. However, both categorical and dimensional approaches raise a vital issue: the differentiation of emotions. People experience different emotions such as sadness and joy, shame and pride, perhaps reflecting a few basic underlying emotions just as the color spectrum is based on three primary colors (Plutchik, 1980).

Categories of basic emotions.   For this reason, many of the principal theories of emotions attempt to draw up lists of basic emotions on rational grounds, with the aim of distinguishing qualitatively different categories of emotions corresponding to fundamental adaptive functions. Modern approaches distinguish emotions that (1) are cross-culturally universal, (2) may be found in higher animals, and (3) correspond to some evolutionary challenge. Plutchik (1980) claims that fear, anger, joy, sadness, acceptance, disgust, anticipation, and surprise are primary emotions that are associated with characteristic stimulus events, inferred cognitions, behaviors, and adaptive effects. Ekman (e.g., 1993), on the basis of universal facial expressions, picks out happiness, fear, surprise, anger, distress, disgust, and contempt. He also cautions, however, that there may be other basic emotions that do not have a unique facial signal (e.g., contentment). Panksepp's (1998) list is based on discrimination of mammalian brain systems for fear, rage, expectancy (behavioral facilitation), and systems for more complex social behaviors such as maternal nurturance.

We could compile many other lists from the corpus of research in this field, but their general style is relatively similar. Although the distinctions between emotions seem sensible, and categorization of some kind is essential, basic emotions have notable problems (see Ben Ze'ev, 2000, for a conceptual critique). In particular:

1. Different theorists disagree on the criteria for deciding what is basic. What appears basic may differ depending on whether we look at brain systems, at facial expressions, or at personal meanings of emotions.

2. Most basic emotions systems emphasize evolved functionality; emotions correspond to specific adaptive tasks linked to evolutionary challenges. Unfortunately, there is no definitive way of deciding what constitutes these key adaptive challenges.

3. It is unclear that there is any simple mapping between emotions and adaptive challenges. For example, joy may be felt in situations involving escape from danger, friendship, nurturance, and personal accomplishment.

4. It is unclear whether some emotions are primary, and others are secondary, perhaps being blends of primaries (Panksepp, 1998). Panksepp (1998), for example, downgrades the status of both low-level, reflex-like responses such as startle and disgust, and higher sentiments found only as subjective human states.

Dimensions of mood and affect.   An alternative perspective investigates the structure of emotional experience in empirical data using a dimensional approach to operationalize affect. Techniques such as factor analysis may indicate how many dimensions need to be differentiated in order to account for covariation in emotions indicators. Strictly speaking, this research usually addresses mood rather than emotions; it is easier to measure feeling states persisting for a few minutes than it is to measure transient states closely tied to changing external events. Various methods, some quite sophisticated psychophysically, have been used in mood assessment (Matthews et al., 2002). There are reliable and valid questionnaires for many emotions/mood states (e.g., Spielberger, Sydeman, Owen, & Marsh, 1999). Also widely used are adjective checklists, on which people rate how well mood descriptors (e.g., tense, tired) apply to their current feelings (e.g., Thayer, 1989).

Most researchers agree that there are only a few dimensions of mood (e.g., Thayer, 1989). In contrast to basic emotions, these dimensions are bipolar, contrasting opposite qualities, such as a continuum of states from energetic to languid. The structure may be as simple as two dimensions: one for positive affects and one for negative affects (Watson & Clark, 1992). Thayer (1989, 1996) offers a similar scheme for self-report arousal distinguishing energetic arousal (vigor vs. tiredness) and tense arousal (nervousness vs. calmness). Dimensional models of this kind have proved very useful for organizing empirical data on the biological and cognitive antecedents of mood, and on their psychological consequences (Thayer, 1989).

Studies of mood are challenging to most basic emotions models. On the one hand, they highlight dimensions that basic emotions theories neglect, such as the energy-tiredness continuum. On the other hand, they suggest that some distinctions are too fine-grained to represent people's actual experience. Fear, anger, and unhappiness may be conceptually distinct, but in actual fact, they tend to co-occur. Anger, for example, is experientially different from other negative emotions, but aversive events often provoke both anger and sadness (Berkowitz, 1993). Clark and Watson (1991) show that the correlation between anxiety and depression measures is often as high as those between alternate measures of anxiety or of depression. Notwithstanding, possible explanations for the mismatch between concepts and data include:

1. Basic emotions research misses an essential level of organization of human feeling states, in terms of two or three dimensions of mood or basic affect. It follows that there is no simple isomorphism between dimensions of basic affect and the more differentiated categories of emotions evident in brain systems, facial expressions, and personal meaning.

2. There may be isomorphism between moods and underlying systems. (Watson & Clark, 1992), for example, relate positive and negative affect to brain systems for reward and punishment, implying that these systems are more basic than the multiple systems identified by Panksepp (1998) and others.

A reasonable solution to such difficulties is to identify a small number of dimensions of basic affects that contribute to both mood and emotions states. Conventional scales seem to do a good job of measuring these affects and the empirical literature shows how these basic affects fit with psychological functioning (see Matthews, Deary, & Whiteman, 2003, for a review). Within the universe of affect, there may be continuous rather than discrete differentiation, such as temporal persistence, intensity, and accessibility to consciousness. Thus construed, mood and emotion might be better seen as rather loosely defined terms that signal the extent of explicit linkage of the feeling state to precipitating events.

Concluding thoughts on emotions theories.   The complexities evidenced in emotions theories have implications for developing theory and measures of EI, as well as determining the efficacy of applications in real-life settings. For example, if developing a measure of emotional perception—a core component in many EI approaches—should one attempt to incorporate dimensions of mood, or basic categories of emotions, and if so, which model? If an intervention is developed, can it really be successful if emotions are primarily a function of neurons and neurochemistry? This brief exposition also suggests that the most

comprehensive theories of EI will minimally attempt to address neurophysiological, information-processing, and adaptive functions. If nothing else, these
passages should also serve to highlight that more popular claims for the EI
construct should be treated with circumspection: understanding the nature of
emotions is clearly a complex scientific enterprize.

1.4   TRAIT MODELS OF PERSONALITY

Personality traits may be defined as stable, dispositional characteristics that influence behavior across a variety of different situations (e.g., sensation-seeking;
see Matthews et al., 2003, for a review). They are typically distinguished from
abilities as representing styles of behavior, rather than efficiency of performance output. Some authors (e.g., Wechsler, 1958) have used *personality* as
a broad umbrella term to cover both intelligence and qualitative styles of behavior, though this approach is certainly not viewed as mainstream.

The scientific study of traits began in the early years of the twentieth century, and has been preoccupied with two questions. The first issue is how
many different traits should be distinguished from one another. Answers to
this question have ranged from two to more than thirty. However, there are
now signs of some limited consensus on the dimensional structure of personality. As with ability theory, trait psychologists typically adopt higher-
order models, with a level of 20–30 relatively narrow primary factors supporting a super-ordinate level of broader secondary factors or super-factors. The
dominant view is that there are five robust super-factors: Extraversion, Neuroticism, Conscientiousness, Agreeableness, and Openness (Costa & McCrae,
1992; Goldberg, 1993; De Raad, 2000).

The second issue is the theoretical basis for traits: what underlying processes
are responsible for individual differences in personal characteristics? The dominant paradigm for studying this issue has been neuroscience models, reflecting the influence of DNA on personality. Eysenck (1967) proposed that traits
were controlled by individual differences in the excitability of key brain systems. Extraversion, for example, was thought to relate to a circuit controlling
arousability of the cerebral cortex in response to stimuli. There is an extensive
psychophysiological literature that provides partial support for such hypotheses (Matthews & Gilliland, 1999). In recent years, there has been growing interest in cognitive psychological accounts of personality traits, which may be related to individual differences in processing and evaluating events, and choice
of action (e.g., Matthews, Schwean, Campbell, Saklofske, & Mohamed, 2000).

The Big Five.   The Big Five or Five Factor Model (FFM) is that model of personality that almost all of the authors contributing to the present book refer.
Indeed, McCrae and John (1992) suggest that researchers "adopt the working
hypothesis that the five-factor model of personality is essentially correct in its
representation of the structure of traits and to proceed to its implications for
personality theory and its applications throughout psychology" (p. 176). While

there are alternative models of personality, notably Eysenck's (e.g., 1992) three-factor model (which discriminates Extraversion, Neuroticism, and Psychoticism), there is some convergence between different models and near-universal consensus on Extraversion and Neuroticism as basic personality dimensions (Zuckerman, 1998). Consequently, we will use the FFM as the basis for discussing trait models of personality, acknowledging that other conceptions also have merit.

The Big Five may be summarized thus:

- *Extraversion (E)* includes dimensions of sociability, liveliness, and talkativeness. This construct has at its core whether the individual likes to be alone (introversion) or with others (extraversion), and whether they are vigorous and energetic (introverts tend to be less so than extraverts).

- *Neuroticism (N)* contrasts people described as emotional, anxious, and highly-strung (neuroticism), with those seen as unemotional, calm, and comfortable with themselves (emotional stability).

- *Agreeableness (A)* is a dimension best perceived as interpersonal in its manifestation, containing aspects of sympathy, compassion, and generosity (as for the other personality factors, individuals have these qualities to greater or lesser extent).

- *Conscientiousness (C)* includes achievement striving, organization, scrupulousness, and responsibility.

- *Openness to new experiences (O)* includes willingness to entertain novel ideas and unconventional values. Openness is also the trait most related to cognitive intelligence, correlating around $r = .30$ with crystallized intelligence (Ackerman & Heggestad, 1997).

Despite several accounts that are critical of some aspects of the FFM (e.g., Block, 1995; Eysenck, 1992), various lines of converging evidence support its scientific credibility. These include:

1. Analyses of personality-descriptive words, in English (and other languages), which suggest that the domain of personality descriptors are almost completely accounted for by five robust factors (e.g., Goldberg, 1993). In short, the Big Five Factors appear to be embedded in natural language.

2. Factor analytic studies of well-established personality questionnaires, either in isolation or when combined, frequently demonstrate the five factors at the item level (e.g., McCrae & Costa, 1995).

3. The five factors relate to psychologically meaningful constructs that emerge from various approaches to studying personality (i.e., genetic research, experimental studies, longitudinal designs, biological studies, and so forth).

4. The five factors appear universal in that, it is claimed that they appear in all cultures (although debate continues on how closely personality models correspond to one another cross-culturally [e.g., De Raad, 2000]).

5. The five factors provide added value in that they predict a variety of characteristics over and above the trait itself. For example, knowing that a person is extraverted tells us not just that she is lively and sociable, but also predicts her vocational interests, her risk of various mental disorders, and her performance on laboratory tasks.

The psychological processes underlying the Big Five is also receiving increasing attention, although there is much more evidence relating to extraversion and neuroticism than to the remaining three factors. Generally these traits appear to be comprised of multiple processes, represented at different levels of abstraction including individual differences in (1) neural function, (2) information-processing, and (3) high-level cognitions of personal meaning (Matthews, 1997). For example, extraversion-introversion relates to (1) arousability of the neocortex and subcortical reward systems, (2) information-processing routines influencing attention, memory, and language use, and (3) a tendency to evaluate situations as challenging, and calling for direct action. The different component processes associated with a trait may be seen as supporting a common adaptation; handling demanding social environments in the case of extraversion (see, e.g., Matthews, 1997).

Concluding thoughts on theories of personality.   As for intelligence, this brief account of trait approaches to personality should suggest to the reader that demonstrating the extent that personality is independent of EI is an important research topic. The Big Five personality factors variously contain elements of sociability (both E and A), require dealing with the personal value of emotions (N), managing one's behavior (C), or thinking about one's private life (O); all of which find parallels in popular approaches to defining EI (e.g., Goleman, 1995). As we shall see, this too then is a topic that many of the contributors will frequently have recourse to address.

1.5   METHODOLOGICAL ISSUES

Almost any published empirical study in the area of EI draws on mathematical-statistical methods to analyze its data. This section is intended to provide a rough guide to facilitate the distillation of useful information from the results of such analyses, as reported in the chapters of this book. It is written for those readers who do not possess elaborate background knowledge on methodological concepts, terminology and procedures, and for those who feel in need of a refresher. Our treatment is, of course, very simplified and cursory due to the limited space that can be devoted to these topics. Hence, readers are encouraged to additionally consult the pertinent literature we refer to in the passages that follow.

Before we begin, consider the following scenario: You are surfing the world wide web, looking for interesting internet sites on EI. After a short time, you find a "Test yourself" website. On the pages of this website you find a test claiming to measure EI. You decide to take the test and are required to respond to a series of questions like "I am known for making other people happy" and "I talk a lot about my feelings" on a graded response scale from "strongly disagree" to "strongly agree". After receiving your result (which enthusiastically points out your very high EI), you begin to wonder if this test measures anything psychologically meaningful and what the idea behind designing such a test might be. For the moment, you assume the test does measure EI (the result is just too good to believe). Now you wonder about the quality of this alleged EI test. More specifically, you are interested in the precision to which your EI score can be estimated with this assessment procedure. You also ask yourself whether it was really your EI that determined your responses or rather some other characteristic that the assessment procedure is not supposed to measure (e.g., your extraversion or even your inclination to give responses that are socially desirable). Questions of this type, pertaining to the concepts behind, and the quality of, psychological assessment are the subject of this section. They are often discussed under the headings of reliability (precision) and validity (relation of the variable of interest to responses). The following subsections provide more details on these (and other terms) that are required for a basic understanding of psychological assessment.

1.5.1   Psychological Assessment: Key Terms and Concepts

Two of the most fundamental questions raised in this book relevant to the assessment[2] of EI are whether EI exists at all as a meaningful psychological characteristic of humans, and if so, how can it be measured. For the example given above, the answers to these questions that might be given by the authors of the questionnaire are: It is assumed that EI exists, it can be measured, and a self-report approach to assessment is obviously the appropriate procedure.

As will become evident throughout the current book, the answer to the first question (i.e., the existence of EI) is a contentious issue in the scientific literature; something you probably have suspected after finishing reading the review of emotions theory. We will not address this question here, preferring instead to leave this issue to the chapter authors. The same is true for a description of the many different assessment procedures, purportedly measuring EI, and which of these might be most appropriate for this purpose. However, to introduce concepts and key terms in psychological measurement we have to presume that there are answers to these questions. We simply assume, for example, that the first question can be answered affirmatively. With regards to the second question (i.e., how EI might be measured), we recognize that there are many different ways. We use self-report as an example, mainly because of its simplicity, and focus on concepts relevant to the evaluation of existing assessment procedures.

---

[2]We use the terms *assessment* and *measurement* rather loosely and interchangeably in this chapter. For an overview and in-depth treatment of measurement approaches and concepts as well as test theories fundamental for psychological measurement, see, for example, Hambleton, Robin, and Xing (2000); Lord and Novick (1968); McDonald (1999); Michell (1990).

Latent variables.   As a first step, we make the following widely adopted assumptions about EI: a) it is a characteristic that varies across humans (i.e., it is a variable), b) it is not directly observable with available assessment procedures (i.e., it is a latent variable), but they allow for inferences about EI, and c) persons with different EI differ to a certain degree and this can be expressed numerically (i.e., it is a quantitative latent variable). Whereas point a) and c) might be intuitively plausible assumptions in the context of assessment, the status of EI as a latent variable requires some additional comments (for general discussions of this topic, see Bollen, 2002; Borsboom, Mellenbergh, & van Heerden, 2003).

An important implication of conceptualizing EI as a latent variable is that items of an EI questionnaire, for example, are considered to be *indicators* of EI. As a latent variable, EI is assumed to determine the responses to an appropriate set of indicators. Any given set of indicators can be more or less appropriate depending on the extent to which responses are determined by the latent variable EI, but a set of indicators does not define what EI is. This means that proponents of self-report assessment approaches assume that agreement with statements (as given above) are a consequence of a person's high EI. Correspondingly, disagreement would be indicative of low EI. In other words, observed responses are assumed to correlate with EI. If the correlation is strong, then an indicator can be considered to be good, because it closely reflects, or is very informative concerning, the underlying latent variable. If EI only weakly determines the responses, then the correlation is also weak. Furthermore, if EI is a determinant common to a set of indicators, then all of the indicators should correlate depending on their strength of relationship with the common cause (i.e., EI).

Correlations.   What does it mean to state that a correlation between two variables is strong? A correlation is numerically expressed as the correlation coefficient, which is symbolized by r. It has a clear definition, intensely studied distributional properties, and a clear (technical) interpretation (see, e.g., Hotelling, 1953; Schulze, 2004). For present purposes, the following interpretative aid should suffice. The correlation coefficient can take on any value in the interval $[-1, 1]$. Three values in this interval are especially important as anchors for interpretation. The minimum and maximum (-1 and 1) represent what can be called "perfect" correlations. That is, the relationship between two variables is such that the relative position of values for one variable maps onto the relative position of values in the other. The difference in interpretation between a positive and negative correlation is that, for the former, high values for one variable are associated with high values in the other. For the latter, high values for one variable are associated with low values in the other. If, for example, the correlation between two EI self-report indicators was $r = 1$, then strong agreement for one indicator would imply strong agreement in the other as well. For the case of $r = -1$, strong agreement for one indicator would imply strong disagreement for the other. This happens, for example, when one of two self-report indicators is negatively worded (e.g., "I can never tell when someone is sad"). Another important value for interpretations is $r = 0$. This value indicates the absence of a linear relationship between two variables, that is, knowing the value for one of the variables does not allow any prediction for the value of the other variable. The correlation coefficient is extremely important to understand in assessing the efficacy of EI research, since in almost all empirical studies correlations are reported.

Constructs and factors.   Before more details are provided concerning concepts and indices for the quality of measures, a comment concerning the use of the terms construct and factor appears in order. Although we can not discuss the many methodological subtleties associated with these two terms, the reader should be aware of the fact that the terms construct, the name of the variable of interest (e.g., EI), factor, and latent variable are often used interchangeably in the literature. This bears certain problems (see, e.g., Borsboom & Mellenbergh, 2002) and blurs the distinction of theoretical terms (constructs and their names) and mathematical-statistical entities (latent variables, factors) that are intended to correspond to theoretical terms to a certain degree. In fact, the issue of this correspondence is at the very heart of the problem of validity, to be addressed in the next subsection. Hence, the reader is advised to bear such a distinction in mind, but to be prepared for use of the terms as synonyms.

Criteria for the evaluation of measurement procedures include their objectivity, reliability, and validity. The first criterion refers to the extent to which results depend on the situation in which assessment takes place, the dependency of the scoring procedure on the person (or device) who (which) translates responses into scores, and the dependency of the score interpretation on the person who arrives at them. Ideally, if none of these dependencies exists, then objectivity is said to be given. The other two criteria of test evaluation are detailed below.

1.5.2   Reliability

According to the definition of classical test theory (see, e.g., Lord & Novick, 1968), reliability is a property of a test that expresses the proportion of observed score variability between respondents that can be attributed to their latent variable scores. If an observed variable (e.g., the sum of responses to a set of items) correlates perfectly with a latent variable (e.g., EI), then the proportion of observed variability attributable to the latent variable is 100%, no error of measurement is present, and therefore the precision of measurement (reliability) is perfect. Of course, this is an unrealistic, extreme, case. Nevertheless, it illustrates the basic concept and, at least partly, enables an interpretation of reliability estimates reported in empirical studies.

There are many ways to estimate reliability (see, e.g. McDonald, 1999), but the range of possible numerical results is the same for all of them. Although technically possible, negative values are not acceptable for any reliability estimate, because reliability is conceptualized as a proportion. Hence, the lowest value for reliability is 0. The case of perfect reliability is ordinarily not expressed as a percentage (as above) but directly as a proportion. Thus, the maximum reliability is 1. Values between zero and one indicate the degree of precision, or reliability. There is no consensus among researchers on a generally accepted threshold value that leads to the conclusion that a measure is reliable. However, for EI research, inspection of the literature seems to indicate that values of .70 or larger are considered as satisfactory by most researchers.

The most often used reliability estimate to be found in EI research is probably Cronbach's α (Cronbach, 1951). Although there are many interpretational issues associated with this coefficient (Cortina, 1993), the general guidelines for interpretation given above apply to this specific coefficient as well.

1.5.3   Validity and Validation

There is much debate in the methodological literature on what test validity actually is (cf. Cronbach, 1988; Lord & Novick, 1968; Messick, 1995). We present a conceptualization that at least partly goes back to the seminal paper by Cronbach and Meehl (1955) and that is widely adopted in the literature as well as in the chapters of this book.[3] Additionally, we find it reasonable to make a distinction between test validity and validation, where the former is a property of a test and the latter designates the process of collecting evidence on test validity (see Borsboom, Mellenbergh, & van Heerden, 2004).

There are different forms of validity: content validity, concurrent or predictive validity, and construct validity. Content validity is said to be given when the test content is a representative sample of the target domain of behaviors. Concurrent validity refers to the association (most often measured by the correlation coefficient) of test results with certain criteria that occur or exist simultaneously to the test situation, whereas predictive validity refers to the association with criteria that occur in the future (e.g., prediction of future academic success with an EI measure). Of course, the choice of criteria is the most critical aspect for this type of validity and has to be theoretically justified.

Lastly, construct validity is closely associated with procedures to develop and test scientific theories (Cronbach & Meehl, 1955). It can not be expressed as a single coefficient, but rather is connected to the analysis of a whole network of associations between the test of interest and other tests, which are supposed to measure different constructs. Theoretical assumptions about these associations have to be available when inspecting such a network and are taken into account to assess the conformity of observed results (i.e., many correlations between several measures) with theoretical assumptions as an indicator of construct validity. It should be noted, however, that there are many more scientific activities, even examination of content and predictive validity, which are sup-

---

[3]Note that it deviates from the latest unified conceptualization presented in the Standards for Educational and Psychological Testing (American Educational Research Association, American Psychological Association, & National Council on Measurement in Education, 1999), where validity is defined as "The degree to which accumulated evidence and theory support specific interpretations of test scores entailed by proposed uses of a test" (p. 184).

posed to inform an assessment of the construct validity of a measure (Cronbach & Meehl, 1955). Nevertheless, assessment of the so-called convergent and discriminant validity of a measure is among the most important activities of construct validation.

Convergent validity is said to be given when theory states that some constructs are related (but not identical) with one another (e.g., EI and other forms of intelligence) and corresponding correlations between test scores at the observational level are in accordance with such statements. Discriminant validity is said to be given when correlations between measures reflect the theoretical assumption of non-related constructs (e.g., EI and extraversion). In this case, correlations of zero between tests should be observed to assign discriminant validity. A systematic way of analyzing entire matrices of correlations and testing the fit of theoretical statements about the relations between constructs, on the one hand, and with relations between tests at the observational level, on the other, is validation with multitrait multimethod (MTMM) matrices (Campbell & Fiske, 1959). Advances in the statistical literature (see, e.g., Schmitt & Stults, 1986) have led to the application of sophisticated analysis techniques, not envisioned by Campbell and Fiske (1959), which can be found in this book. Readers not familiar with the required statistical background can nevertheless profit from inspecting these results when bearing in mind the overall purpose of such analyses as briefly sketched in the present chapter.

In sum, the process of establishing a high quality measure that is reliable and valid involves a larger number of effortful activities (for an EI related overview, see, e.g., Matthews et al., 2002; Matthews, Emo, Zeidner, & Roberts, in press). It is highly unlikely that for any of the currently available public, and free, EI tests on the internet, evidence of the qualities described above is available. Hence, if you find yourself asking the types of questions described at the beginning of this section, there is likely to be no definitive answer to them. In fact, as will be evidenced by the content of the chapters of this book, even in the scientific literature evidence is still in the process of being collected, and to date there are not as many high quality measures of EI available as we might wish.

1.6   GENERAL DESIGN AND ANALYSIS ISSUES

Most studies in the field of EI research use so-called correlational designs. As its name implies, the correlation coefficient plays a central role in this methodology. It also refers to so-called *observational studies*, where phenomena of interest are only observed and no purposeful manipulation of them is implemented. This type of design is often contrasted to experimental research, where manipulation is a defining feature. However, it might be argued that this distinction is too strict and has a far too strong influence on thinking about design and analysis, which is deeply rooted in the history of psychological research (Cronbach, 1957, 1975). Nevertheless, what is important to bear in mind, is that experimental designs clearly do have their virtues over correlational designs with respect to inferences about causal relationships. Thus, the reader is advised to be critical when confronted with causal inferences on the basis of results from correlational studies. It should also be borne in mind that the simple fact of carrying out an experiment is not sufficient to draw causal inferences (see Shadish, Cook, & Campbell, 2002).

The main analysis strategy in the literature is to compute correlations (see above) and use multiple regression analysis (see Draper & Smith, 1998). The latter goes beyond correlations in that variables are categorized into those that predict (also called *independent variables*) and the one that is predicted (also called criterion or *dependent variable*). Among the most often focused statistics in regression analysis is the coefficient of determination (symbolized by R^2), which represents the proportion of observed variance explained in the criterion by a set of predictors. When examining a set of predictors, it is often of interest whether an additional predictor (e.g., EI) does add a significant portion of variance explained in the criterion (e.g., academic success). This is assessed by the difference between R^2 without the additional predictor and R^2 with the predictor. This strategy is of importance and often used in EI research in the context of assessing the so-called incremental predictive validity of a predictor. The incremental (i.e., added) predictive validity is simply the difference between the two coefficients of determination.

Finally, it should be mentioned that in a regression model, the regression coefficients are frequently a basis for interpreting the results. These coefficients are weights attached to the predictors. Especially in their standardized form, they are often interpreted as "measures of variable importance" or as if they were correlations. Except for some special cases, rarely given in individual differences research, such interpretations are at least problematic and often are plainly wrong (see Holling & Schulze, 2004). When predictors are intercorrelated, interpretation of regression weights is an intricate subject. The reader is referred to the pertinent literature (e.g., Draper & Smith, 1998) for clarification of this issue.

1.7   APPLICATIONS OF EMOTIONAL INTELLIGENCE

Before closing, a comment on applied applications, which is also a major focus of the current volume, would appear in order. For many, a central element underlying EI is the impetus to improve psychological functioning in real life. Individuals may enjoy richer, more fulfilling, lives if they have better awareness and control of their own emotions, and those of others. Organizations benefit from the increased productivity, satisfaction, teamwork, and organizational commitment of emotionally intelligent persons. Society, in general, gains from alleviation of problems that may result from poor emotion-management skills, such as violent crime, drug abuse, and some forms of mental illness. And in the education context, inculcating self-awareness, self-control, conflict resolution, empathy, and cooperation might not only create better citizens (Goleman, 1995), but also impact considerably on academic achievement.

As in the case of theory, there is a considerable body of scientific knowledge that is not always adequately acknowledged by proponents of EI. Clinical psychology offers a range of therapeutic techniques for improved emotion-management, especially in the fields of anxiety, stress, and mood disorders. Occupational psychology offers life-skills coaching, stress management techniques, and training programs for motivational enrichment. Dealing with the emotional problems of students has been a central part of school psychology since its inception. Again, as you read through the chapters you must confront an important question: Can EI add to these efforts? We preface this open question with two possibilities (see also Matthews et al., 2002). First, *emotional dysregulation* may define a specific set of problems that have not been sufficiently recognized in existing practice. Second, practitioners in applied fields may have been improving EI without necessarily realizing it. If so, an explicit understanding of EI as a focus for real-world interventions may improve existing practice and suggest new techniques for hitherto intractable problems.

1.8 CONCLUDING COMMENTS

We trust that this brief overview of these vast fields of psychological enquiry has left the reader with a set of critical tools to evaluate each of the chapters that follow. Equally, we trust that you may choose to explore them in more depth, since we could easily have written a book length treatment on any of these topics. Hopefully, each overview should have given you a sense of the many issues that need to be resolved in developing a scientifically sound program of research into understanding the nature of EI, should it actually exist.

Author Note

The ideas expressed in this manuscript are those of the authors and not necessarily of ETS. While both of the first two authors are currently at ETS, they would like to acknowledge the support of both Sydney University and the Westfälische Wilhelms-Universität Münster where they first conceptualized the idea of this volume (and ensuing chapters), and remain affiliated.

REFERENCES

Ackerman, P. L., & Heggestad, E. D. (1997). Intelligence, personality, and interests: Evidence for overlapping traits. *Psychological Bulletin, 121,* 219–245.

American Educational Research Association, American Psychological Association, & National Council on Measurement in Education. (1999). *Standards for educational and psychological testing.* Washington, DC: American Educational Research Association.

Averill, J. R. (1980). A constructivist view of emotion. In R. Plutchik & H. Kellerman (Eds.), *Emotion: Theory, research, and experience. Vol. 1. Theories of emotion* (pp. 305–339). San Diego, CA: Academic Press.

Beck, A. T. (1967). *Depression: Causes and treatment.* Philadelphia: University of Pennsylvania Press.

Ben Ze'ev, A. (2000). *The subtlety of emotions.* Cambridge, MA: MIT Press.

Berkowitz, L. (1993). *Aggression: Its causes, consequences, and control.* New York: McGraw-Hill.

Block, J. (1995). A contrarian view of the five-factor approach to personality description. *Psychological Bulletin, 117,* 187–215.

Bollen, K. A. (2002). Latent variables in psychology and the social sciences. *Annual Review of Psychology, 53,* 605–634.

Borsboom, D., & Mellenbergh, G. J. (2002). True scores, latent variables, and constructs: A comment on Schmidt and Hunter. *Intelligence, 30,* 505–514.

Borsboom, D., Mellenbergh, G. J., & van Heerden, J. (2003). The theoretical status of latent variables. *Psychological Review, 110,* 203–219.

Borsboom, D., Mellenbergh, G. J., & van Heerden, J. (2004). The concept of validity. *Psychological Review, 111,* 1061–1071.

Campbell, D. T., & Fiske, D. W. (1959). Convergent and discriminant validation by the multitrait- multimethod matrix. *Psychological Bulletin, 56,* 81–105.

Carroll, J. B. (1993). *Human cognitive abilities: A survey of factor-analytic studies.* New York: Cambridge University Press.

Cattell, R. B. (1971). *Abilities: Their structure, growth, and action.* Boston: Houghton Mifflin.

Clark, L. A., & Watson, D. (1991). Tripartite model of anxiety and depression: Psychometric evidence and taxonomic implications. *Journal of Abnormal Psychology, 100,* 316–336.

Cortina, J. M. (1993). What is coefficient alpha? An examination of theory and applications. *Journal of Applied Psychology, 78,* 98–104.

Costa, P. T., Jr., & McCrae, R. R. (1992). Normal personality assessment in clinical practice: The NEO Personality Inventory. *Psychological Assessment, 4,* 5–13.

Cronbach, L. J. (1951). Coefficient alpha and the internal structure of tests. *Psychometrika, 16,* 297–335.

Cronbach, L. J. (1957). The two disciplines of scientific psychology. *American Psychologist, 12,* 671–684.

Cronbach, L. J. (1975). Beyond the two disciplines of scientific psychology. *American Psychologist, 30,* 116-127.

Cronbach, L. J. (1988). Five perspectives on the validity argument. In H. Wainer & H. I. Braun (Eds.), *Test validity* (pp. 3–17). Hillsdale, NJ: Lawrence Erlbaum.

Cronbach, L. J., & Meehl, P. E. (1955). Construct validity in psychological tests. *Psychological Bulletin, 52,* 281–303.

Damasio, A. R. (1999). *The feeling of what happens: Body and emotion in the making of consciousness.* San Diego, CA: Harcourt.

De Raad, B. (2000). *The big five personality factors: The psycholexical approach to personality.* Kirkland, WA: Hogrefe & Huber.

Draper, N. R., & Smith, H. (1998). *Applied regression analysis* (3rd ed.). New York: John Wiley.

Ekman, P. (1993). Facial expression and emotion. *American Psychologist, 48,* 384–389.

Eysenck, H.-J. (1967). *The biological basis of personality*. Springfield, IL: Thomas.

Eysenck, H.-J. (1992). Four ways five factors are not basic. *Personality and Individual Differences, 13*, 667–673.

Gardner, H. (1993). *Frames of mind: The theory of multiple intelligences* (2nd ed.). New York: Basic Books.

Goldberg, L. R. (1993). The structure of phenotypic personality traits. *American Psychologist, 48*, 26–34.

Goleman, D. (1995). *Emotional intelligence: Why it can matter more than IQ*. New York: Bantam Books.

Guilford, J. P. (1967). *The nature of human intelligence*. New York: McGraw-Hill.

Guilford, J. P. (1988). Some changes in the structure-of-intellect model. *Educational and Psychological Measurement, 48*, 1–4.

Hambleton, R. K., Robin, F., & Xing, D. (2000). Item response models for the analysis of educational and psychological test data. In H. E. A. Tinsley & S. D. Brown (Eds.), *Handbook of applied multivariate statistics and mathematical modeling*. San Diego, CA: Academic Press.

Hedlund, J., & Sternberg, R. J. (2000). Too many intelligences? Integrating social, emotional and practical intelligence. In R. Bar-On & J. D. A. Parker (Eds.), *The handbook of emotional intelligence: Theory, development, assessment, and application at home, school, and in the workplace* (pp. 136–167). San Francisco: Jossey-Bass.

Holling, H., & Schulze, R. (2004). Statistische Modelle und Auswertungsverfahren in der Organisationspsychologie [Statistical models and ananlysis procedures in organizational psychology]. In H. Schuler (Ed.), *Enzyklopädie der Psychologie. Organisationspsychologie 1—Grundlagen und Personalpsychologie* (pp. 75–129). Göttingen: Hogrefe.

Horn, J. L., & Noll, J. (1994). A system for understanding cognitive capabilities: A theory and the evidence on which it is based. In D. K. Detterman (Ed.), *Current topics in human intelligence: Volume IV* (pp. 151–203). New York: Springer.

Hotelling, H. (1953). New light on the correlation coeffcient and its transforms. *Journal of the Royal Statistical Society, Series B, 15*, 193–232.

Izard, C. E., Libero, D. Z., Putnam, P., & Haynes, O. M. (1993). Stability of emotion experiences and their relations to traits of personality. *Journal of Personality and Social Psychology, 65*, 847–860.

Jensen, A. R. (1998). *The g factor*. Westport, CT: Praeger Publishers.

Lazarus, R. S. (1991). *Emotion and adaptation*. New York: Oxford University Press.

Lazarus, R. S., & Alfert, E. (1964). Short-circuiting of threat by experimentally altering cognitive appraisal. *Journal of Abnormal and Social Psychology, 65*, 195–205.

Lord, F. M., & Novick, M. R. (1968). *Statistical theories of mental test scores*. Reading, MA: Addison-Wesley.

Matthews, G. (1997). Extraversion, emotion and performance: A cognitive-adaptive model. In G. Matthews (Ed.), *Cognitive science perspectives on personality and emotion* (pp. 339–442). Amsterdam: Elsevier.

Matthews, G., Deary, I. J., & Whiteman, M. C. (2003). *Personality traits* (2nd ed.). Cambridge, UK: Cambridge University Press.

Matthews, G., Emo, A., Zeidner, M., & Roberts, R. D. (in press). What is thing called "emotional intelligence"? In K. R. Murphy (Ed.), *The EI bandwagon: The struggle between science and marketing for the soul of emotional intelligence.* Mahwah, NJ: Lawrence Erlbaum.

Matthews, G., & Gilliland, K. (1999). The personality theories of H. J. Eysenck and J. A. Gray: A comparative review. *Personality and Individual Differences, 26,* 583–626.

Matthews, G., Roberts, R. D., & Zeidner, M. (2004). Seven myths about emotional intelligence. *Psychological Inquiry, 15,* 179–196.

Matthews, G., Schwean, V. L., Campbell, S. E., Saklofske, D. H., & Mohamed, A. A. R. (2000). Personality, self-regulation and adaptation: A cognitive-social framework. In M. Boekarts, P. R. Pintrich, & M. Zeidner (Eds.), *Handbook of self-regulation* (pp. 171–207). New York: Academic Press.

Matthews, G., Zeidner, M., & Roberts, R. D. (2002). *Emotional intelligence: Science and myth.* Cambridge, MA: MIT Press.

Mayer, J. D., Salovey, P., & Caruso, D. R. (2000). Models of emotional intelligence. In R. J. Sternberg (Ed.), *Handbook of intelligence* (pp. 396–420). New York: Cambridge University Press.

McCrae, R. R., & Costa, P. T., Jr. (1995). Positive and negative valence within the five-factor model. *Journal of Research in Personality, 29,* 443–460.

McCrae, R. R., & John, O. P. (1992). An introduction to the five-factor model and its applications. *Journal of Personality, 60,* 175–215.

McDonald, R. P. (1999). *Test theory: A unified treatment.* Mahwah, NJ: Lawrence Erlbaum.

Messick, S. (1995). Validity of psychological assessment: Validation of inferences from persons' responses and performances as scientific inquiry into score meaning. *American Psychologist, 50,* 741–749.

Michell, J. (1990). *An introduction to the logic of psychological measurement.* Mahwah, NJ: Lawrence Erlbaum.

Neisser, U., Boodoo, G., Bouchard, T. J., Jr., Boykin, A. W., Brody, N., Ceci, S. J., et al. (1996). Intelligence: Knowns and unknowns. *American Psychologist, 51,* 77–101.

Ortony, A., Clore, G., & Collins, A. (1988). *The cognitive structure of emotion.* New York: Cambrige University Press.

O'Sullivan, M., & Guilford, J. P. (1975). Six factors of behavioral cognition: Understanding other people. *Journal of Educational Measurement, 12,* 255–271.

Panksepp, J. (1998). *Affective neuroscience: The foundations of human and animal emotions.* New York: Oxford University Press.

Parkinson, B. (1996). Emotions are social. *British Journal of Psychology, 87,* 663–683.

Plutchik, R. (1980). A general psychoevolutionary theory of emotion. In R. Plutchik & H. Kellerman (Eds.), *Emotion: Theory, research and experience. Vol. 1. Theories of emotion* (pp. 3–33). San Diego, CA: Academic Press.

Pylyshyn, Z. W. (1999). What's in your mind? In E. Lepore & Z. W. Pylyshyn (Eds.), *What is cognitive science?* (pp. 1–25). Malden, MA: Blackwell.

Roberts, R. D., Markham, P. M., Zeidner, M., & Matthews, G. (2005). Assessing intelligence: Past, present, and future. In O. Wilhelm & R. W. Engle (Eds.), *Understanding and measuring intelligence* (pp. 333–360). Thousand Oaks, CA: Sage.

Schmidt, F. L., & Hunter, J. E. (1998). The validity and utility of selection methods in personnel psychology: Practical and theoretical implications of 85 years of research findings. *Psychological Bulletin, 124,* 262–274.

Schmitt, N., & Stults, D. M. (1986). Methodology review: Analysis of multitrait-multimethod matrices. *Applied Psychological Measurement, 10*, 1–22.

Schulze, R. (2004). *Meta-analysis: A comparison of approaches.* Seattle, WA: Hogrefe & Huber.

Schulze, R. (2005). Modeling structures of intelligence. In O. Wilhelm & R. W. Engle (Eds.), *Understanding and measuring intelligence* (pp. 241–263). Thousand Oaks, CA: Sage.

Schulze, R., & Wittmann, W. W. (2003). On the moderating effect of the principle of compatibility and multidimensionality of beliefs: A meta-analysis of the theory of reasoned action and the theory of planned behavior. In R. Schulze, H. Holling, & D. Böhning (Eds.), *Meta-analysis: New developments and applications in medical and social sciences.* Seattle, WA: Hogrefe & Huber Publishers.

Shadish, W. R., Jr., Cook, T. D., & Campbell, D. T. (2002). *Experimental and quasi-experimental designs for generalized causal inference.* Boston, MA: Houghton Mifflin.

Simon, H. A. (1967). Motivational and emotional controls of cognition. *Psychological Review, 74,* 29–39.

Spearitt, D. (1996). Carroll's model of cognitive abilities: Educational implications. *International Journal of Educational Research, 25,* 107–197.

Spearman, C. (1923). *The nature of intelligence and the principles of cognition.* London: MacMillan.

Spielberger, C. D., Sydeman, S. J., Owen, A. E., & Marsh, B. J. (1999). Measuring anxiety and anger with the State-Trait Anxiety Inventory (STAI) and the State-Trait Anger Expression Inventory (STAXI). In M. E. Maruish (Ed.), *The use of psychological testing for treatment planning and outcomes assessment* (2nd ed., pp. 993–1021). Mahwah, NJ: Lawrence Erlbaum.

Sternberg, R. J. (1985). *Beyond IQ: A triarchic theory of human intelligence.* New York: Cambridge University Press.

Thayer, R. E. (1989). *The biopsychology of mood and arousal.* New York: Oxford University Press.

Thayer, R. E. (1996). *The origin of everyday moods: Managing energy, tension, and stress.* New York: Oxford University Press.

Thurstone, L. L. (1938). *Primary mental abilities.* Chicago: University of Chicago Press.

Watson, D., & Clark, L. A. (1992). On traits and temperament. General and specific factors of emotional experience and their relation to the five-factor model. *Journal of Personality, 60,* 441–476.

Wechsler, D. (1958). *The measurement and appraisal of adult intelligence* (4th ed.). Baltimore: Williams & Wilkins.

Zuckerman, M. (1998). Psychobiological theories of personality. In D. F. Barone, M. Hersen, & V. B. Van Hasselt (Eds.), *Advanced personality* (pp. 123–154). New York: Plenum Press.

2

Models of Emotional Intelligence

Aljoscha C. Neubauer
H. Harald Freudenthaler
Institute of Psychology
University of Graz, Austria

Summary

Stimulated by Daniel Goleman's bestseller, the concept of Emotional Intelligence (EI) has become enormously popular in recent years. Originally formulated by Peter Salovey and John Mayer in 1990, three major components of EI were postulated: appraisal and expression of emotion, regulation of emotions, and utilization of emotions (with further subdivisions of each of these branches). Seven years later these authors presented a modified version of EI and the first performance test (i.e., Multifactor Emotional Intelligence Scale, MEIS). Models and measures provided by Mayer and colleagues are hitherto the only published *ability models* of EI. In the present review of EI models these are contrasted with more recently developed mixed models of EI (like Bar-On's) and the trait EI concept (developed by Petrides and Furnham). The term *mixed* describes the fact that EI is viewed as a collection of (partially already well-known) abilities and non-ability traits. In addition to elaborating conceptual differences between EI models, fundamental differences regarding measurement approaches are demonstrated. Finally, critical issues regarding the status of ability and mixed models are discussed.

2.1   INTRODUCTION

Human intelligence is among the most frequently studied constructs in the field of individual differences. The sound theoretical foundation and empirically demonstrated usefulness of cognitive ability tests are well documented (e.g., Schmidt & Hunter, 1998). However, some researchers argue that the IQ is a rather narrow concept. From this perspective it is suggested that while cognitive intelligence is a potent predictor of educational and professional success, it is nonetheless an imperfect predictor of successful functioning in everyday life (Brody, 1992). According to this viewpoint, this functioning relies not simply on cognitive intelligence but rather on the relatively new (and emerging) construct of emotional intelligence (EI).

Historically, at least part of this suggestion may be traced to Daniel Goleman who, in 1995, published *Emotional Intelligence: Why it Can Matter More Than IQ*. This book became a bestseller in many countries. It also generated enormous popular interest, typified by a plethora of popular books, magazine and newspaper articles, comic strips, and even the occasional talk show program. In Goleman's rather simplistic view, EI is much more important than cognitive intelligence. Since classical IQ scores explain only about 20% of success in life, Goleman argues that a significant proportion of the rest should be determined by EI. Although Goleman's claims are based on a priori assumptions rather than empirical data, it nonetheless seems plausible that EI might have incremental validity beyond cognitive intelligence and personality. Although the "raw" science in Goleman's book is sparse, it served to spark increased scientific study of EI. Recently, numerous studies on the conceptualization, operationalization, validity, and utility of EI have emerged in the peer-reviewed scientific literature and in a range of academic and quasi-academic books.

However, rather than a consensus of opinion on what EI is, several alternative models of EI have been proposed (e.g., Bar-On, 1997; Cooper & Sawaf, 1997; Goleman, 1995; Mayer & Salovey, 1997; Salovey & Mayer, 1990; Weisinger, 1998). These models can be classified into two fairly distinct groups, that is, *ability models* and *mixed models* (see Mayer, Salovey, & Caruso, 2000a, 2000b; cf. also Freudenthaler & Neubauer, 2001). With the exception of Mayer and Salovey's ability model, existing conceptualizations of EI are mixed, and so expand the meaning of this construct by explicitly incorporating a wide range of personality characteristics. However, ability versus mixed models of EI not only vary considerably regarding the (scope of) conceptualizations but also with respect to the proposed instruments used to measure EI. Thus, mixed models rely on self-report measures of EI, while the ability model centers on performance-based measures of emotional abilities.

In this chapter, Salovey and Mayer's (1990) original model of emotional intelligence (referred to as EI90), Mayer and Salovey's (1997) modified ability model of emotional intelligence (referred to as EI97), and Bar-On's (1997) non-cognitive mixed model of emotional (and social) intelligence are reviewed. Moreover, two approaches within the organizational context (i.e., Boyatzis, Goleman, & Rhee, 2000; Dulewicz & Higgs, 2000) are briefly described to broaden the analysis of the conceptual underpinnings of EI. Notably, other EI models, such as those mentioned above (e.g., Goleman, Cooper & Sawaf, and Weisinger) have evoked little commentary in the scientific literature. Consequently, these models shall be dealt with only in passing, though the reader interested in exploring them further may consult the previously cited sources (see also Table 9.3 on Page 196f. in Chapter 9 by Pérez, Petrides, & Furnham).

2.2 SALOVEY AND MAYER'S (1990) ORIGINAL MODEL OF EMOTIONAL INTELLIGENCE

The question of the relationship between intelligence and emotion is a long-lasting and controversial topic at the societal as well as the scientific level (see Mayer, 2002; Mayer et al., 2000a). In 1990, Peter Salovey and John Mayer drew together the existing psychological literature on general contributions of emotion and emotionality to personality and suggested a new concept of how to synthesize the two psychological concepts of intelligence and emotion. They proposed the first published, formal concept of EI as a guiding framework for the integration of an exciting but scattered body of research on individual differences in the capacity to *process*, and to *adapt to*, emotional information.

According to this framework, the main details of which are represented in Figure 2.1, EI comprises three conceptually related mental processes involving emotional information. These processes are: (a) the appraisal and expression of emotion, (b) the regulation or control of emotion, and (c) the utilization of emotion in adaptive ways. As can be ascertained from Figure 2.1, two branches are further subdivided into *self* and *other*. Thus, Salovey and Mayer distinguish between the two perspectives of perceiving and regulating one's own emotions or the emotions of another person. In the lower branch (appraisal and expression) the self and other perspective are further subdivided according to a content factor, that is, a verbal versus a nonverbal domain. The model seeks to incorporate a number of well-established constructs from emotions research. The appraisal of others' emotions in the verbal domain, for example, is equated with the well-known construct of *empathy*.

Figure 2.1 also shows that the upper left branch comprises four sub-factors, which assume high EI persons to be more flexible in their utilization of emotions due to flexible planning, more creative thinking, the ability to (re-)direct attention, and a propensity to motivate themselves and others. Furthermore, this model assumes that emotionally intelligent individuals should be especially adept in certain domains. These include (a) perceiving and appraising their own emotions accurately, (b) expressing and communicating them accurately to others when appropriate, (c) recognizing the emotions in others accurately and responding to them with socially adaptive behaviors, (d) regulating emotions in themselves and others effectively in order to meet particular goals (e.g., to enhance their own and others mood), and (e) using their own emotions in order to solve problems by motivating adaptive behaviors (cf. Mayer & Salovey, 1993).

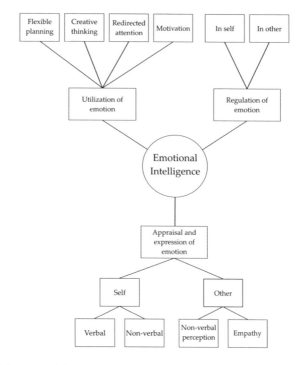

Figure 2.1   Salovey and Mayer's 1990 model of emotional intelligence.

2.2.1   Operationalization and Conceptual Validation

In order to assess the components of EI that they identified, Salovey and Mayer (1990) proposed several approaches that can be divided into self-report versus ability measures (cf. Neubauer & Freudenthaler, 2001). Notably Salovey and Mayer had demonstrated how aspects of EI might be measured as an ability (e.g., Mayer, DiPaolo, & Salovey, 1990; see also Mayer & Geher, 1996), even at this early point in time. However, in this initial work, they also considered self-report measures of related constructs (e.g., empathy, emotional expressivity, or mood regulation) as ancillary measures of emotion-related abilities.

At the time of writing, only one self-report measure (and no performance-based measure) had been explicitly designed to measure EI as *originally* conceptualized by Salovey and Mayer (1990). This measure is the Schutte et al. (1998) trait measure of emotional intelligence (SEI; see also the Trait Meta Mood Scale proposed by Salovey, Mayer, Goldman, Turvey, & Palfai, 1995, for a related, but conceptually more restricted, questionnaire). Factor analyses that have been employed on data provided by the SEI, by different authors (e.g., Ciarrochi, Deane, & Anderson, 2002; Petrides & Furnham, 2000, Schutte et al., 1998) have so far yielded different factor solutions. Moreover, these findings demonstrate neither the structure of emotion-related mental abilities proposed by Salovey and Mayer (1990) nor the existence of a coherent domain of emotional intelligence.

2.2.2   Criticism and Response

The status of two branches of EI90 (appraisal and expression, regulation) within the domain of emotion ability related constructs remains largely undisputed. However, the third branch has been criticized, in part, for the vagueness of concepts employed. For example, what does "flexible planning", "redirected attention", and the like mean? Equally, it appears that the upper left branch in Figure 2.1 introduces "fuzziness" to well-known psychological constructs, like attention and motivation, that might otherwise clarify the role of EI. Moreover, liberally borrowing established constructs has prompted questions of whether EI is a new form of intelligence at all (cf. Neubauer & Freudenthaler, 2002; Weber & Westmeyer, 2001).

Despite these problems, Mayer and Salovey argue that EI clearly represents a meaningful new type of intelligence because the series of emotion-related abilities they posit does fit well within the boundaries of widely acknowledged conceptual definitions of intelligence. Consider, for example, correspondence with Wechsler's (1958) definition of *intelligence* as "the aggregate or global capacity of the individual to act purposefully, to think rationally, and to deal effectively with his environment" (p. 7). Although EI shows important convergence with other ability concepts like *social intelligence*, Mayer and Salovey (1993) argue that EI is not a mere re-description of social intelligence. Instead, because EI primarily focuses on the emotional problems embedded in personal and social problems, it is argued to be a narrower descriptor than social intelligence. Thus, EI should display better discriminant validity with respect to cognitive intelligence (cf. Mayer & Salovey, 1997). Indeed, EI is broader, as it also covers the perception of, and reasoning about, *internal* emotions (Mayer, Caruso, & Salovey, 1999).

Finally, Mayer and Salovey (1993) argue that EI represents unique mechanisms that might underlie the processing of affective information. In so doing, they also contend that EI should not be considered as a collection of socially desired personality traits and talents, but rather as an intelligence that enhances the processing of certain types of information. In some ways, this account thus represents the first demarcation of the domain, in turn leaving the research community to decide between ability-based and mixed models of EI.

2.3   MAYER AND SALOVEY'S (1997) REVISED ABILITY MODEL OF EMOTIONAL INTELLIGENCE

In 1997, Mayer and Salovey presented a revised and refined conceptualization of EI (here referred to as EI97) that strictly constrains EI to a mental ability concept and separates it from classical social-emotional personality traits like the Eysenckian PEN factors, the Big Five personality traits, and many others. The revised model omits the upper left branch of the 1990 model (EI90) in Figure 2.1, and includes a new, performance-related domain, referred to as *thinking about emotions* (Mayer & Salovey, 1997). In EI97, the authors define

EI as a collection of emotional abilities that can be divided into four classes, facets, or (in their terminology) branches. These four classes of emotion-related abilities are arranged from more basic to higher-level skills (see also Mayer et al., 1999, 2000b). Within each branch, four representative abilities are described which differ in their developmental antecedents (see Figure 2.2).

Branch I (*Perception, Appraisal and Expression of Emotion*) involves the receiving and recognizing of emotional information and comprises the most basic emotion-related skills. These components range from the ability to identify emotions in one's self to the ability to discriminate between emotions, for example, honest versus dishonest expression of feelings (cf. Figure 2.2). These basic input processes are necessary preconditions for the further processing of emotional information in order to solve problems (Mayer, Salovey, Caruso, & Sitarenios, 2001).

Branch II (*Emotional Facilitation of Thinking*) describes the use of emotions to enhance reasoning and proposes various emotional events that assist in intellectual processing. Included under this branch are emotions that direct attention to important information and different kind of moods that may facilitate different forms of reasoning (e.g., deductive vs. inductive reasoning).

Branch III (*Understanding and Analyzing Emotions*) involves cognitive processing of emotions and comprises four representative abilities involving abstract understanding and reasoning about emotions. These components range from the ability to label emotions and recognize relations among the words and the emotions themselves, to the ability to recognize likely transitions among emotions.

Branch IV (*Reflective Regulation of Emotions*) refers to the ability to manage emotions in oneself, and in others, in order to enhance emotional and intellectual growth. This ability comprises the most advanced skills, ranging from the ability to stay open to feelings—both pleasant and unpleasant ones—to the ability to manage emotions in oneself and others by enhancing pleasant emotions and moderating negative ones. This highest branch represents an interface of many factors including motivational, emotional, and cognitive factors that must be recognized and balanced in order to manage and cope with feelings successfully (Mayer, 2001; Mayer et al., 2001).

2.3.1   Convergence of EI with Standard Criteria for an Intelligence

Mayer and colleagues claim, in a series of recent papers (e.g., Mayer & Salovey, 1997; Mayer et al., 1999, 2000a, 2001), that their revised conceptualization now meets important criteria that moves EI firmly into the domain of intelligence constructs. The criteria they cite are conceptual, correlational, and developmental. In the passages that follow, we briefly exposit these criteria.

Conceptual criterion.   The authors argue that EI is composed of a series of conceptually related mental abilities, referring to various aspects of reasoning about emotions that can be clearly distinguished from personality traits and talents. Moreover, their proposed branches of EI involve those mental

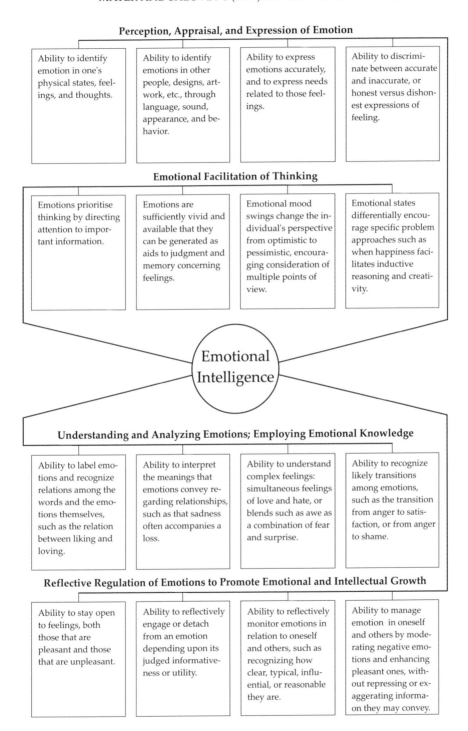

Perception, Appraisal, and Expression of Emotion

Ability to identify emotion in one's physical states, feelings, and thoughts.	Ability to identify emotions in other people, designs, artwork, etc., through language, sound, appearance, and behavior.	Ability to express emotions accurately, and to express needs related to those feelings.	Ability to discriminate between accurate and inaccurate, or honest versus dishonest expressions of feeling.

Emotional Facilitation of Thinking

Emotions prioritise thinking by directing attention to important information.	Emotions are sufficiently vivid and available that they can be generated as aids to judgment and memory concerning feelings.	Emotional mood swings change the individual's perspective from optimistic to pessimistic, encouraging consideration of multiple points of view.	Emotional states differentially encourage specific problem approaches such as when happiness facilitates inductive reasoning and creativity.

Emotional
Intelligence

Understanding and Analyzing Emotions; Employing Emotional Knowledge

Ability to label emotions and recognize relations among the words and the emotions themselves, such as the relation between liking and loving.	Ability to interpret the meanings that emotions convey regarding relationships, such as that sadness often accompanies a loss.	Ability to understand complex feelings: simultaneous feelings of love and hate, or blends such as awe as a combination of fear and surprise.	Ability to recognize likely transitions among emotions, such as the transition from anger to satisfaction, or from anger to shame.

Reflective Regulation of Emotions to Promote Emotional and Intellectual Growth

Ability to stay open to feelings, both those that are pleasant and those that are unpleasant.	Ability to reflectively engage or detach from an emotion depending upon its judged informativeness or utility.	Ability to reflectively monitor emotions in relation to oneself and others, such as recognizing how clear, typical, influential, or reasonable they are.	Ability to manage emotion in oneself and others by moderating negative emotions and enhancing pleasant ones, without repressing or exaggerating information they may convey.

Figure 2.2   Mayer and Salovey's 1997 model of emotional intelligence.

processes that are widely acknowledged as central parts of an intelligence system. These include abstract understanding or reasoning as a core feature of a system that is assisted by several adjunct functions of input processing, knowledge processing, and meta-processing (Mayer et al., 2000a, 2001). Thus, according to Mayer and Salovey, EI can be operationalized as a set of emotion-related abilities that have clearly defined performance components.

Correlational criterion.   Mayer et al. propose that EI describes a set of mental ability components that are rather closely related to each other and moderately correlated with other intelligences. Moderate correlations suggest that the new intelligence belongs to the domain of intelligences and that it is distinct from those already identified and measured. The finding is important since if the correlations are too high it would raise the possibility that the new intelligences are not sufficiently distinct from traditional intelligence conceptions.

Developmental criterion.   If EI follows the model of traditional intelligences, it should vary with age and experience. To this end, Mayer and Salovey's EI-model predicts that an individual's level of EI should rise with age and experience. Mayer and Salovey assume, then, that EI reflects a set of acquired skills which develop through experience and social interaction (cf. Davies, Stankov, & Roberts, 1998; Schaie, 2001) rather than reflecting innate or static skills. Moreover, the third branch (understanding of emotions) mainly reflects the processing of emotions through reference to an acquired emotional knowledge base (see Mayer et al., 2001). On the basis of these assertions, one would expect EI to be particularly related to crystallized intelligence.

2.3.2   Operationalization and Conceptual Validation

Mayer and Salovey (1997) claim that only psychometric performance tests of the proposed emotion-related abilities, enabling discrimination between correct and incorrect responses, can demonstrate and prove the existence of EI. To fill the measurement void surrounding this claim, Mayer et al. (1999) developed the Multifactor Emotional Intelligence Scale (MEIS), which consists of 12 performance tasks designed to measure the four branches of EI97:

1. Branch I consists of four tests that measure the ability to identify emotions in faces, music, designs, and stories.
2. Branch II comprises two tasks designed to measure the ability to assimilate emotions into perceptual and cognitive processes.
3. Branch III consists of four tasks assessing the ability to reason about and understand emotions.
4. For Branch IV, two tasks measure the participants' abilities to manage their own emotions and the emotions of others.

Unlike the domain of cognitive intelligence, where the correctness of responses can usually be determined fairly easily on logical grounds, this has proven difficult in the case of emotions (see Zeidner, Matthews, & Roberts, 2001, for a discussion). Currently, three approaches are followed:

1. Group consensus: Each response is scored according to the proportion of participants who gave the same answer.

2. Expert scoring: The correct answer is determined by asking experts in the field what the best/correct answer is (for the MEIS the first two authors served as experts).

3. Target criterion: The correct response is determined by correspondence with a target person experiencing the emotion. For the subtests *perception of emotions in music, designs, and stories* of the MEIS, the composers/designers/authors identified the best response alternatives.

To validate the MEIS empirically (thereby validating the underlying EI model), Mayer et al. (1999) employed an exploratory factor analysis that yielded a three-factor solution: emotion perception, assimilation and understanding of emotions, and managing of emotions). As the correlations of these factors were substantial (from $r = .33$ to $r = .49$), the authors conducted a hierarchical factor analysis. Here a single second-order *general EI* factor was extracted, with salient loadings from each of the primary factors.

An exploratory factor analysis of consensus subscale scores conducted by Roberts, Zeidner, and Matthews (2001) also yielded three interpretable factors (perception, understanding, management). However, contrary to Mayer et al.'s findings, the two assimilation subscales loaded about equally on the three extracted factors. Thus, the utilization of emotion to facilitate thought and action seems to represent a (factorially) complex domain encompassing or requiring emotion-related abilities of all other three branches. Nevertheless, confirmatory factor analyses conducted by Roberts et al. (2001), on both consensus and expert scores, identified the proposed four-factor structure to be the most plausible model tested.

A further evaluation was conducted by Ciarrochi, Chan, and Caputi (2000). Consistent with Mayer et al. (1999), they found that all measures of the MEIS loaded on the first principal component, which provides further evidence for an emotional g. However, below the g-factor they could only extract two factors labeled *Emotional Perception* and *Emotion Regulation/Management*. The tasks designed to measure emotional assimilation and understanding loaded substantially on both the perception and the regulation factors.

Generally, these findings provide support for the assumption of a general factor of EI and for the conceptual validity of at least Branches I and IV (perception and management/regulation of emotions). However, the conceptual validity remains rather equivocal for Branches II and III. Moreover, Roberts et al.'s (2001) comprehensive evaluation of the MEIS also reveals various problems related to measurement issues and scoring. Some of the ability measures are problematic because of low reliabilities (Ciarrochi et al., 2000). The cross-correlations between consensus- and expert-scored subscales are much too low to demonstrate satisfactory convergence between these two scoring-methods.

Moreover, consensus- and expert-scored EI measures show different relation-ships to other criterion variables. Thus, it seems rather questionable whether the same personal qualities are assessed by these two scoring procedures.

To resolve some of these problems, as well as to improve the psychomet-ric qualities of the MEIS, Mayer and colleagues developed the Mayer-Salovey-Caruso Emotional Intelligence Test (MSCEIT; Mayer et al., 2000b; see also Mayer, Salovey, Caruso, & Sitarenios, 2003). Two scoring procedures are used for the MSCEIT: (a) a general consensus criterion which is based on the an-swers of more than 2,000 participants, and (b) an expert-consensus criterion which is based on the assessments of 21 members of the International Society of Research in Emotion (see Mayer et al., 2003). In this latter instance, each response is scored according to the proportion of experts who gave the same answer. In a recent analysis of the correlation of the two sets of scores, Mayer et al. (2003) report a surprisingly high correlation coefficient of $r = .91$, as well as improved reliabilities (relative to the MEIS).

However, as Zeidner et al. (2001) point out, it is up to Mayer and col-leagues to show that this new measure has conceptual overlap (i.e., correlates highly) with its predecessor MEIS (as it is has been done with most other well-established psychological tests, like the Wechsler, Kaufmann, and Stanford-Binet scales). Without such a demonstration, as Zeidner et al. claim, "it is entirely possible that what is being assessed each time is something entirely dissimilar, rendering it impossible to compile a corpus of knowledge around which a concept like EI might coalesce" (Zeidner et al., 2001, p. 268).

In concluding this section, it should be acknowledged that the research group around Mayer represents the first, and hitherto also the only published, efforts towards the development of EI performance tests. Nevertheless, the MEIS seems problematic in several respects and the actual empirical status of the MSCEIT requires the emergence of a body of independent research sup-porting its psychometric properties and construct validity.

2.4   BAR-ON'S MIXED MODEL OF EMOTIONAL INTELLIGENCE

In contrast to Mayer and Salovey's ability conceptualization of EI, mixed mod-els (e.g., Bar-On, 1997; Cooper & Sawaf, 1997; Goleman, 1995, 1998; Weisinger, 1998) do not exclusively refer EI to emotion or intelligence. Instead, they claim that EI is often used as a label for a diverse group of personality characteris-tics that might predict success in professional and everyday domains. Because among the mixed models Bar-On's (1997) broad conceptualization of EI has re-ceived most attention in the scientific literature, and is the only one for which empirical findings have been reported, it is the main model discussed here.

In contrast to Salovey and Mayer, who argue that EI is ability-based, Bar-On (1997) defines EI as "an array of noncognitive capabilities, competencies, and skills that influence one's ability to succeed in coping with environmental de-mands and pressures." (p. 14). For Bar-On, a clinical psychologist, EI becomes highly relevant since it answers the question "Why are some individuals more able to succeed in life than others?".

Bar-On reviewed personality characteristics supposed to determine life-success beyond cognitive intelligence, and identified five broad dimensions. He regards these dimensions, which are further subdivided into 15 subscales, as key factors of EI. They are:

1. Intrapersonal skills, comprising

   - self-regard (being aware of, understanding and accepting oneself),
   - emotional self-awareness (being aware of and understanding one's emotions),
   - assertiveness (expressing one's emotions, ideas, needs, and desires),
   - self-actualization (realizing one's potential capacities),
   - independence (being self-directed, self-controlled and free of emotional dependency);

2. Interpersonal skills, comprising

   - empathy (being aware of and understanding others' emotions),
   - social responsibility (demonstrating oneself as a constructive member of one's social group),
   - interpersonal relationships (forming and maintaining intimate relationships);

3. Adaptability, comprising

   - problem solving (solving personal and social problems constructively),
   - reality testing (validating one's thinking and feelings),
   - flexibility (adjusting one's feelings, thoughts, and behavior to changing conditions);

4. Stress management, comprising

   - stress tolerance (actively and positively coping with stress),
   - impulse control (resisting or delaying an impulse or drive, and controlling one's emotions); as well as

5. General mood, comprising

   - happiness (feeling satisfied with one's life),
   - optimism (maintaining positive attitudes).

In 2000, Bar-On presented a revised conceptualization of this EI model. This modified conceptualization, which these authors labeled "a model of emotional and social intelligence", comprises 10 components from the original model. These components are self-regard, emotional self-awareness, assertiveness, empathy, interpersonal relationship, stress tolerance, impulse control, reality testing, flexibility, and problem-solving. The other five subcomponents of the original model (i.e., self-actualization, independence, social responsibility, optimism, and happiness) are now considered as *facilitators* rather than *constituent components* of emotional and social intelligence.

2.4.1 Operationalization and Conceptual Validation

Like Mayer and Salovey's model, Bar-On's model required a new assessment tool. To assess his 1997 mixed model of EI, he developed the Emotional Quotient Inventory (EQ-i; 1997), which consists of 133 items. By means of factor analyses, the proposed model was more or less empirically confirmed (see Bar-On, Brown, Kirkcaldy, & Thomé, 2000; Petrides & Furnham, 2001). Bar-On postulated that the total item score represents an indicator of an individual's overall (i.e., general) EI.

For the criterion-related validity, Bar-On (1997) reported correlations of up to $r = .52$ between EQ-i factors and self-report measures of job performance and work satisfaction. In response to this study, Petrides and Furnham (2001) examined the relationships of the EQ-i scales to measures of well-known personality traits in two of their own studies. Their findings, which are based on factor analyses of several additional personality measures, yielded the isolation of an EI factor in Eysenckian factor space (Study 1) as well as within the Five-Factor-Model (Study 2). However, other authors reported a high multi-collinearity among the EQ-i factors and personality traits. Dawda and Hart (2000) observed moderate to high correlations of EQ-i scores with neuroticism, extraversion, agreeableness, and conscientiousness, as well as negative correlations of the EQ-i with depression, somatic symptomatology, and increased experience of somatic symptoms under stress. Similarly, Newsome, Day, and Catano (2000) obtained a very high correlation of $r = -.77$ between the EQ-i score and the anxiety factor of the 16PF. In contrast, they found no correlations between the EQ-i and cognitive abilities or with academic achievement (but academic achievement was significantly correlated with cognitive abilities, extraversion, and self-control). On the basis of these findings, especially the high correlation with anxiety, Newsome et al. concluded that the EQ-i can largely be regarded as a measure of (lack of) neuroticism.

2.4.2 Limitations and Critical Issues

Bar-On's conceptualization includes not only emotion-related mental abilities, but also broader social skills (e.g., assertiveness) and non-ability traits that refer to personality traits (e.g., impulse control) and chronic mood (happiness, optimism). Therefore, to some, the appropriateness of the term *emotional intelligence* seems rather questionable (cf. Neubauer & Freudenthaler, 2002). Indeed, some of the components suggested by Bar-On at best indirectly relate to *emotional* processes (e.g., problem solving or reality testing), therefore, the construct cannot be emotional. Other components do not label an ability but rather traits that refer to peoples' preferred way of behaving (e.g., social responsibility), likewise the construct cannot be an intelligence. Although there is strong agreement among intelligence researchers that other traits beyond intelligence can predict success, most of them strongly object to classifying these characteristics as intelligence components. The critique on the fuzziness of the (original) EI concept by Salovey and Mayer (e.g., Weber & Westmeyer, 2001) applies even much more strongly to Bar-On's model. If *abilities and traits* and *emotional as well as non-emotional* constructs can be labeled emotional intelligence, where are the (necessary) borders of such a psychological construct? Is then the whole domain of personality psychology simply a domain of emotional intelligence?

2.5 CONCEPTUAL APPROACHES TO EMOTIONAL INTELLIGENCE WITHIN AN ORGANIZATIONAL CONTEXT

Boyatzis et al. (2000) proposed an EI conceptualization encompassing four competence clusters (i.e., self-awareness, self-management, social awareness, and social skills) which differ from each other with respect to two dimensions, namely (a) self versus other, and (b) recognition versus regulation or management (see also Goleman, 1998, 2001). Similar to Bar-On's mixed model, the four competence cluster involve various components that are not exclusively restricted to emotion-related competencies (e.g., emotional self-awareness) but are rather related to broader social skills (e.g., leadership, conflict management, developing others) or to personality and motivational constructs (e.g., self-confidence, service orientation, initiative, achievement orientation). However, empirical analyses of the proposed conceptualization of EI by means of the so-called Emotional Competence Inventory (designed to assess the proposed competence components from an organizational perspective; see also Chapter 9 by Pérez et al.), have yielded inconsistent findings and failed to confirm the proposed structure of competencies (see also Matthews, Zeidner, & Roberts, 2002).

Regarding the impact of EI on success and performance in the organizational context, Dulewicz and Higgs (2000) presented another relatively broad conceptual approach. For several years, Dulewicz and Herbert (e.g., Dulewicz, 1998; Dulewicz & Herbert, 1999) have been working on the identification of competencies that are related to success in organizational life and developed a job competencies survey (JCS). For each of the 40 competencies, a single score was calculated by aggregating the performance-ratings of the evaluated manager and his/her boss. In a recent study, Dulewicz and Higgs (2000) subdivided these competencies by means of content analyses into three different groups, that is emotional (EQ), intellectual (IQ), and managerial (MQ) competencies. Sixteen of the 40 competencies (supposed to be related to various components of existing, mixed models of EI) have been classified into six clusters of EQ-competencies (i.e., sensitivity vs. achievement, resilience, influence and adaptability, decisiveness and assertiveness, energy vs. integrity, leadership). Similar to other existing mixed models of EI, the selected EQ-competencies address a relatively broad combination of individual traits, values, and (social) behaviors. However, in order to test the predictive/incremental validity of the three different types of competencies, aggregate scores of the EQ, IQ, and MQ competence-scales as well as composite measures of $EQ + IQ$ and $EQ + IQ + MQ$ competencies have been correlated with long-term managerial advancement. Using multiple regression analyses, the authors report that all three types of competencies (EQ, IQ, MQ considered separately as well as two composite scales $[EQ + IQ, EQ + IQ + MQ]$ contribute significantly to managers' rate of advancement within their organization over a period of seven years (purportedly accounting for 71 percent of the total variance on the dependent variable). According to Dulewicz and Higgs, these findings provide evidence for the incremental validity of EI as well as the proposed usefulness of combining different types of competencies with respect to the prediction of success.

2.6   GENERAL DISCUSSION

Thirteen years after the first mention of a concept of EI by Salovey and Mayer, we are finally seeing some small, albeit important, steps towards the development of a coherent model of EI. Goleman's popular assertions about EI, though not empirically proven themselves, spurred scientific inquiry into the construct. Recent work on EI follows two paths:

1. As is highlighted throughout this book, the importance of distinguishing two fundamentally different types of models is apparent. These two types of models have been assigned different labels, for example, ability versus mixed EI models (Mayer et al., 1999). Whereas models of the first type refer to EI strictly as an ability construct, models of the second type allow for a much broader combination of diverse (partially older and well-established) personality traits under the umbrella term EI. With regard to the different measurement approaches to EI, Petrides and Furnham (2001) emphasize a conceptual differentiation between *trait EI* and *ability/information processing EI*. The authors propose that the trait approach places EI in the domain of personality, encompassing various behavioral dispositions and self-assessed abilities that ought to be measured by self-report tests. Taking into account that intelligence and personality represent independent constructs, trait EI should be exclusively related to personality dimensions and not to cognitive intelligence. Petrides and Furnham suggest their formal concept of *trait EI* as a guiding framework for the integration and systematization of research on the different facets of EI encompassed by existing mixed models. By contrast, *ability EI* is viewed as a cognitive-emotional ability within an ability framework that ought to be measured by means of maximum perfor-

mance tests. Therefore, ability EI should primarily be related to cognitive intelligence components.

2. Although there are fundamental differences between ability and mixed (or trait) EI, regarding conceptualization and operationalization, these two approaches are not mutually exclusive but rather tend to be complementary with respect to emotion-related components (see Ciarrochi et al., 2000; Petrides & Furnham, 2001). Almost all existing concepts and measures of EI cover at least four emotion-related areas that result from the factorial combination of the two dimensions of self versus other and recognition/awareness versus regulation/management: (a) recognition or awareness of one's own emotions, (b) recognition or awareness of the emotions of others, (c) regulation or management of one's own emotions, (d) regulation or management of the emotions of others. Although self-report measures of emotion-related competencies might be influenced by personality traits, some authors (e.g., Mayer et al., 2000b; Neubauer & Freudenthaler, 2001) think they have their own merits and should not be completely disregarded. They (a) can provide relevant information about internal processes and experiences that can hardly be assessed by performance tests, (b) might be used to assess the validity of performance tests, and (c) might contribute either directly or indirectly to the prediction of life-success.

3. Currently, there is debate about the appropriateness of using the term EI for mixed or trait EI models. Proponents of ability models, as well as most researchers from the domain of cognitive intelligence, hold the view that the term *intelligence* should be reserved for strictly performance related psychological constructs (some theorists even argue that *intelligence* should stay a reserved term for the classical cognitive intelligence concept). Proponents of mixed or trait models allow for EI as a new umbrella term for various (old and new) personality traits. Nevertheless, Petrides and Furnham (2001) also emphasize the importance of using different terms for the verbal description of ability- versus trait-related constructs via the following alternative labels: *cognitive-emotional ability* for the former and *emotional self-efficacy* for the latter.

4. Also in the realm of ability concepts, some progress has been achieved concerning the subfactors that should be included in the domain of EI. The literature on model development and recent empirical data suggests that components like *emotion perception* and *emotion management/regulation* can be operationalized via performance tests and show up clearly in factor analyses. The usefulness of other components suggested by Mayer and Salovey (1997), namely *Emotional Facilitation of Thinking* and *Understanding and Analyzing Emotions*, has been undermined by several studies; the current status of these factors (or at least their operationalizations via the MEIS), is largely equivocal.

5. Clearly, many questions about EI have been raised in the last two decades. Many of these are highlighted in a special issue of *Emotion*, that examined EI. Some of the more intriguing points made there are:

(a) Maybe the most important issue regarding the new concept of EI is the question of convergent and discriminant validity: Where does EI fit in the space of the plethora of already existing psychological constructs? For convergent validity some correlations with (components of) cognitive ability as well as with some personality traits have been demonstrated. But with respect to discriminant validity the question must be raised: How does EI relate to other construct like for instance wisdom, social intelligence, ego resiliency and so forth? As Schaie (2001) says, we are awaiting proof that the MEIS and MSCEIT "are not simply performance measures of well-established personality traits" (p. 244).

From the viewpoint of Izard, a luminary in the field of emotion research, we must question if EI does not overlap largely with well-established concepts from emotions research. Concepts such as *emotional knowledge* (itself composed of emotion perception and emotion labelling) and *emotional adaptiveness*, have actually been extensively studied, albeit predominantly in children.

(b) Directly related to the question of convergent versus discriminant validity is the question of incremental validity, which may be the pivotal issue in EI studies. Roberts et al. (2001) noted that while Mayer and colleagues have so far reported a number of meaningful correlates of EI, we are still awaiting a demonstration that EI can predict real life criteria after statistically controlling for "rival predictors" (Izard, 2001), namely intellectual ability and personality.

(c) As already noted by Mayer and colleagues, the postulation of a new construct also requires developmental evidence, that is, the ontogenetic development of EI must be demonstrated. Some evidence on this issue was reported by Mayer et al. (1999), but Schaie (2001) points to deficiencies in this study. Further, Schaie (2001) argues that the development of the interrelationships between EI subcomponents must be studied, that is, "how does their structure unfold or in late life converge once again" (p. 245). If similar to the domain of general intelligence maybe we could also observe a process of differentiation and dedifferentiation of EI abilities (Schaie, 2001).

(d) With respect especially to concerns raised about Branches II and III of the EI97-model, Zeidner et al. (2001) note that, in fact, much of emotional and social knowledge can be implicit and procedural. They argue that humans have acquired emotional and social skills (especially nonverbal ones) that are often difficult to verbalize. An individual might have excellent academic knowledge about emotions without behaving with emotional intelligence in social interactions. If this is the case, current assessments may be missing an important array of implicit components of EI.

A compounding problem in the field is the lack of psychometrically sound measures. It has yet to be determined whether the MEIS and MSCEIT, the only available measurements of the EI97 model, really represent competency or if they rather reflect knowledge cumulated over varying learning opportunities (Zeidner et al., 2001). Current measures of EI are mainly of a crystallized kind; the question remains open if more fluid tests of EI, that is, for *emotional reasoning* might be devised in the future. Again, we can observe here the strong interdependence between theorizing and measurement; in this case, the measurement tools (MEIS and MSCEIT) strongly moved EI in one direction without having a priori resolved whether EI should more resemble *Gf* or *Gc* forms of ability. This also has important implications for the issue of cultural relativity and cultural fairness. Thus, Zeidner et al. (2001) point to the fact that crystallized tests/conceptions of EI (like MEIS/MSCEIT) might be extremely cultural dependent. Many Western cultural beliefs might not apply to Eastern cultures, while changes over time are easily conceivable (in times of totalitarian regimes probably different social-emotional behavior can be considered emotionally intelligent than in more democratic times and so forth). As Zeidner et al. (2001) have stated: "The weakness of EI and similar adaptive constructs is that emotional situations or ... interpersonal situations may be too broad and ill-defined to constitute a coherent adaptive challenge" (p. 273) and "at present it is unclear what is meant exactly by the term EI" (p. 273).

2.7   CONCLUSIONS

Currently, we face several conceptual approaches to modeling EI, which—roughly classified—belong either to the ability or the trait/mixed model domain. However, with the possible exception of the integrative approach by Petrides and Furnham (2001), EI conceptions and models seem rather self-contained in that their development is mainly psychometrically driven (i.e., strongly connected to the instruments designed to measure them). Since research on cognitive intelligence started in similar fashion, this approach cannot be considered wrong in and of itself. Nevertheless, as pointed out by Matthews et al. (2002) the models presented so far are lacking from integrating theories and results from related fields like the psychology of emotions and biological approaches. Research on cognitive intelligence took this path. Starting from the psychometric perspective many decades of IQ research have seen a strong emphasis on structural aspects, with research on developmental aspects, on biological, psychological, and sociological correlates showing up later. For example, for biopsychological correlates it was not before the 1970s before serious efforts were taken to explain IQ biologically (Neubauer & Fink, 2005). Viewed from this perspective, there is a long way for EI to travel: On the input side (the causes) the construct must be better connected to, or grounded in, the psychology of emotions; biological correlates should be established; the influence of nature and nurture assessed through behavior genetic research; and so forth. Regarding the output side (the effects) researchers must inquire into psychological as well as sociological correlates of EI. As pointed out by Matthews et al. (2002) such research should help also in answering what are probably the most important questions: "Is EI an underlying competence? Is EI an outcome of more basic psychological factors?" (p. 531).

These questions refer to possibly the most fundamental issue: In view of the enormous variety of existing psychological constructs and their fundamental theories, the question remains open if EI really describes a new meaningful psychological characteristic of human beings, or if it is only a new label for existing constructs. In a similar vein, the study of EI could also be viewed as an attempt towards reanimation of the related, but historically rather unsuccessful, concept of social intelligence. Once the relation between these two concepts have been clarified and integrative attempts have both demarcated the boundaries of EI and its subcomponents, all efforts should head towards the development of reliable and valid performance measures of EI. If these can be shown to have incremental validity beyond established constructs, from both the ability and the trait domains, the concept of EI will have served its purpose.

REFERENCES

Bar-On, R. (1997). *BarOn Emotional Quotient Inventory (EQ–i): Technical manual.* Toronto, Canada: Multi-Health Systems.

Bar-On, R. (2000). Emotional and social intelligence: Insights from the Emotional Quotient inventory. In R. Bar-On & J. D. A. Parker (Eds.), *The handbook of emotional intelligence: Theory, development, assessment, and application at home, school, and in the workplace* (pp. 363–388). San Francisco: Jossey-Bass.

Bar-On, R., Brown, J. M., Kirkcaldy, B. D., & Thomé, E. P. (2000). Emotional expression and implications for occupational stress; An application of the Emotional Quotient inventory (EQ–i). *Personality and Individual Differences, 28,* 1107–1118.

Boyatzis, R. E., Goleman, D., & Rhee, K. S. (2000). Clustering competence in emotional intelligence: Insights from the Emotional Competence Inventory. In R. Bar-On & J. D. A. Parker (Eds.), *The handbook of emotional intelligence: Theory, development, assessment, and application at home, school, and in the workplace* (pp. 343–362). San Francisco: Jossey-Bass.

Brody, N. (1992). *Intelligence* (2nd ed.). London: Academic Press.

Ciarrochi, J., Chan, A. Y. C., & Caputi, P. (2000). A critical evaluation of the emotional intelligence construct. *Personality and Individual Differences, 28,* 539–561.

Ciarrochi, J., Deane, F. P., & Anderson, S. (2002). Emotional intelligence moderates the relationship between stress and mental health. *Personality and Individual Differences, 32,* 197–209.

Cooper, R. K., & Sawaf, A. (1997). *Executive EQ: Emotional intelligence in leadership and organizations.* New York: Grosset/Putnam.

Davies, M., Stankov, L., & Roberts, R. D. (1998). Emotional intelligence: In search of an elusive construct. *Journal of Personality and Social Psychology, 75,* 989–1015.

Dawda, D., & Hart, S. D. (2000). Assessing emotional intelligence: Reliability and validity of the Bar-On Emotional Quotient inventory (EQ-i) in university students. *Personality and Individual Differences, 28,* 797–812.

Dulewicz, S. V. (1998). *Personal Competency Framework Manual.* Windsor, UK: ASE.

Dulewicz, S. V., & Herbert, P. J. A. (1999). Predicting advancement to senior management from competencies and personality data: A 7-year follow-up study. *British Journal of Management, 10*, 13–22.

Dulewicz, S. V., & Higgs, M. J. (2000). Emotional intelligence: A review and evaluation study. *Journal of Managerial Psychology, 15*, 341–372.

Freudenthaler, H. H., & Neubauer, A. C. (2001). Emotionale Intelligenz [Emotional intelligence]. In B. B. Seiwald, J. Guthke, H. Petermann, J. F. Beckmann, & M. Roth (Eds.), *6. Arbeitstagung der Fachgruppe für Differentielle Psychologie, Persönlichkeitspsychologie und Psychologische Diagnostik der Deutschen Gesellschaft für Psychologie* (pp. 46–48). Leipzig, Germany: Leipziger Universitätsverlag.

Goleman, D. (1995). *Emotional intelligence: Why it can matter more than IQ*. New York: Bantam Books.

Goleman, D. (1998). *Working with emotional intelligence*. New York: Bantam.

Goleman, D. (2001). An EI-based theory of performance. In C. Cherniss & D. Goleman (Eds.), *The emotionally intelligent workplace: How to select for, measure, and improve emotional intelligence in individuals, groups, and organizations* (pp. 27–44). San Francisco: Jossey-Bass.

Izard, C. E. (2001). Emotional intelligence or adaptive emotions? *Emotion, 1*, 249–257.

Matthews, G., Zeidner, M., & Roberts, R. D. (2002). *Emotional intelligence: Science and myth*. Cambridge, MA: MIT Press.

Mayer, J. D. (2001). A field guide to emotional intelligence. In J. Ciarrochi, J. P. Forgas, & J. D. Mayer (Eds.), *Emotional intelligence and everyday life* (pp. 3–24). New York: Psychology Press.

Mayer, J. D. (2002). Foreword. In L. F. Barrett & P. Salovey (Eds.), *The wisdom in feeling: Psychological processes in emotional intelligence*. New York: Guilford Press.

Mayer, J. D., Caruso, D. R., & Salovey, P. (1999). Emotional intelligence meets traditional standards for an intelligence. *Intelligence, 27*, 267–298.

Mayer, J. D., DiPaolo, M., & Salovey, P. (1990). Perceiving affective content in ambiguous visual stimuli: A component of emotional intelligence. *Journal of Personality Assessment, 54*, 772–781.

Mayer, J. D., & Geher, G. (1996). Emotional intelligence and the identification of emotion. *Intelligence, 22*, 89–113.

Mayer, J. D., & Salovey, P. (1993). The intelligence of emotional intelligence. *Intelligence, 17*, 433–442.

Mayer, J. D., & Salovey, P. (1997). What is emotional intelligence? In P. Salovey & D. J. Sluyter (Eds.), *Emotional development and emotional intelligence: Educational implications* (pp. 3–31). New York: Basic Books.

Mayer, J. D., Salovey, P., & Caruso, D. R. (2000a). Emotional intelligence as zeitgeist, as personality, and a mental ability. In R. Bar-On & J. D. A. Parker (Eds.), *The handbook of emotional intelligence: Theory, development, assessment, and application at home, school, and in the workplace* (pp. 92–117). San Francisco: Jossey-Bass.

Mayer, J. D., Salovey, P., & Caruso, D. R. (2000b). Models of emotional intelligence. In R. J. Sternberg (Ed.), *Handbook of intelligence* (pp. 396–420). Cambridge: Cambridge University Press.

Mayer, J. D., Salovey, P., Caruso, D. R., & Sitarenios, G. (2001). Emotional intelligence as a standard intelligence. *Emotion, 1*, 232–242.

Mayer, J. D., Salovey, P., Caruso, D. R., & Sitarenios, G. (2003). Measuring emotional intelligence with the MSCEIT V2.0. *Emotion, 3,* 97–105.

Neubauer, A. C., & Fink, A. (2005). Basic information processing and the psychophysiology of intelligence. In R. J. Sternberg & J. Pretz (Eds.), *Cognition and intelligence: Identifying the mechanisms of mind* (pp. 68–87). Cambridge, UK: Cambridge University Press.

Neubauer, A. C., & Freudenthaler, H. H. (2001). Emotionale Intelligenz: Ein Überblick [Emotional intelligence: A review]. In E. Stern & J. Guthke (Eds.), *Perspektiven der Intelligenzforschung* (pp. 205–232). Lengerich, Germany: Pabst.

Neubauer, A. C., & Freudenthaler, H. H. (2002). Sind emotionale traits als Fähigkeiten messbar [Can emotional traits be measured as abilities]? *Zeitschrift für Personalpsychologie, 1,* 177–178.

Newsome, S., Day, A. L., & Catano, V. M. (2000). Assessing the predictive validity of emotional intelligence. *Personality and Individual Differences, 29,* 1005–1016.

Petrides, K. V., & Furnham, A. (2000). On the dimensional structure of emotional intelligence. *Personality and Individual Differences, 29,* 313–320.

Petrides, K. V., & Furnham, A. (2001). Trait emotional intelligence: Psychometric investigation with reference to established trait taxonomies. *European Journal of Personality, 15,* 425–448.

Roberts, R. D., Zeidner, M., & Matthews, G. (2001). Does emotional intelligence meet traditional standards for an intelligence? Some new data and conclusions. *Emotion, 1,* 196–231.

Salovey, P., & Mayer, J. D. (1990). Emotional intelligence. *Imagination, Cognition and Personality, 9,* 185–211.

Salovey, P., Mayer, J. D., Goldman, S., Turvey, C., & Palfai, T. (1995). Emotional attention, clarity, and repair: Exploring emotional intelligence using the Trait Meta–Mood Scale. In J. W. Pennebaker (Ed.), *Emotion, disclosure, and health* (pp. 125–154). Washington, DC: American Psychological Association.

Schaie, K. W. (2001). Emotional intelligence: Psychometric status and developmental characteristics—Comment on Roberts, Zeidner, and Matthews (2001). *Emotion, 1,* 243–248.

Schmidt, F. L., & Hunter, J. E. (1998). The validity and utility of selection methods in personnel psychology: Practical and theoretical implications of 85 years of research findings. *Psychological Bulletin, 124,* 262–274.

Schutte, N. S., Malouff, J. M., Hall, L. E., Haggerty, D. J., Cooper, J. T., Golden, C. J., et al. (1998). Development and validation of a measure of emotional intelligence. *Personality and Individual Differences, 25,* 167–177.

Weber, H., & Westmeyer, H. (2001). Die Inflation der Intelligenzen [The inflation of intelligences]. In E. Stern & J. Guthke (Eds.), *Perspektiven der Intelligenzforschung* (pp. 251–266). Lengerich, Germany: Pabst Science Publisher.

Wechsler, D. (1958). *The measurement and appraisal of adult intelligence* (4th ed.). Baltimore: Williams & Wilkins.

Weisinger, H. (1998). *Emotional intelligence at work: The untapped edge for success.* San Francisco: Jossey-Bass.

Zeidner, M., Matthews, G., & Roberts, R. D. (2001). Slow down, you move too fast: Emotional intelligence remains an "elusive" intelligence. *Emotion, 1,* 265–275.

3

The Emotion Systems and the Development of Emotional Intelligence

David Schultz
University of Maryland–Baltimore County, USA

Carroll E. Izard
University of Delaware, USA

Jo Ann A. Abe
Southern Connecticut State University, USA

Summary

The starting point for considering the development of emotional intelligence is this: Emotions themselves are intelligent. Much of what some call *emotional intelligence* (EI) reflects direct functioning of the emotion systems. Other aspects of EI are shaped over time by a person's emotion experiences. In the present chapter we examine this last hypothesis by considering children's abilities to recognize how others' feel. We believe that those aspects of EI that influence children's social and behavioral adjustment most strongly will be aspects most closely associated with emotion systems functioning.

3.1   THE EMOTION SYSTEMS AND THE DEVELOPMENT OF EMOTIONAL INTELLIGENCE

The starting point for considering the development of emotional intelligence (EI) is this: Emotions themselves are intelligent. In a sense, the development of EI began with the genesis and evolution of the emotion systems (e.g., the amygdala, the hippocampal-entorhinal complex, the hypothalamic-pituitary-adrenal axis). The emotion systems seem to have functioned and continue to function, at least in part, to promote species survival (cf. Damasio, 1994; Darwin, 1872/1965; Ekman, 1999; Izard, 1971). Clearly, emotion responses are not adaptive at all times or in all situations. Almost everyone wishes that anger had not motivated her or him to say or do something at one point in time. We often overlook, however, that throughout our daily lives our emotion responses—including anger—help us to respond intelligently and adaptively to our world. The adaptive function of emotions includes:

1. focusing attention on important aspects of our environment (e.g., threatening messages and approaching vehicles),
2. provision of internal cues about our current or future status with our environments (e.g., angry feelings tell us when someone has infringed upon us; anticipatory feelings of fear inform us that we should not say something critical to our bosses),
3. priming of certain parts of our bodies to respond (e.g., anger at a bully sends internal signals to increase blood flow to appendages), and
4. motivation of facial and bodily expressions that communicate important information to others (e.g., smiles that tell others how much we appreciate their friendships).

In general, emotions serve us well. Many authors have raised concerns about the cohesiveness of the construct of EI (Zeidner, Roberts, & Matthews, 2002). Many components of EI seem to overlap with established dimensions of temperament and intelligence and, overall, do not seem to cohere into a single, measurable construct. We share these concerns. We believe that many of the components of what is being called emotional "intelligence" actually reflect functioning of the emotion systems.

In this chapter, we will discuss ways in which the emotion systems influence one component common to many models of EI, emotion recognition. Recognition of others' emotions refers to the ability to identify how others feel based on facial expressions, knowledge of situational triggers, observed behaviors, vocal tones, and other signals. It represents a basic emotion ability that has received much empirical attention and that lays a foundation for other components of EI, as many theorists suggest. We distinguish between declarative emotion (recognition) knowledge and emotion (recognition) processing patterns.

Declarative emotion knowledge has been researched extensively. Investigators typically assess it by examining how often children can associate expressions, situations, behaviors, or vocal tones with the emotion label that a consensus of other people do (e.g., Jill's cat ran away, how do you think Jill feels?). Emotion processing patterns have received increased attention in recent years and refer to tendencies some children have to attribute particular discrete emotion states to others. For example, we have found that some children tend to attribute anger to others more often than do other children (Schultz, Izard, & Bear, 2004). Declarative emotion knowledge and emotion processing patterns overlap conceptually to some extent. If children have strong processing tendencies toward a particular emotion, for example, they may perform less well on declarative knowledge tasks. As we will present and discuss later, they seem to differ somewhat in their antecedents, however, and processing patterns exhibit unique variance in the prediction of social outcomes even after controlling for declarative emotion knowledge.

In this chapter, we first present a brief overview of the emotion systems and emotionality. We then provide an overview of developmental transitions that occur in emotion recognition in infancy and childhood. We then review and discuss literature that suggests ways in which the emotion systems influence the development of emotion recognition. The emotion systems play an influential role in the development of declarative emotion knowledge (Abe & Izard, 1999a). We believe that the individual differences in emotion recognition that are most meaningful for social interactions, however, reflect differences not in declarative knowledge but in emotion processing patterns. These processing patterns are strongly influenced by previous interpersonal emotion experiences and current emotion states. In different sections of the current chapter, we review the literature for these claims. We believe the distinction we draw between declarative emotion knowledge and emotion processing patterns applies not only to emotion recognition but also to many other components of EI. To the extent that emotion processing patterns—influenced by emotion traits and experiences—influence social interactions strongly, a central role for the emotion systems is implied by the term emotional *intelligence*.

3.2 THE EMOTION SYSTEMS

Emotions "contain the wisdom of the ages" (Lazarus, 1991, p. 820). One important function of the evolution of emotions is to allow rapid processing of, and organized response to, external and internal stimuli. For example, we do not have to decide consciously if a quickly approaching bus deserves our attention. Our emotion systems will likely focus our gaze on the bus and motivate the central nervous system to prepare a bodily response before we can consciously think to ourselves, "That bus sure is big". We may (or may not) process our behavioral response consciously (e.g., "Step back onto the sidewalk!"), but the emotion systems have already prepared us to make that decision and to enact it. In this way, we may consider our discrete emotions evolutionary "best guesses" as to how we should respond when certain categories of events (e.g., object loss, object gain, goal blocking) occur (Tooby & Cosmides, 1990).

Knowledge of specific brain mechanisms involved in emotions has been described as "bleak" (LeDoux, 2000, p. 159). Although brain imaging techniques have identified specific areas of the brain that are activated when emotion perception or arousal occurs, an understanding of the roles many of these neural connections play within emotion experiences remains unknown. At least five anatomically distinct networks exist in the human brain (for a review, see Mesulam, 1998). One of these is considered the emotion/memory network and contains epicenters in the anterior cingulated cortex, hippocampal-entorhinal complex, and the amygdala. This network plays a critical role in the development of conditioned associations between various stimuli and emotions. Many people with amygdala damage have deficits in understanding the emotional signals in facial expressions (Adolphs, Tranel, Damasio, & Damasio, 1995; Calder et al., 1996) and tones of voice (Scott et al., 1997). Lesions within this network, in both humans and other primates, have led to a failure to react emotionally to typically arousing stimuli, including Playboy photographs (Bauer, 1982), and a blunted ability to learn new conditioned responses, especially fear responses (Bechara et al., 1995; Downer, 1962; Gloor, Olivier, Quesney, Andermann, & Horowitz, 1982; Rosen & Schulkin, 1998).

Throughout this chapter, we will refer to the emotion systems. When we do, we refer to the preceding neural complex and others (e.g., the hypothalamic-pituitary-adrenal axis) that have been linked closely with emotion functioning.

3.3   EMOTIONALITY/TEMPERAMENT

People differ in the frequency and intensity with which they experience different discrete emotions. Some of the most reliably measured temperament traits include behavioral inhibition or shyness (Kagan, Reznick, & Snidman, 1987), negative affectivity, extraversion, and effortful control (Rothbart, Ahadi, Hershey, & Fisher, 2001). Most of these dimensions reflect emotion systems functioning. For example, inhibited infants and children are shy- or fear-prone as exhibited by wariness when presented with strangers or other novel stimuli. Children with negative affectivity are sad- and anger-prone as shown by frequent distress in response to environmental events (Abe & Izard, 1999b). Extraverted children are happy- and interest-prone (Abe & Izard, 1999b), approaching novel stimuli with positive affect.

Emotionality has shown moderate stability across time and predicts behavioral and social functioning. Distinct patterns of emotion expressions at 18 months of age, for example, have predicted maternal ratings of children's personality at three and a half years (Abe & Izard, 1999b). Negative emotion expressions at 18 months correlated robustly with neuroticism at three and a half years, and intense positive expressions at 18 months predicted Extraversion. In other work, infant negative emotionality (i.e., irritability) predicted aggression at 7 years of age (Rothbart, Ahadi, & Hershey, 1994).

Twin studies have suggested that temperament traits exhibit considerable heritability. Estimates typically suggest genes account for around half of the variation in temperament (Davis, Luce, & Kraus, 1994; DiLalla & Jones, 2000; Plomin & Stocker, 1989). For the development of positive emotionality, however, shared environmental experiences seem very important (Goldsmith & Campos, 1986; Goldsmith, Lemery, Buss, & Campos, 1999; Lytton, 1990). In one study with adult twins, shared environment accounted for 22% of the variance in positive affectivity (Tellegen et al., 1988).

In addition to genetic constraints, early emotion experiences, even within the womb, seem to play a critical role in determining levels of emotionality. Pregnant monkeys exposed to repeated but unpredictable noise in the dark, for example, have produced offspring who exhibit heightened levels of anxious behavior. Compared to offspring not exposed to prenatal stress, these offspring clung to other monkeys and self-stimulated more often, and displayed less exploratory behaviors (Schneider, 1992). Similar results have been found in rats (Fameli, Kitraki, & Stylianopoulou, 1994). In both of these examples, prenatal stress seems to have affected the level of negative emotionality and/or inhibition in offspring.

Early postnatal experiences also impact the development of emotionality. Experimental studies with rats suggest that maternal behavior during this period affects levels of emotionality not only in infancy but also adulthood. For example, infant rats separated from, or deprived of, their mothers have, in adulthood, exhibited elevated adrenocorticotropin hormone levels (i.e., the hormone associated with stress) both at baseline and during stressful conditions (Ladd, Owens, & Nemeroff, 1996; Plotsky & Meaney, 1993).

Non-experimental studies involving humans suggest that both maternal separation and/or deprivation and, generally, chronic stress can produce similar outcomes. Children who had been institutionalized in Romanian orphanages for more than 8 months as infants and young children displayed, six years later, elevated hypothalamic-pituitary-adrenal (HPA) axis activation compared to matched controls and other children, who had only experienced 4 or less months of institutionalization (Gunnar, Morison, & Chisholm, 2001). Moreover, other forms of chronic stress exposure have been associated with increased levels of physiological reactivity (Fleming, Baum, Davidson, Rectanus, & McArdle, 1987; Kaufman et al., 1997; Ockenfels et al., 1995). These studies suggest that recurring stressors, such as maternal deprivation, seem to have a potentially profound effect on levels of negative emotionality across the life span.

3.4   DEVELOPMENT OF EMOTION RECOGNITION

A rudimentary ability to recognize others' emotions appears soon after birth, if not at birth (Izard, 1971). Studies with infant monkeys, for example, suggest that emotion perception skills develop rapidly following birth. Some cells in the temporal cortex, an area implicated in facial recognition, appear mature as early as 6 weeks into the postnatal period (Rodman, Skelly, & Gross, 1991), and other areas of the temporal cortex associated with facial recognition complete maturation at 6 months of postnatal age (Rodman, 1994). One study with human infants exhibited their ability to distinguish between happiness, sadness, and anger at 10 weeks of age (Haviland & Lelwica, 1987). When mothers posed happy expressions, for example, infants tended to gaze forward happily. When mothers posed sad expressions, infants tended to look down. Interestingly, high levels of testosterone, more common in males, may impede the development of temporal cortical areas, leaving infant males slightly less able on average to recognize facial expressions than females (Bachevalier, Hagger, & Bercu, 1989; Hagger, Bachevalier, & Bercu, 1987).

In addition to innate and/or rapidly unfolding capacities, through modeling and exposure, the socialization of emotion recognition occurs immediately following birth. Infants imitate facial expressions and gestures from the first few days of life (Field, Woodson, Greenberg, & Cohen, 1982; Meltzoff & Moore, 1983). At three months, mothers who more often encouraged infants to attend to their facial expressions had infants that exhibited greater abilities to discriminate between subtle variations in facial expressions (Kuchuk, Vibbert, & Bornstein, 1986).

A classic study exhibited not only the ability of infants to recognize emotion expressions and interpret their meanings but also the power of caregiver emotion expressions to influence infant behaviors. One-year-old infants were placed on a platform that contained a plexiglass floor and a visible floor immediately below. Mothers stood on the opposite end of the platform and encouraged infants to come toward them. Halfway across the platform, however, the visible floor dropped several feet (the actual plexiglass floor continued). When infants reached this visual cliff, if mothers posed smiling faces, a majority of the infants continued to crawl. When mothers posed fearful facial expressions, however, no infant ventured forward (Sorce, Emde, Campos, & Klinnert, 1985).

The development of language in the second and third years of life changes the nature of the emotion socialization landscape. By 3 years of age, approximately 93% of children use the primary emotion labels of happy, sad, angry, and scared regularly (Ridgeway, Waters, & Kuczaj, 1985). At this age, verbally mediated socialization of emotion recognition, through such processes as coaching and induction, become important components of parental socialization. Through discussions with their sons and daughters, parents help children develop and strengthen associations between environmental events, emotion experiences, and emotion labels. This discourse seems helpful to children's development beyond the effects of cognitive development. In one study, parental emotion discourse predicted children's emotion recognition even after controlling for their age and cognitive ability (Denham, Zoller, & Couchoud, 1994).

In early grade school children develop a more complex understanding of how others feel. For one, they begin to appreciate that others may feel multiple and conflicting emotion responses to a single event. Early studies of mixed emotions focused on charting normative age-related changes and emphasized the role of cognitive development in children's appreciation of mixed emotions (e.g., Donaldson & Westerman, 1986; Harris, Olthof, & Terwogt, 1981). These studies typically found that not until well into middle-childhood do children readily acknowledge that the same event or person can evoke contradictory and conflicting emotions. More recent research has revealed, however, that by early school years children demonstrate at least a rudimentary or partial understanding of mixed emotions (Kestenbaum & Gelman, 1995; Peng, Johnson, Pollock, Glasspool, & Harris, 1992).

An important socializing agent for understanding mixed emotions seems to be parents and other family members who fit the description of good emotion coaches (Gottman, Katz, & Hooven, 1996). Whereas some parents view negative emotions as harmful to children and in need of extinction as quickly as possible, other parents identify and accept these expressions and view them as opportunities for discussion. Studies that examine the early correlates of mixed emotion understanding suggest the beneficial effects of expression and discussion of emotion experiences within the family. Positive affective bonds between family members seem to lay a critical foundation for these expressions and discussions. Family discussions about the causes of behavior and positive interactions with older siblings, measured when children were 3 years of age, predicted their appreciation of mixed emotions 3 years later, even after controlling for verbal ability (Brown & Dunn, 1996). Strikingly, in another study, the affective bond between 1-year-old infants and their mothers—as measured by security of attachments—predicted understanding of mixed emotions by children 5 years later (Steele, Steele, Croft, & Fonagy, 1999). Mothers of secure infants exhibited greater flexibility in communicating a wide range of feelings than mothers of insecurely attached dyads. This communicative flexibility related to emotions may have played a mediating role in the development of mixed emotion understanding.

Finally, several theorists have asserted that emotion recognition provides a foundation for the development of other components of EI. A couple of studies support this theory. In one, children's accurate labeling of discrete emotions in experimental tasks at age 3 predicted their understanding of more complex emotion experiences, including mixed emotion reactions, at age 6 (Dunn, Brown, & Maguire, 1995). In another, declarative emotion knowledge assessed following kindergarten predicted aggression in third-grade. Importantly, however, the data fit a model in which early declarative emotion knowledge had both a direct effect on later aggression and an indirect effect mediated by other, more complex aspects of emotion processing. These more complex aspects, assessed following second-grade, included attributions of hostile intent, production of maladaptive responses, positive evaluations of aggression, and holding instrumental goals (Dodge, Laird, Lochman, & Zelli, 2002).

The preceding data are correlational and therefore cannot establish causality. Future experimental studies will need to establish with certainty whether other emotion-related abilities indeed build upon emotion recognition or whether all of these skills simply share a similar lineage. Along with others (e.g., Fox, 2003), we believe that children's declarative emotion knowledge and, especially, emotion processing patterns—influenced by their past and current emotion experiences—will prove to have great influence upon their future social cognitive development.

3.5   THE EMOTION SYSTEMS INFLUENCE ON DECLARATIVE EMOTION KNOWLEDGE

Over time, positive emotionality may have a beneficial influence on the development of declarative emotion knowledge. Happiness is known to foster creativity and the ability to make associations between stimuli (Isen, 1999). Furthermore, children with positive affect who approach new and different situations eagerly may expose themselves more often to learning moments for understanding the causes and nuances of emotion experience. Conversely, negative emotion experiences may impede the development of declarative emotion knowledge. Negative emotion arousal often motivates a focus on the self and alleviation of arousal (Eisenberg et al., 1996). Because of this, children in negative emotion states may miss opportunities to learn from emotion-eliciting events.

Only recently have researchers begun to examine the relationship between emotionality and declarative emotion knowledge. These studies have established initial support that higher levels of positive emotionality and extraversion are associated with greater declarative emotion knowledge, albeit weakly (Matsumoto et al., 2000; Schultz et al., 2004; cf. Arsenio, Cooperman, & Lover, 2000). It also appears that children's anger-proneness and/or neuroticism correlate with lower levels of declarative emotion knowledge (Arsenio et al., 2000; Matsumoto et al., 2000).

3.6   THE EMOTION SYSTEMS AND EMOTION PROCESSING PATTERNS

As stated at the outset, in addition to examining children's declarative emotion knowledge, several researchers have recently focused on specific patterns in children's emotion attributions (Barth & Bastiani, 1997; Pollak, Cicchetti, Hornung, & Reed, 2000; Schultz et al., 2004). Initial findings suggest that emotion experiences strongly influence the development of these patterns. In our work, we have shown that some young children have a tendency to interpret emotion cues as representing anger more often than other children (Schultz, Izard, & Ackerman, 2000; Schultz et al., 2004). Studies examining the origins of these tendencies implicate hostile and chaotic family environments, such as homes characterized by abuse (Pollak et al., 2000; Pollak, Klorman, Thatcher, & Cicchetti, 2001), instability (Schultz et al., 2000), and maternal depression (Schultz et al., 2000). Some evidence suggests that anger-prone children also tend to attribute anger to others' emotion states (Schultz et al., 2004). Researchers have suggested that this atypical processing pattern may serve adaptive purposes for children within certain family environments (Pollak & Sinha, 2002; Schultz et al., 2004). Failure to interpret parental cues as hostile may sometimes lead to severe consequences for some children. Abusive experiences or other experiences characterized by threat or pain to the child will likely elicit intense fear in them. These fear experiences may condition the emotion systems both to respond to threatening cues more quickly and to associate a variety of cues that are loosely related to anger or hostility (e.g., ambiguous facial expressions) with threat.

We believe that idiosyncratic appraisal tendencies associated with intense negative emotion experiences may influence social interactions more greatly than whether or not children have developed general declarative knowledge of typical emotion reactions. Three published studies have included assessments of both declarative emotion knowledge and the frequency with which children attribute anger to others. In two of these, children's anger attribution tendencies predicted social functioning after controlling for declarative emotion knowledge, but declarative emotion knowledge failed to predict functioning after controlling for anger expectancy tendencies (Barth & Bastiani, 1997; Schultz et al., 2000). In the third study, declarative emotion knowledge and anger attribution tendencies predicted aggression equally strongly, though the researchers did not analyze the predictive ability of each component after controlling for the other (Schultz et al., 2004). In daily interactions, people do not pose prototypic facial expressions a majority of the time, and dynamics within social events are often complex. Because of this, expressions and situations rarely have a single emotion that necessarily corresponds with them. Children, influenced by their past emotion experiences and their emotion systems responses to these experiences, are constantly left to fill in the blanks to interpret how others feel. Their emotion processing tendencies, influenced by the emotion systems, may influence these interpretations in more meaningful ways than declarative emotion knowledge.

3.7   THE EMOTION SYSTEMS, EMOTION STATES, AND EMOTION PERCEPTIONS

Children with negative emotionality will likely exhibit particular patterns of emotion processing. A large body of research documents that arousal of negative emotions will influence interpretations of social stimuli (for a review, see Rusting, 1998). Several studies provide direct evidence that emotion arousal influences patterns of emotion attributions. College students who previously heard an irritating noise attributed more negative emotions to others; those who previously heard a disgusting tape attributed more disgust to others; and those who previously heard a comedy tape attributed more positive emotions to others (Schiffenbauer, 1974; cf. Carlson, Felleman, & Masters, 1983). When induced to feel anxious, children tend to attribute hostility toward hypothetical peers in vignettes (Dodge & Somberg, 1987). Anger induced through role play tends to cause participants to perceive expressions of anger when exposed stereoscopically to expressions of anger and joy (Izard, Wehmer, Livsey, & Jennings, 1965). Finally, emotion arousal speeds the perception and judgment of emotion-congruent cues (e.g., facial expressions, words) (Niedenthal, Setterlund, & Jones, 1994). Because of their greater frequency of experiencing certain discrete emotions, in their actual peer interactions children with negative emotionality will attend to and attribute particular emotions to others.

3.8   THE EMOTION SYSTEMS AND THE VALUE OF EMOTION RECOGNITION

Finally, a key ingredient to effective social adjustment is not just having declarative knowledge of emotions but also consistently applying this knowledge to one's interactions. Individual differences in emotionality and reinforcement histories mediated by the emotion systems likely play an important role in the application of declarative emotion knowledge. Many theorists predict that lower levels of declarative emotion knowledge will lead to conflicted social interactions. For example, failing to recognize anger in others may lead to contextually inappropriate behaviors toward them, leading to conflict. In our own research, however, we have found inconsistent and weak associations between assessments of declarative emotion knowledge and how frequently children fight. Many aggressive children may know how others feel when forced to consider the question on an experimental task but may not value and/or spontaneously apply this knowledge in their social interactions. Levels of empathy and reinforcement histories for applying declarative emotion knowledge probably combine to influence whether or not children actually use their declarative emotion knowledge. The extent to which children value and/or use their declarative emotion knowledge is probably as critical an element in predicting social interactions as the level of declarative knowledge itself. Some evidence suggests that individual differences in emotionality may influence this valuation. Positive emotionality has been related to empathy, for example, and certain negative emotion experiences such as sadness and anger are often characterized by focus on the self (Eisenberg, Fabes, & Bernzweig, 1993; Eisenberg et al., 1996; Young, Fox, & Zahn-Waxler, 1999).

3.9   ADDITIONAL COMMENTS ON THE DEVELOPMENT OF EMOTION RECOGNITION

Several writers have pointed out that some aspects of EI may reflect goodness of fit between children and their environments (Chess & Thomas, 1999; Zeidner, Matthews, Roberts, & MacCann, 2003). The tendency to attribute anger to others is a good example of this. Although the development of appraisal processes conditioned toward assuming anger and hostility may serve adaptive purposes within certain family environments, multiple correlational studies suggest that this processing tendency may lead to greater numbers of aggressive encounters with peers and dislike by them (Barth & Bastiani, 1997; Schultz et al., 2000, 2004).

Second, although we have focused almost exclusively on the influence of the emotion systems, we certainly do not mean to suggest that individual differences in emotion recognition, especially declarative emotion knowledge, can be completely accounted for by different aspects of emotion systems functioning. Declarative emotion knowledge varies depending upon an individual's level of intelligence; children who can process information more quickly will tend to have developed more associations between emotion cues, labels, and situational events. We consistently find moderate correlations (i.e., r's ranging from .16 to .63 but typically from .30 to .50) between declarative emotion knowledge scores and verbal ability. The contribution of verbal ability to declarative emotion knowledge seems independent of effects of certain temperamental traits. First-grade children's verbal ability predicted both emotion expression knowledge and emotion situation knowledge even after controlling for attentional persistence and behavioral control (Schultz, Izard, Ackerman, & Youngstrom, 2001). In contrast to the associations between intelligence and declarative emotion knowledge, in our work children's tendencies to attribute anger to others fails to correspond with their verbal ability.

Emotion recognition is one of the few components of EI that has shown a capacity to predict social and behavioral adjustment after controlling for both specific temperamental traits and intelligence. Individual differences in a composite of emotion expression and situation knowledge predicted first-grade children's social problems and social withdrawal after controlling for preschool attentional persistence, behavioral control, and verbal ability (see Schultz et al., 2001). In the same sample of children, preschool facial expression knowledge predicted teacher ratings of social skills, behavior problems, and academic competence in third-grade after controlling for difficult temperament and verbal ability in preschool (Izard et al., 2001). Other investigators have confirmed these findings. Children's anger-proneness and happiness both predicted aggression and peer acceptance in predicted directions, after which declarative emotion knowledge added significantly to the prediction of both aggression and peer acceptance (Arsenio et al., 2000). Emotion recognition seems to be a construct shaped in part by temperament and intelligence but which also retains independence both as a construct and as a predictor of social and behavioral functioning. As outlined in this chapter, we believe this independence is largely influenced by emotion experiences and subsequent emotion processing patterns mediated by the emotion systems.

Finally, it is noteworthy that many schools now take a more deliberate and active role in the development of their students' EI. Psychologists and educators have developed a variety of curricula available to principals and teachers that focus on the promotion of children's emotion and social skills (e.g., recognizing emotions, anger regulation, taking turns). One of the most research-based of these programs is entitled Promoting Alternative Thinking Strategies (PATHS; Greenberg & Kusche, 1998). Randomized trials have found the PATHS program to promote many individual aspects of EI, such as the size of children's emotion vocabularies and understanding of others' abilities to hide feelings (Greenberg, Kusche, Cook, & Quamma, 1995), to enhance classroom atmospheres (Conduct Problems Prevention Research Group, 1999), and to reduce student levels of externalizing behaviors such as aggression (Greenberg & Kusche, 1998). We do not yet know, however, what the active ingredients are within these programs that promote change in children's behaviors. Do children's newly acquired thinking skills by themselves cause changes in their behavior? Through the process of learning and delivering the lessons, many teachers also likely experience growth, becoming more skilled coaches and managers of their students' emotions. These teacher changes may play as critical a role in promoting adaptive behaviors in children as changes in children's thinking skills.

3.10   CONCLUSIONS

We have seen that we can conceptualize individual differences in emotion recognition in at least two overlapping ways: (a) declarative emotion knowledge, and (b) emotion processing patterns. The emotion systems influence the development of both of these components, especially the latter. Emotion experiences and emotionality may facilitate or impede the acquisition of declarative emotion knowledge (Abe & Izard, 1999a), and emotion processing patterns reflect emotion experiences and dispositional traits more directly.

We believe the distinctions we have outlined between declarative emotion knowledge and emotion processing patterns apply to other components of EI. For example, much research attention has focused on children's abilities to generate response options to social situations. A child who responds to peer teasing by calling the teaser a bad name, however, likely knows that she could ignore the teaser, ask the teaser to stop, or tell the teacher. These responses probably have not been sufficiently reinforced in the child to cause her emotion systems to motivate her to use them. Possibly, through seeing respected siblings or peers call others' bad names, she may in fact have been reinforced to use name calling as a strategy. She may have a tendency toward generating angry and hostile responses, especially when scared or angry, rather than a deficit in declarative knowledge related to social responses. Future research on EI should delineate between these aspects, as they likely have somewhat distinct antecedents and may predict social functioning differentially.

REFERENCES

Abe, J. A., & Izard, C. E. (1999a). The developmental functions of emotions: An analysis in terms of differential emotions theory. *Cognition and Emotion, 13*, 523–549.

Abe, J. A., & Izard, C. E. (1999b). A longitudinal study of emotion expression and personality relations in early development. *Journal of Personality and Social Psychology, 77*, 566–577.

Adolphs, R., Tranel, D., Damasio, H., & Damasio, A. R. (1995). Fear and the human amygdala. *Journal of Neuroscience, 15*, 5879–5891.

Arsenio, W. F., Cooperman, S., & Lover, A. (2000). Affective predictors of preschoolers' aggression and peer acceptance: Direct and indirect effects. *Developmental Psychology, 36*, 438–448.

Bachevalier, J., Hagger, C., & Bercu, B. B. (1989). Gender differences in visual habit formation in 3-month-old rhesus monkeys. *Developmental Psychobiology, 22*, 585–599.

Barth, J. M., & Bastiani, A. (1997). A longitudinal study of emotion recognition and preschool children's social behavior. *Merrill-Palmer Quarterly, 43*, 107–128.

Bauer, R. M. (1982). Visual hypoemotionality as a symptom of visual-limbic disconnection in man. *Archives of Neurology, 39*, 702–708.

Bechara, A., Tranel, D., Damasio, H., Adolphs, R., Rockland, C., & Damasio, A. R. (1995). Double dissociation of conditioning and declarative knowledge relative to the amygdala and hippocampus in humans. *Science, 269*, 1115–1118.

Conduct Problems Prevention Research Group. (1999). Initial impact of the fast track prevention trial for conduct problems: II. Classroom effect. *Journal of Consulting and Clinical Psychology, 67*, 648–657.

Brown, J. R., & Dunn, J. F. (1996). Continuities in emotion understanding from 3–6 yrs. *Child Development, 67*, 789–802.

Calder, A. J., Young, A. W., Rowland, D., Perrett, D., Hodges, J. R., & Etcoff, N. L. (1996). Facial emotion recognition after bilateral amygdala damage: Differentially severe impairment of fear. *Cognitive Neuropsychology, 13*, 699–745.

Carlson, C. R., Felleman, E. S., & Masters, J. C. (1983). Influence of children's emotion states on the recognition of emotion in peers and social motives to change another's emotional state. *Motivation and Emotion, 7*, 61–79.

Chess, S., & Thomas, A. (1999). *Goodness of fit: Clinical applications from infancy through adult life.* Philadelphia: Brunner/Mazel.

Damasio, A. R. (1994). *Descartes' error: Emotion, reason, and the human brain.* New York: Grosset/Putnam.

Darwin, C. (1965). *The expression of the emotions in man and animals.* Chicago: University of Chicago Press. (Original work published 1872)

Davis, M. H., Luce, C., & Kraus, S. J. (1994). The heritability of characteristics associated with dispositional empathy. *Journal of Personality, 62*, 369–391.

Denham, S. A., Zoller, D., & Couchoud, E. A. (1994). Socialization of preschoolers' emotion understanding. *Developmental Psychology, 30*, 928–936.

DiLalla, L. F., & Jones, S. (2000). Genetic and environmental influences on temperament in preschoolers. In V. J. Molfese & D. L. Molfese (Eds.), *Temperament and personality development across the life span* (pp. 33–55). Mahwah, NJ: Lawrence Erlbaum.

Dodge, K. A., Laird, R., Lochman, J. E., & Zelli, A. (2002). Multidimensional latent-construct analysis of children's social information processing patterns: Correlations with aggressive behavior problems. *Psychological Assessment, 14*, 60–73.

Dodge, K. A., & Somberg, D. R. (1987). Hostile attributional biases among aggressive boys are exacerbated under conditions of threat to the self. *Child Development, 58*, 213–224.

Donaldson, S. K., & Westerman, M. A. (1986). Development of children's understanding of ambivalence and causal theories of emotions. *Developmental Psychology, 22*, 655–662.

Downer, C. L. C. (1962). Interhemispheric integration in the visual system. In V. B. Mountcastle (Ed.), *Interhemispheric relations and cerebral dominance* (pp. 87–100). Baltimore: Johns Hopkins University Press.

Dunn, J. F., Brown, J. R., & Maguire, M. (1995). The development of children's moral sensibility: Individual differences and emotion understanding. *Developmental Psychology, 31,* 649–659.

Eisenberg, N., Fabes, R. A., & Bernzweig, J. (1993). The relations of emotionality and regulation to preschoolers' social skills and sociometric status. *Child Development, 64,* 1418–1438.

Eisenberg, N., Fabes, R. A., Karbon, M., Murphy, B. C., Wosinski, M., Polazzi, L., et al. (1996). The relations of children's dispositional prosocial behavior to emotionality, regulation, and social functioning. *Social Development, 5,* 330–351.

Ekman, P. (1999). Basic emotions. In T. Dalgleish & M. J. Power (Eds.), *Handbook of cognition and emotion* (pp. 45–60). New York: John Wiley.

Fameli, M., Kitraki, E., & Stylianopoulou, F. (1994). Effects of hyperactivity of the maternal hypothalamic-pituitary-adrenal (HPA) axis during pregnancy on the development of the HPA axis and brain monoamines of the offspring. *International Journal of Developmental Neuroscience, 12,* 651–659.

Field, T. M., Woodson, R., Greenberg, R., & Cohen, D. (1982). Discrimination and imitation of facial expressions by neonates. *Science, 218,* 179–181.

Fleming, I., Baum, A., Davidson, L. M., Rectanus, E., & McArdle, S. (1987). Chronic stress as a factor in physiologic reactivity to challenge. *Health Psychology, 6,* 221–237.

Fox, N. A. (2003). Not quite ready to invest. *Human Development, 46,* 104–108.

Gloor, P., Olivier, A., Quesney, L. F., Andermann, F., & Horowitz, S. (1982). The role of the limbic system in experiential phenomena of temporal lobe epilepsy. *Annals of Neurology, 12,* 129–144.

Goldsmith, H. H., & Campos, J. J. (1986). Fundamental issues in the study of early temperament: The Denver twin temperament study. In M. E. Lamb, A. L. Brown, & B. Rogoff (Eds.), *The development of attachment and affiliative systems* (pp. 161–193). New York: Plenum Press.

Goldsmith, H. H., Lemery, K. S., Buss, K. A., & Campos, J. J. (1999). Genetic analyses of focal aspects of infant temperament. *Developmental Psychology, 35,* 972–985.

Gottman, J. M., Katz, L. F., & Hooven, C. (1996). Parental meta-emotion philosophy and the emotional life of families: Theoretical models and preliminary data. *Journal of Family Psychology, 10,* 243–268.

Greenberg, M. T., & Kusche, C. A. (1998). Preventive intervention for school-aged deaf children: The PATHS curriculum. *Journal of Deaf Studies and Deaf Education, 3,* 49–63.

Greenberg, M. T., Kusche, C. A., Cook, E. T., & Quamma, J. P. (1995). Promoting emotional competence in school-aged children: The effects of the PATHS curriculum. *Development and Psychopathology, 7,* 117–136.

Gunnar, M. R., Morison, S. J., & Chisholm, K. (2001). Salivary cortisol levels in children adopted from romanian orphanages. *Development and Psychopathology, 13,* 611–628.

Hagger, C., Bachevalier, J., & Bercu, B. B. (1987). Sexual dimorphism in the development of habit formation: Effects of perinatal steroidal gonadal hormones. *Neuroscience, 22*, 520.

Harris, P. L., Olthof, T., & Terwogt, M. M. (1981). Children's knowledge of emotion. *Journal of Child Psychology and Psychiatry and Allied Disciplines, 22*, 247–261.

Haviland, J. M., & Lelwica, M. (1987). The induced affect response: 10-week-old infants' responses to three emotion expressions. *Developmental Psychology, 23*, 97–104.

Isen, A. M. (1999). Positive affect. In T. Dalgleish & M. J. Power (Eds.), *Handbook of cognition and emotion* (pp. 521–539). New York: John Wiley.

Izard, C. E. (1971). *The face of emotion*. New York: Appleton-Century-Crofts.

Izard, C. E., Fine, S., Schultz, D., Mostow, A., Ackerman, B. P., & Youngstrom, E. A. (2001). Emotion knowledge as a predictor of social behavior and academic competence in children at risk. *Psychological Science, 12*, 18–23.

Izard, C. E., Wehmer, G. M., Livsey, W., & Jennings, J. R. (1965). Affect, awareness, and performance. In S. S. Tomkins & C. E. Izard (Eds.), *Affect, cognition, and personality* (pp. 2–41). New York: Springer.

Kagan, J., Reznick, S. J., & Snidman, N. (1987). The physiology and psychology of behavioral inhibition in children. *Child Development, 58*, 1459–1473.

Kaufman, J., Birmaher, B., Perel, J., Dahl, R. E., Moreci, P., Nelson, B., et al. (1997). The corticotropin-releasing hormone challenge in depressed abused, depressed nonabused, and normal control children. *Biological Psychiatry, 42*, 669–679.

Kestenbaum, R., & Gelman, S. A. (1995). Preschool children's identification and understanding of mixed emotions. *Cognitive Development, 10*, 443–458.

Kuchuk, A., Vibbert, M., & Bornstein, M. H. (1986). The perception of smiling and its experiential correlates in three-month-old infants. *Child Development, 57*, 1054–1061.

Ladd, C. O., Owens, M. J., & Nemeroff, C. B. (1996). Persistent changes in cortiocopropin-releasing factor neuronal systems induced by maternal deprivation. *Endocrinology, 137*, 1212–1218.

Lazarus, R. S. (1991). Progress on a cognitive-motivational relational theory of emotion. *American Psychologist, 46*, 819–834.

LeDoux, J. E. (2000). Emotion circuits in the brain. *Annual Review of Neuroscience, 23*, 155–184.

Lytton, H. (1990). Child and parent effects in boys' conduct disorder: A reinterpretation. *Developmental Psychology, 26*, 683–697.

Matsumoto, D., LeRoux, J., Wilson-Cohn, C., Raroque, J., Kooken, K., Ekman, P., et al. (2000). A new test to measure emotion recognition ability: Matsumoto and Ekman's Japanese and Caucasian Brief Affect Recognition Test (JACBART). *Journal of Nonverbal Behavior, 24*, 179–209.

Meltzoff, A. N., & Moore, M. K. (1983). Newborn infants imitate adult facial gestures. *Child Development, 54*, 702–709.

Mesulam, M.-M. (1998). From sensation to cognition. *Brain, 121*, 1013–1052.

Niedenthal, P. M., Setterlund, M. B., & Jones, D. E. (1994). Emotional organization of perceptual memory. In P. M. Niedenthal & S. Kitayama (Eds.), *The heart's eye: Emotional influences in perception and attention* (pp. 87–113). San Diego, CA: Academic Press.

Ockenfels, M. C., Porter, L., Smyth, J., Kirschbaum, C., Hellhammer, D. H., & Stone, A. A. (1995). Effect of chronic stress associated with unemployment on salivary cortisol: Overall cortisol levels, diurnal rhythm, and acute stress reactivity. *Psychosomatic Medicine, 57*, 460–467.

Peng, M., Johnson, C., Pollock, J., Glasspool, R., & Harris, P. L. (1992). Training young children to acknowledge mixed emotions. *Cognition and Emotion, 6*, 387–401.

Plomin, R., & Stocker, C. (1989). Behavioral genetics and emotionality. In J. S. Reznick (Ed.), *Perspectives on behavioral inhibition* (pp. 219–240). Chicago: University of Chicago Press.

Plotsky, P. M., & Meaney, M. J. (1993). Early, postnatal experience alters hypothalamic corticotropin-releasing factor (CRF) mRNA, median eminence CRF content and stress-induced release in adult rats. *Molecular Brain Research, 18*, 195–200.

Pollak, S. D., Cicchetti, D., Hornung, K., & Reed, A. (2000). Recognizing emotion in faces: Developmental effects of child abuse and neglect. *Developmental Psychology, 36*, 679–688.

Pollak, S. D., Klorman, R., Thatcher, J. E., & Cicchetti, D. (2001). P3b reflects maltreated children's reactions to facial displays of emotion. *Psychophysiology, 38*, 267–274.

Pollak, S. D., & Sinha, P. (2002). Effects of early experience on children's recognition of facial displays of emotion. *Developmental Psychology, 38*, 784–791.

Ridgeway, D., Waters, E., & Kuczaj, S. A. (1985). Acquisition of emotion-descriptive language: Receptive and productive vocabulary norms for ages 18 months to 6 years. *Developmental Psychology, 21*, 901–908.

Rodman, H. R. (1994). Development of inferior temporal cortex in the monkey. *Cerebral Cortex, 5*, 484–498.

Rodman, H. R., Skelly, J. P., & Gross, C. G. (1991). Stimulus selectivity and state dependence of activity in inferior temporal cortex of infant monkeys. *Proceedings of the National Academy of Sciences, 88*, 7572–7575.

Rosen, J. B., & Schulkin, J. (1998). From normal fear to pathological anxiety. *Psychological Review, 105*, 325–350.

Rothbart, M. K., Ahadi, S. A., & Hershey, K. L. (1994). Temperament and social behavior in childhood. *Merrill-Palmer Quarterly, 40*, 21–39.

Rothbart, M. K., Ahadi, S. A., Hershey, K. L., & Fisher, P. (2001). Investigations of temperament at three to seven years: The children's behavior questionnaire. *Child Development, 72*, 1394–1408.

Rusting, C. L. (1998). Personality, mood, and cognitive processing of emotional information: Three conceptual frameworks. *Psychological Bulletin, 124*, 165–196.

Schiffenbauer, A. (1974). Effect of observer's emotional state on judgments of the emotional state of others. *Journal of Personality and Social Psychology, 30*, 31–35.

Schneider, M. L. (1992). Prenatal stress exposure alters postnatal behavioral expression under conditions of novelty challenge in rhesus monkey infants. *Developmental Psychobiology, 25*, 529–540.

Schultz, D., Izard, C. E., & Ackerman, B. P. (2000). Children's anger attribution biases: Relations to family environment and social adjustment. *Social Development, 9*, 284–301.

Schultz, D., Izard, C. E., Ackerman, B. P., & Youngstrom, E. A. (2001). Emotion knowledge in early childhood: Self-regulatory antecedents and relations to social difficulties and withdrawal. *Development and Psychopathology, 13,* 53–67.

Schultz, D., Izard, C. E., & Bear, G. (2004). Children's emotion processing: Relations to emotionality and aggression. *Development and Psychopathology, 16,* 371–387.

Scott, S. K., Young, A. W., Calder, A. J., Hellawell, D. J., Aggleton, J. P., & Johnson, M. (1997). Impaired auditory recognition of fear and anger following bilateral amygdala lesions. *Nature, 385,* 254–257.

Sorce, J. F., Emde, R. N., Campos, J. J., & Klinnert, M. D. (1985). Maternal emotional signaling: Its effect on the visual cliff behavior of 1-year-olds. *Developmental Psychology, 21,* 195–200.

Steele, H., Steele, M., Croft, C., & Fonagy, P. (1999). Infant-mother attachment at one year predicts children's understanding of mixed emotions at six years. *Social Development, 8,* 161–178.

Tellegen, A., Lykken, D. T., Bouchard, T. J., Jr., Wilcox, K., Segal, N. S., & Rich, S. (1988). Personality similarity in twins reared apart and together. *Journal of Personality and Social Psychology, 54,* 1031–1039.

Tooby, J., & Cosmides, L. (1990). The past explains the present: Emotional adaptations and the structure of ancestral environment. *Ethology and Sociobiology, 11,* 375–424.

Young, S. K., Fox, N. A., & Zahn-Waxler, C. (1999). The relations between temperament and empathy in 2-year-olds. *Developmental Psychology, 35,* 1189–1197.

Zeidner, M., Matthews, G., Roberts, R. D., & MacCann, C. (2003). Development of emotional intelligence: Towards a multi-level investment model. *Human Development, 46,* 69–96.

Zeidner, M., Roberts, R. D., & Matthews, G. (2002). Can emotional intelligence be schooled? A critical review. *Educational Psychologist,* 215–231.

4

Mindfulness-Based Emotional Intelligence: A Theory and Review of the Literature

Joseph Ciarrochi
Claire Godsell
University of Wollongong, Australia

Summary

We present a theory of the source of human suffering, and then describe an emotional intelligence (EI) framework that is based on this theory. We illustrate how a wide variety of EI-relevant measures can be understood in terms of this framework. Finally, we describe an intervention approach that is specifically designed to undermine the theorized causes of suffering. EI-relevant measures can be used to evaluate the efficacy of this intervention and to provide feedback about how to improve it.

4.1   INTRODUCTION

"The single most remarkable fact of human existence is how hard it is for human beings to be happy" (Hayes, Strosahl, & Wilson, 1999, p. 1). At any given time, a substantial number of people report feeling moderately to severely anxious or depressed (Ciarrochi, Deane, & Anderson, 2002; Ciarrochi, Scott, Deane, & Heaven, 2003). Up to one third of people have a diagnosable mental disorder. In addition, about half of the population will face moderate to severe levels of suicidality sometime in their lives (Hayes et al., 1999). Add up all the people who are hostile, depressed, alcoholic, fearing intimacy, suicidal, self-destructive, addicted, workaholic, and desperate. One can not help but acknowledge the first of the Buddhist noble truths: Suffering is the human condition (Kapleau, 1989).

What is the cause of human suffering and what can be done to reduce it? Is emotional intelligence (EI) the answer?

4.2   A DIFFERENT STARTING POINT FOR EI

A substantial amount of research focuses on developing new EI measures and evaluating whether these measures are distinctive from personality and IQ. One goal of this research is prediction. For example, we know that IQ and personality can predict workplace outcomes (Schmidt & Hunter, 1998; Tokar, Fischer, & Subich, 1998). An important question is whether EI measures can predict variance over and above these well-established measures. If not, then why would we need the EI measure (if our goal is incremental prediction)?

Our primary purpose in this chapter is not to argue for new and unique EI measures. Rather, it is to understand the causes of human suffering and how it can be alleviated. Our chapter has three goals: 1) to present a theory of human suffering (Hayes et al., 1999), 2) to utilize this theory to provide a framework for the vast number of EI-relevant measures, and 3) to suggest ways that suffering can be alleviated. Our goal is prediction-and-control as a single thing (Hayes, Hayes, & Reese, 1988), rather than just prediction. This goal dictates what measures we review. For example, if someone's primary goal was solely to predict future negative affectivity, then the best predictor of this would be likely to be past negative affectivity (Clark, Watson, & Mineka, 1994). However, knowing that past negativity predicts future negativity would not necessarily serve our goals, since it would not help us to reduce future negativity (the goal of control).

Similarly, EI measures that assess "stress tolerance" or "impulse control" (Bar-On, 1997) do not necessarily aid us in the goal of control and therefore are not discussed here. Saying that someone gets stressed because they have low stress tolerance does not seem to tell us anything about what one does to increase stress tolerance. As a final example, saying that personality traits such as extraversion (or positive affectivity) and neuroticism (or negative affectivity) are related to depression (Clark et al., 1994) again suggests nothing about what one does about depression. Do we seek to increase extraversion? Do we seek to reduce neuroticism? How?

We are not arguing that the goal of prediction-and-control is better than a primary goal of prediction. Both goals are clearly important. What we are arguing is that what one focuses on depends upon ones goals (Laudan, 1981).

The EI-relevant measures we review here have two important features. First, they can be clearly connected to and understood via the proposed theory of human suffering. Second, they can at least in principle be used as process measures in an EI intervention. That is, they can be used to help evaluate why an EI intervention works, and to provide feedback so that such interventions can be improved.

4.3   DEFINITIONS

Emotional well-being refers to a broad category of phenomena that includes peoples affective responses (e.g., state levels of guilt, depression, anger, joy, and self assurance) and global judgments of life satisfaction (Diener, Suh, Lucas, & Smith, 1999). There are negative indices (e.g., anger, stress, anxiety) and positive indices (joy, vigor). Each of the specific aspects of well-being warrant study in their own right, yet they all tend to correlate, suggesting the need for a higher order well-being construct (Diener et al., 1999).

We find it useful to utilize the words "pain" and "suffering" in a specific way (Hayes et al., 1999). Pain is what occurs during the course of just living one's life. Painful emotions are often labelled as sadness, annoyance, and remorse (Ellis, 2001). In contrast, suffering is emotional discomfort that is created from our ineffective reactions to pain. For example, the label "depression" can describe a state of suffering, if it is the result of feeling bad about a loss (sadness) and believing a negative evaluation about the entire future (e.g., "the future is hopeless").

Emotional intelligence is defined here in terms of four dimensions (see Table 4.1) that involve the ability to act effectively in the context of emotions and emotionally charged thoughts, and use emotions as information. We will talk much more about these dimensions throughout the chapter, but one example might be clarifying. The first dimension of EI is effective emotional orientation. People who have an ineffective orientation tend to repress or avoid their emotions. For example, they may attempt to repress feelings of anger towards a colleague. They may even pretend that they do not have angry feelings. Unfortunately, anger might be providing them with valuable information about the colleague (e.g., that the person is behaving unfairly). Thus, killing the messenger (e.g., the anger) also kills the message (the colleague is behaving unfairly). Without this valuable information, the person may also lose the ability to act effectively (e.g., respond with assertion to the injustice).

4.4   A THEORY OF UNIVERSAL HUMAN SUFFERING
F.E.A.R.: FUSION AND RELATIONAL FRAME THEORY

We now describe a theory that seeks to explain why suffering is so universal. We then use this theory to generate a framework for EI-relevant measures. Finally, we will review evidence suggesting that being high in each dimension is associated with lower suffering and increased vitality.

Language is essential to our survival. However, it also appears to have a dark side (Hayes, Barnes-Holmes, & Roche, 2001). The problems of language and how we use it can be captured in the acronym F.E.A.R.: Fusion, Evalu-

Table 4.1   The Components of Internally Focused Emotional Intelligence

EI component	Description
Defusing Unhelpful Self-Concepts (i.e., undermining the power of unhelpful self-concepts to act as barriers to effective action)	– Looking *at* self-evaluations, rather than *through* them – Escaping the perceived need to defend self-esteem – Recognizing that emotionally charged evaluations of the self do not have to stop us from pursing our goals – Making contact with the "observer self"; finding the safe place from which to accept all negative emotions, self-doubts, and other unpleasant inner experiences
Defusing Unhelpful Thoughts and Emotions (i.e., undermining the power of unhelpful thoughts and emotions to act as barriers to effective action)	– Looking *at* emotionally charged verbal content, rather than *through* it – Seeing that emotionally charged thoughts about life are not equivalent to life – Being able to be mindful of moment to moment experience (either internal or external)
Using Emotion as Information	– Identifying emotions – Understanding the appraisals that activate different emotions – Understanding the consequences of emotions on cognition, health, and so forth – Understanding how emotions progress over time – Distinguishing between helpful and unhelpful emotions and emotionally charged thoughts
Effective Emotional Orientation	– Willingness to have emotionally charged private experiences (thoughts, images, emotions) when doing so fosters effective action – Accepting the inevitably of a certain amount of unpleasant affect and negative self-evaluation – Understand that private experiences do not have to stop one from pursuing a valued direction (and therefore one does not have to get rid of them)

ation, Avoidance, and Reason giving. The F.E.A.R. framework is presented in more detail by its creators, namely, Hayes and his colleagues (Hayes et al., 1999, 2001).

Relational Frame Theory (RFT) has been used to account for the pervasiveness of human suffering and to suggest how it can be reduced. It has been tested in the lab under highly controlled conditions, and has found substantial experimental support during the last two decades (Hayes et al., 1999). We have only a small space here to discuss RFT, but please see Hayes et al. (1999) for a book length treatment of it.

4.4.1   Implication 1: Language Makes Monsters Present

Research has shown that language tends to be bi-directionally related to experience (Hayes et al., 2001). For example, the word "shock" will carry with it some of the aversive functions of shock itself. This bi-directionality appears to be unique in humans (Hayes et al., 2001). A pigeon can be taught to peck a key if it has been shocked (by giving it food) and peck another key if it has not been shocked. Essentially, the pigeon is reporting whether it has been shocked. This report will never become aversive for the bird, because it has never predicted shock. Indeed, it predicts reinforcement (food). In contrast, human verbal reports of past painful experience can bring forth much of the pain experienced in the trauma. This occurs even when the reports do not predict the trauma, and indeed even when the report has never been made before (Hayes et al., 1999).

This discussion leads us to one of the defining characteristics of RFT. The act of relating stimuli leads to the transformation of stimulus functions. When two stimuli are related, some of the functions of each stimulus change according to what stimulus it is related to, and how it is related to that stimulus. In the above example, the word "shock" started out as a neutral sound, but became transformed into something aversive because it became related to actual shock.

4.4.2   Implication 2: Language Processes Are Dominant

A substantial number of verbal relations can be derived outside of experience. For example, if we know that A is good and B is like A, then we can derive that B is good. If C is like B, we can further derive that B is good and B is like A, and so forth. As a further example, consider the following question: "How is a mouse like a bag or oranges?" Although you may never have been asked this question, you are probably now able to derive relations between mice and oranges. Indeed, humans have the ability to derive relations between just about any two things. And each derivation may lead to further transformation of stimulus functions (Blackledge, 2003).

RFT research confirms that if people are taught just a few links via experience, they can derive a substantial number of links without experience. For example, one study demonstrated that for each link between two stimuli that was learned via experience, 15 new links could be derived (Wulfert & Hayes,

1988). Thus, the percentage of our understanding that is based on experience can be quite small compared to the percentage that is derived. RFT-related research also suggests that when our verbal constructions are inconsistent with our experience, the verbal constructions can dominate. For example, experimental studies have compared the performance of people who learned a task either by directly following a verbal rule or by experience (Hayes, Brownstein, Haas, & Greenway, 1986). The task requirements were later changed. All of the participants who learned the task by experience where sensitive to the change. In contrast, only half of the participants who learned the task by rules were sensitive to the change. In general, overreliance on verbal rules can lead to rigid, inflexible behavior (Hayes et al., 1999).

4.4.3   Implication 3: Language Processes Are Controlled by Context and Reinforcement

RFT premises that the reason we constantly derive relations, or engage in relational framing, is because the verbal community reinforces such relating. For example, a child may be trained to connect the letters "C" "A" "T" with an actual cat and with the sound "CAT". When a cat actually walks by, a parent might say to the child, "what is that?". Without ever being taught the link between the sound and the actual cat, the child will correctly respond "CAT". The parent might reinforce the child by saying "good!". There is now strong evidence that relating is under the influence of reinforcement and context, as suggested by RFT (see Hayes et al., 1999).

There are numerous contexts in which relational framing is reinforced. For example, in the context or "reason giving", the social community reinforces people for providing reasons for their behavior (Hayes et al., 1999). If you ask a person with social anxiety, "why didn't you give the speech?", they might respond, "I don't know". Many people would actively discourage this response. If the person said, "I couldn't give the speech because I was anxious", the community would be more likely to find this acceptable. Thus, the person was reinforced for creating a causal "frame" between anxiety and not engaging in a particular behavior (Hayes et al., 2001). As discussed above, people tend to believe these rules, even when it is destructive to do so.

4.4.4   Fusion

This discussion brings us to the notion of cognitive fusion. Fusion involves symbols becoming functionally equivalent, to some extent, with the event it symbolizes (Hayes et al., 1999). In the above example, the word "shock" can have similar effects to an actual shock. Fusion means that our verbal world can become even more psychologically powerful than reality at times. Verbal reports of painful experience can be as painful as the actual experience.

Fusion is hypothesized to be the beginning of suffering (Hayes et al., 1999). It allows us to create symbolic worlds and do battle with them in order to vanquish the "bad" thoughts and feelings. As we shall see soon, such attempts to control our private worlds often fail, and indeed can makes things worse. Fusion also allows us to live almost entirely in our interpreted world and to become insensitive to experience that is inconsistent with this world (Hayes et al., 1999).

4.4.5   Evaluation

One of the goals of a primitive human was to avoid getting eaten. We evolved a "critical mind", which refers to our natural tendency to evaluate the external environment for threats (Bless, 2001; Forgas, 1995). Evaluation is certainly essential for surviving, but it can also be turned against us. Language allows us to create an abstracted concept of "I". Our critical mind can then be turned on this "I", just as it would be turned on the external world. It evaluates "I", compares "I" to others, and sometimes finds "I" to be bad or inadequate.

Language also allows us to create names for our internal states. We create labels like "anxiety" and "stress". The critical mind can then evaluate these states and declare them to be bad. We may then try to avoid the internal states just as we avoid genuinely threatening external events. We also create abstract labels like "our life." Critical mind can evaluate our life as "worthless" and "unbearable", and thereby provide the impetus for suicide. Finally, language allows us to create ideals about ourselves, other people, and the world around us. Critical mind can than compare the ideal to present reality, and find the present to be unacceptable.

Consistent with this view, evidence suggests that social comparison and negative self-evaluation are pervasive and linked to suffering (Blascovich & Tomaka, 1991; Lyubomirsky, 2001). We shall have more to say about this later.

4.4.6   Avoidance

It is often adaptive to avoid threats in the outside world. Humans create an internal, private world of symbols, and learn to avoid aspects of it. Such avoidance can be attempted by directly suppressing unpleasant experiences or by seeking to modify such experiences. Experiential avoidance may work in the short run, but often not in the long run. Indeed, it can have a paradoxical rebound effect. The more one tries to avoid the experience , the more it can dominate one's life (Hayes et al., 1999; Wegner, 1994).

The downsides to experiential avoidance are now well documented. Research has shown that when participants are asked to suppress a thought, they later show an increase in this suppressed thought as compared with those not given suppression instructions (Wenzlaff & Wegner, 2000). Indeed, the suppression strategy may actually stimulate the suppressed mood in a kind of self-amplifying loop (Feldner, Zvolensky, Eifert, & Spira, 2003). Similar results have been found in the coping literature. Avoidant coping strategies predict negative outcomes for substance abuse, depression, and effects of child sexual abuse (for review, see Hayes et al., 1999).

4.4.7   Reason Giving/Rule Creation

People learn to put forth reasons as valid and sensible causes of behavior (Hayes et al., 1999). You might ask somebody, "Why didn't you leave the house?". They might respond with something like "I was too anxious". This seems perfectly reasonable to us. If, in contrast, they respond with, "I have no idea", we are likely to find this explanation unacceptable and insist that they give us a reason. This is an example of how the social community tends to reinforce reason giving.

Unfortunately, people begin to believe their own reasons and stories (Hayes et al., 1999), even when they are harmful if followed. People tell themselves, "I am worthless" and behave accordingly. They might tell themselves "I must have other people's approval", and waste a great deal of energy trying to get approval from every significant other. Or they might think, "I can't take a risk, because I am too anxious". They act as if they really can not take a risk, although experience will quickly show them that they can take risks and be anxious (Bourne, 2000).

4.5   EI COMPONENTS DERIVED FROM THE THEORY

We now turn our attention to the different dimensions of EI that we believe undermine the harmful influence of F.E.A.R.. For a book length treatment of how to undermine F.E.A.R., please see Hayes et al. (1999) and other work under the heading of "Acceptance and Commitment Therapy". After describing each EI dimension, we will review a number of individual difference measures that appear to tap into the dimensions, and discuss their relationship to well-being.

4.5.1   Effective Emotional Orientation (EEO)

Defining EEO.   Effective emotional orientation involves willingness to have private experiences (e.g., anxiety), when doing so fosters effective action (Table 4.1). It also involves accepting the inevitability of unpleasant affect and negative self-evaluation, and recognizing that these private experiences do not have to stop us from pursuing a valued direction (Hayes et al., 1999).

People quite reasonably avoid things in the world that are aversive. Cognitive fusion means that the thoughts about things are also aversive. People naturally evaluate their aversive thoughts as bad and seek to avoid them. As discussed above, avoidance often does not work and indeed can make matters worse. The rule of private experience is: If you are not willing to have it, you have it (Hayes et al., 1999). This is completely different from the rule of public experience. If you are not willing to have something unpleasant in the public world (say an ugly sofa), you usually can get rid of it.

The link between well-being and individual differences in EEO.   EEO is more of a family of constructs, rather than a single construct. The "family" members are interrelated, yet sometimes statistically separable. In general, all of the measures of EI described in this chapter have this family property. This chapter will focus on measures that have found empirical support from multiple, independent laboratories. Our purpose is not simply to re-label these old measures as EI. We refer to them by their original labels. Our main purpose is to look at what the last four decades of individual difference research tells us about effective emotional orientation.

The first individual difference we discuss—effective problem orientation—reflects the tendency to see emotional problems as a challenge rather than a threat, and the tendency to face problems, rather than avoid them. There is considerable evidence supporting the link between problem orientation and negative indices of well-being. It has been associated with low depression, anxiety, hopelessness, suicidal ideation, health complaints, and neuroticism (Ciarrochi et al., 2003; D'Zurilla, Chang, Nottingham, & Faccini, 1998; Elliott, Herrick, MacNair, & Harkins, 1994; Elliott & Marmarosh, 1994). It has been shown to be associated with low psychological distress and positive coping strategies, even when controlling for optimism, pessimism, positive affectivity, negative affectivity, and stressful life events (Chang & D'Zurilla, 1996; Ciarrochi et al., 2003). Other research provides some evidence that problem orientation is causally related to well-being. Davey and his colleagues have shown that experimentally induced reductions in effective orientation lead to increases in subsequent catastrophic worrying (Davey, Jubb, & Cameron, 1996).

The White Bear Suppression Inventory measures poor orientation, in that people who score high on it seek to avoid or suppress their private experiences. It has been found to correlate with measures of obsessional thinking and depressive and anxious affect (Wegner & Zanakos, 1994).

The Acceptance and Action Questionnaire (AAQ) measures the willingness to experience thoughts, feelings, and physiological sensations without having to control them, or let them determine one's actions (Bond & Bunce, 2003; Hayes et al., 2003). It has been associated with a range of negative emotional states (Hayes et al., 2003). A longitudinal study found that the AAQ predicts mental health and an objective measure of performance, over and above job control, negative affectivity, and locus of control (Bond & Bunce, 2003). In another study utilizing the AAQ, participants high in emotional avoidance showed more anxiety in response to CO_2 poisoning (biological challenge), particularly when instructed to suppress their emotions (Feldner et al., 2003).

4.5.2   Using Emotion as Information (UEI)

The second dimension of EI involves the ability to use emotions as information to inform effective action (see Table 4.1). Emotions are messengers. They usually tell us something about the world and about our own desires. For example, anxiety results from the appraisal that something undesirable might happen. Anger results from the appraisal that someone has acted unfairly and this has resulted in something undesirable (Ortony, Clore, & Collins, 1988).

The F.E.A.R. framework suggests that we tend to evaluate our unpleasant private experiences as bad and subsequently try to avoid them. Unfortunately, avoiding the messenger (the emotion) does not change the message. Importantly, if we do not know what the message is, we will find it difficult to act effectively. If we do not know that we are anxious, then we may mistakenly think our anxious sensations are due to a physical sickness (Taylor, 2000). Or we may mistakenly blame our anxiety on some irrelevant event (our colleague's behavior), and seek to change this irrelevant event, rather than focusing effectively on the real problem. Essentially, we need to be able to utilize emotions as information if we are to effectively solve our emotional problems.

The link between well-being and individual differences in using emotional information.   The measures discussed here focus on people's ability to identify their emotions, which is essential to being able to use emotional information.

Alexithymia refers to people who have trouble identifying and describing emotions and who tend to minimize emotional experience and focus attention externally (see also Chapter 13 by Parker). This construct appears to be a mix of Using Emotional Information and Effective Emotional Orientation. The Toronto Alexithymia Scale (TAS-20) is one of the most commonly used measures of alexithymia. It has been shown to be related to Bar-On's self-report EI measure (Taylor, Bagby, & Luminet, 2000), and to a number of important life outcomes. For example, people high in alexithymia are more prone to drug addiction, eating disorders, and to report medically unexplained symptoms (Taylor, 2001). The alexithymia subscales—difficulty identifying and describing emotions—are related to a variety of negative indices of well-being (e.g., depression), even after controlling for other measures of emotional intelligence (Ciarrochi et al., 2003). A longitudinal study found that alexithymia predicts persistent somatization at two year follow-up (Bach & Bach, 1995).

The emotional clarity subscale of the Trait Meta-Mood Scale (TMMS) also appears to measure an aspect of Using Emotion as Information (see Salovey, Mayer, Goldman, Turvey, & Palfai, 1995). This scale predicts how much people seem to dwell unproductively on sad thoughts (Salovey et al., 1995). In general, just about every measure of emotional intelligence appears to have a subscale that assesses skill at emotional identification. Such measures include the Mayer-Salovey-Caruso Emotional Intelligence Test (MSCEIT; Mayer, Salovey, and Caruso, 2002) and the Schutte et al. Emotional Intelligence Scales (SEIS; Schutte et al., 1998).[1]

Defusing from unhelpful emotions and thoughts.   The third dimension of EI involves the ability to undermine fusion with unhelpful emotions and thoughts. Table 4.1 lists the key components of this skill (see also Subsection 4.4.4). When language processes dominate,

---

[1]We acknowledge that there are rather substantial differences between self-report and ability based measures of emotion perception. However, discussion of these differences is beyond the scope of this chapter. Please see other chapters in this volume (e.g., Chapter 7 by Wilhelm).

humans fuse with the psychological contents of verbal events. The distinction between thinking and the referent of thought is diminished. As a result, emotionally charged thoughts or feelings (particularly those with provocative or pejorative meanings) become connected to powerful and predictable behavior patterns.
(Hayes et al., 1999, p. 149)

In other words, language has the power to bring forth its own reality. The word "milk" brings forth tastes and images of frothy white. It is as if the word has made the milk present. Language is so powerful that people come to see their verbal constructions of life as equivalent to life itself (Hayes et al., 1999). People fail to distinguish between the verbal products and the experience. We sometimes see life through "horrible" colored glasses (Ellis, 2001, Hayes et al., 1999).

One key to undermining fusion is to learn to look *at* our emotionally charged thoughts, rather than *through* them. It is as if there is a sign that says "Bad Mountain" and then a mountain in front of it. Fusion means that people often do not distinguish the sign from the mountain. They see the mountain through the sign "bad mountain." Defusing means stepping back and looking at the sign as just a sign.

Defusion involves a fundamental shift in context. It involves looking at the feelings, thoughts, sensations, and memories that show up from moment to moment and watching them as they go by. It involves a context shift from the "here and now" ("I am depressed") to the "there and then" (I have had the evaluation that "I am depressed"). Such shifts help people to see their private experience for what it is—streams of thought, fleeting sensations—rather than what it says it is—facts, dangers that must be avoided (Hayes et al., 1999; Kabat-Zinn, 1990).

Mindfulness is on the opposite side of "fusion". Mindfulness can be broken down into a number of components, including "what" skills (i.e., observing things as they come and go, describing them, and participating fully in life), and "how" skills (i.e., taking a non-judgmental stance, one-mindfully focus on what you are doing, doing what works [Linehan, 1993]). Essentially, mindfulness helps people to look at their private experience, rather than through it, and to see their moment-to-moment experience as it is (not as it seems to be when seen through language or intense emotion).

Mindlessly seeing life through unhelpful thoughts is expected to be a major source of suffering (Ellis, 2001). Ellis has proposed four major classes of unhelpful thoughts (Ellis, 2001). These include demandingness ("Things *must* be a certain way"), low distress tolerance ("I can't stand it"), "awfulizing" ("My life is awful"), and global evaluations ("I am completely good or bad; work is completely bad"). The key goal in mindfulness training is not to get rid of the thoughts (they are unhelpful but not necessarily harmful). Rather the key is to accept whatever thoughts show up during the course of pursing goals (effective orientation) and to learn to look at thoughts, rather than through them. The key is to be willing to have the unhelpful thoughts, but not necessarily believe them.

The last two decades have found substantial support for interventions that are designed to increase mindfulness. Acceptance and Commitment Therapy (ACT) is a mindfulness approach that is directly derived from the F.E.A.R. framework described above. There are now nearly two decades of work specifically supporting the efficacy of ACT. Published randomized control trials provide evidence that ACT may do as well or better than traditional cognitive behavioral therapy in reducing depression and anxiety, and that it is effective in the treatment of substance abuse, pain, and psychosis (Hayes, Strosahl, & Wilson, 2002; Zettle, 2003). ACT has also been shown to be effective at reducing stress and sick leave utilization in "normal" populations (Bond & Bunce, 2000; Dahl, Wilson, & Nilsson, 2004).

There is also substantial support for other mindfulness-based interventions, including Dialectic Behavior Therapy (Linehan, 1993), Mindfulness-Based Cognitive Therapy for Depression (Segal, Williams, & Teasdale, 2002), Mindfulness Based Meditation (Cormier & Cormier, 1998), and Mindfulness-Based Stress Reduction (Kabat-Zinn, 1990). Many other approaches have benefited by adding mindfulness and acceptance components to their inventions (for a review see Hayes et al., 1999).

Individual differences in mindfulness and fusion with particular types of unhelpful thoughts.   There are several scales related to this EI dimension. The Mindfulness Attention Awareness Scale (MAAS) measures people's tendency to be mindful of moment to moment experience. This scale has been shown to relate to various aspects of well-being and to how effectively people deal with stressful life events (Brown & Ryan, 2003).

The Demanding Perfection subscale of the Common Belief Survey (CBS-III; Thorpe, Walter, Kingery, & Nay, 2001) measures the extent that people believe unhelpful, demanding thoughts (e.g., people and things should turn out better than they do). This scale has been linked to poor mental health (Ciarrochi & West, 2004).

Another group of measures reflect unhelpful beliefs about uncertainty (e.g., "that uncertainty is awful or intolerable"). These include measures of intolerance of uncertainty (Dugas, Gagnon, Ladouceur, & Freeston, 1998), rigidity (Neuberg & Newson, 1993), and intolerance of ambiguity (Frenkel-Brunswik, 1949). These measures have been shown to relate to depression and anxiety in both clinical and normal populations (Dugas et al., 1998; Freeston, Rheaume, Letarte, Dugas, & Ladouceur, 1994).

Finally, individual differences in rumination seem to reflect high fusion. Rumination can be measured using self-reports measures such as the Emotion Control Questionnaire (Roger & Najarian, 1989). Ruminators seem to be stuck in their thoughts, engaging in repetitive and passive thinking about a problem (Nolen-Hoeksema, 1987). Rumination involves mindlessly bouncing from one negative thought to another, perhaps in an attempt to escape unpleasant affect by controlling the uncontrollable (e.g., uncertainty; Dugas et al., 1998). It has been associated with a range of emotional difficulties, including anger and depression (Nolen-Hoeksema, Larson, & Grayson, 1999; Rusting & Nolen-

Hoeksema, 1998). Longitudinal studies have established that people who engage in more rumination have higher levels of depressive symptoms over time and perceive themselves to be receiving less social support, even when controlling for their baseline levels of depressive symptoms (Nolen-Hoeksema & Davis, 1999; Nolen-Hoeksema, Parker, & Larson, 1994). High rumination has also been associated with delayed recovery from stress, as indicated by delayed heart-rate and physiological (cortisol) recovery (Roger & Jamieson, 1988; Roger & Najarian, 1998).

Rumination might also be seen as an ineffective emotional orientation, since it appears to involve attempts to use reasoning to escape from unpleasant private experiences (Dugas, Freeston, & Ladouceur, 1997). However, we include it here because it seems to involve a mindless absorption in the content of thought (fusion), rather than looking at thought, and a focus on the future or the past, whilst the present goes unnoticed.

The measures may seem quite different from each other in this section, and to some extent they are. However, there is also some evidence that they interrelate. For example, Brown and Ryan (2003) found that higher mindfulness scores were modestly associated with higher self-reported EI and lower rumination. Dugas and his colleagues found that intolerance of uncertainty is related to ruminative activity (Dugas et al., 1997).

These measures also tend to correlate with neuroticism, or the tendency to experience negative affect (Ciarrochi, Forgas, & Mayer, 2001; Ciarrochi & West, 2004; Dugas et al., 1997). This overlap with personality is sometimes seen as a problem in EI research, as it suggests that the measure may not predict variance over and above personality. We should emphasize again that our goal is not primarily incremental prediction or the creation of new EI measures. Thus, for our purposes, it is not a problem if these measures correlate with neuroticism or other personality measures. In fact, we expect that all the measures reviewed in this chapter reflect processes that *lead* to neuroticism. Thus, it would be absurd to posit that they are independent of this variable.

Again, our goal is pragmatic. We seek to reduce suffering. To a large extent, the two personality traits, positive and negative affectivity, or extraversion and neuroticism, are just two indices of suffering. They do not necessarily provide clues as to what one does about suffering. We will soon discuss how one might intervene to reduce suffering and how the measures discussed here can help assess the processes involved in the intervention.

Defusing self-concepts.   The last aspect of EI involves the ability to free oneself, at least briefly, from fusion with unhelpful self-concepts (see Table 4.1). Humans develop a concept of self. The mind then proceeds to evaluate it. We readily evaluate this "self" as "good", "bad", "kind", "flawed", "incomplete", "special", and/or "unethical". Cognitive fusion means we tend to treat these evaluations as literal properties of our self. For example, we can evaluate a cup as "bad", but this badness is not a property of the cup. Ceramic is a property of the cup. Similarly, badness or goodness cannot be a property of the self. It is merely a transient reaction. Everybody in the world can suddenly believe you are flawed, and you would still be exactly the same person. Everybody could believe you were perfect, and you would be the same person. Yet humans tend to confuse evaluations ("I'm bad") with primary properties ("I'm made up of about 70% water"). If you believe badness was a primary property of your self, then it would be very difficult, if not impossible, to change (Ellis, 2001; Hayes et al., 1999).

Problems arise when people come to identify with unhelpful self-concepts. The concept of "me" becomes equal to me. People are then drawn into protecting the concept of self as if it is part of the self (Hayes et al., 1999). They seek to feed it, or defend it against attack. People talk about "building self-esteem" or repairing "damage" done to it. They become "hurt" when someone "attacks" their self-esteem.

Low self-esteem seems to involve at least two parts: negative evaluations of the entire self ("I am worthless") and fusion with this evaluation. Thus, one could have the negative self-evaluation and not believe (fuse with) it. Undermining fusion with self-concepts is very different from "building self-esteem". The goal in undermining fusion is not to get rid of the negative evaluations and replace them with positive evaluations. Rather, it is to accept the negative self-evaluations as they inevitably show up, and to look *at* them, rather than *through* them.

Individual differences in fusing with unhelpful self-concepts and well-being. It appears to be reasonably well established that low self-esteem is associated with higher levels of negative affect (Blascovich & Tomaka, 1991). Self-esteem is often measured using a self-report scale by Rosenberg (1965). It also appears to be measured by the Bar-On emotional quotient inventory (EQ-i; Bar-On, 1997).

What is somewhat more surprising is that some aspects of high self-esteem have been associated with poor well-being, at least in some circumstances (Kernis, Grannemann, & Barclay, 1989; Rhodewalt, 2001). For example, the Narcissist Personality Inventory (NPI) assesses a person's sense of grandiosity, self-importance, and specialness (Raskin & Terry, 1988). Narcissists scan the social context for evidence that supports their elevated sense of self and tend to construct high self-esteem in the absence of objective evidence. Their self-esteem is fragile, and they are prone to respond to threatening feedback with shame, humiliation, anger, and interpersonal aggression (Rhodewalt & Eddings, 2002).

A related line of research has examined individual differences in the stability of self-esteem. Stability can be measured by administering a standard self-esteem inventory at multiple times, and then using the variance between different measurements to predict outcomes (Kernis et al., 1989). People who have unstable high self-esteem have been shown to experience more anger and hostility, perhaps because they feel the "need" to defend their self-worth (Kernis et al., 1989). Other research shows that unstable self-esteem is associated with goal-related affect characterized by greater tenseness and less interest (Kernis, Paradise, Whitaker, Wheatman, & Goldman, 2000).

4.6   REDUCING SUFFERING: LESSONS FROM ACCEPTANCE AND COMMITMENT THERAPY

Now that we have placed a wide variety of EI-relevant measures into the F.E.A.R. framework, we turn to what one might do with knowledge of this framework.

The EI theory proposed here is grounded firmly in what has been termed the "third wave" of cognitive-behavioral therapy (CBT; Hayes, 2004). The second wave of CBT focused on eliminating irrational thoughts or pathological schemas and replacing them with more functional ones (Beck, 1995; Meichenbaum, 1985). In contrast, third-wave CBT does not seek to directly change the content of thought or emotion. Rather, it focuses on acceptance of thoughts and feelings. The goal is to change one's relationship to such private experiences.

EI research and interventions are meant to apply to all humans, not just clinical populations. The third-wave CBT, Acceptance and Commitment Therapy (ACT), appears to be grounded in principles that apply to all humans. For example, it is based on techniques that have been used for centuries by Buddhists (as opposed to clinical groups), who developed the techniques to relieve humans from the universal causes of suffering. It has also been grounded in the RFT theory of language, thus making it relevant to all language-able beings (Hayes et al., 2001).

ACT is a theoretically driven intervention that is specifically designed to improve three of the four EI dimensions listed in Table 4.1. These include effective emotional orientation, defusing from unhelpful thoughts and emotions, and defusing from unhelpful self-concepts (Hayes et al., 1999). We hypothesize that the ACT intervention should also indirectly improve the ability to utilize emotions as information. For example, if ACT successfully improves emotional orientation, then people will be less likely to repress or avoid unpleasant emotions. Instead, people will be mindfully present to whatever emotions are showing up. We hypothesize that this should make it more likely for these people to be able to utilize this emotion as information (since they are fully aware of it).

How does ACT seek to reduce suffering? We will provide a brief example here (see Hayes et al., 1999, for more detailed treatment). ACT views language processes as the cause of suffering. Thus, the intervention techniques in ACT minimize the use of language and reasoning. Instead , they tend to involve metaphors and exercises that attempt to put people in touch with their own experiences (Hayes et al., 1999). The exercises also tend to shift people into the present moment, and away from excessive reasoning about the past or future.

For example, consider the following ACT intervention for improving emotional orientation (Hayes et al., 1999). It is designed to help people make experiential contact with paradoxical nature of emotion control strategies. People are asked to imagine that they are hooked up to a polygraph that measures exactly how anxious they are feeling. They are told that all they have to do is not feel anxious for the next three minutes. To make sure they are sufficiently motivated, and to exaggerate the point, we then tell them we will point a gun at their head. If they show any signs of anxiety, then we will pull the trigger. So all they have to do is not get anxious.

People very quickly see the problems of trying to control private experience. ACT has a substantial number of similar exercises that help people to defuse from unhelpful verbal rules (e.g., "I must get rid of my anxiety") and to discover what works in experience.

Everything done within ACT is in the service of the person's values (Hayes et al., 1999; Wilson & Murrel, 2004). For example, letting go of emotional control strategies would be encouraged if such letting go would help the person achieve their goals. Defusing from a particular private experience (e.g., the verbal statement "I am worthless") would only be done if the private experience was acting as a barrier to valued action.

There is substantial evidence that ACT reduces suffering in clinical populations (Hayes et al., 1999). There is increasing evidence that it can be of benefit to "normal" populations. For example, Dahl and colleagues investigated the effects of a brief ACT intervention in the treatment of caretakers and nurses working in the public health sector (Dahl et al., 2004). The participants had chronic stress/pain and were at-risk for high sick-leave utilization. Participants were randomly assigned to ACT or Medical-Treatment-As-Usual (MTAU). Results indicated that ACT participants took fewer sick days and used less medical treatment resources than those in the MTAU condition.

In another study, Bond and Bunce (2000) investigated the effects of ACT in a large media organization (Bond & Bunce, 2003). Participants were randomly assigned to an ACT group, an Innovation Promotion Program (IPP) that helped participants to identify and then change causes of occupational strain, or a waitlist control group. Improvements in mental health and innovation were found following both interventions compared to the waitlist. However, the change processes differed in the two groups. Changes in outcome variables in the ACT condition were mediated only by the acceptance of undesirable thoughts and feelings (EI dimension 1). Changes in the IPP condition were mediated only by attempts to modify stressors. Thus, ACT appeared to improve mental health and behavior through increases in acceptance of unpleasant thoughts, feelings, and sensations.

4.7   CONCLUSIONS AND FUTURE DIRECTIONS

The present EI framework is quite different from the EI ability framework proposed by Mayer and his colleagues (Mayer, Caruso, & Salovey, 1999). Mayer has been interested in creating an EI measure that is similar to intelligence measures (e.g., it has right and wrong answers). His approach has been reasonably successful, in that the EI test predicts such things as job performance, social problem behavior, and relationship quality. The test has also proven to be largely distinctive from self-report measures of EI and personality (Ciarrochi, Chan, & Caputi, 2000; Mayer et al., 2002).

Our approach has focused on self-report, and therefore will tend to be reasonably distinct from that of Mayer and his colleagues. Thus, we do not see ourselves as competitors. Importantly, our focus on currently existing measures is not an attempt to re-label old measures as EI. We encourage people to use the original labels. We focus on these older measures and the decades of research associated with them in order to get a better understanding of what it means to be emotionally intelligent. Our EI framework will hopefully help organize these measures into coherent groups and suggest new directions for research. For example, it would be worth investigating whether the measures described here capture four separate factors, as would be suggested by our four factor model.

There has been ongoing debate about what EI "ought" to be. Some argue that it ought to be similar to cognitive intelligence and it ought to be measured with ability tests. We start with a different set of assumptions. The F.E.A.R. framework is based on how people manage personally-relevant private experiences. Self-reports seem to allow people to answer questions about personally relevant experiences. When asked the question, "To what extent do you have feelings that you can't quite identify?", people can look into the context of their lives and provide a reasonably accurate report (Taylor & Bagby, 2000). In contrast, ability EI measures appear to ask questions about stimuli with which participant are unfamiliar (e.g., unfamiliar faces and stories). We believe it is possible to be emotionally intelligent with regards to the processing of unfamiliar emotional information, but not be emotionally intelligent when it comes to processing emotional information in the context of our everyday life. Future research needs to investigate this possibility, and to evaluate if an ability-based EI measure can be designed that contains personally relevant content.

One thing is strikingly different about our model compared to others. Our model does not posit that emotionally intelligent people are better able to directly modify and improve their emotions. Indeed, we have argued that emotional control strategies are often the problem, not the solution. Thus, in our framework, the emotionally intelligent person is often willing to have whatever emotions show up, in the service of doing what they value. They accept the emotions and let them pass or stay. This acceptance approach is expected to have a paradoxical effect: By not struggling to eliminate our unpleasant emotions, we are less likely to experience unpleasant emotions. To use a metaphor, by not struggling in quicksand, we are less likely to sink into it.

We do not mean to imply that emotional control strategies are always bad, or that people can not be taught to engage in some effective control strategies. Rather, the prediction is that if people let go of unhelpful attempts to get rid of the pain, they will be less likely to suffer. We seek to undermine unhelpful control moves rather than teaching people new control moves. Research is needed to determine the value of this strategy, though the initial evidence is quite promising (Bond & Bunce, 2000; Dahl et al., 2004; Hayes et al., 1999).

In closing, EI research is thriving, as evidenced by the chapters in this volume and the substantial number of publications that are appearing in peer reviewed journals. We believe that the human desire for self-improvement will keep the field thriving for more years to come. People seem to recognize that some of their suffering is unnecessary. They often realize that they "sweat the small things" and wreck havoc on their most cherished relationships. In our experience, people strongly desire to become more effective with their emotions. We hope that the next decade of EI research will help people to achieve this important goal.

REFERENCES

Bach, M., & Bach, D. (1995). Predictive value of alexithymia: A prospective study in somatizing patients. *Psychotherapy and Psychosomatics, 64,* 43–48.

Bar-On, R. (1997). *BarOn Emotional Quotient Inventory (EQ–i): Technical manual.* Toronto, Canada: Multi-Health Systems.

Beck, J. S. (1995). *Cognitive therapy: Basics and beyond.* New York: Guilford Press.

Blackledge, J. T. (2003). An introduction to relational frame theory: Basics and applications. *The Behavior Analyst Today, 3,* 421–433.

Blascovich, J., & Tomaka, J. (1991). Measures of self-esteem. In J. P. Robinson & P. R. Shaver (Eds.), *Measures of personality and social psychological attitudes* (Vol. 1, pp. 115–160). San Diego, CA: Academic Press.

Bless, H. (2001). Mood and the use of general knowledge structures. In L. L. Martin & G. L. Clore (Eds.), *Theories of mood and cognition: A user's guidebook* (pp. 9–26). Mahwah, NJ: Lawrence Erlbaum.

Bond, F. W., & Bunce, D. (2000). Mediators of change in emotion-focused and problem-focused worksite stress management interventions. *Journal of Occupational Health Psychology, 5,* 156–163.

Bond, F. W., & Bunce, D. (2003). The role of acceptance and job control in mental health, job satisfaction, and work performance. *Journal of Applied Psychology, 88,* 1057–1067.

Bourne, E. J. (2000). *The anxiety and phobia workbook.* Oakland, CA: New Harbinger Publications.

Brown, K. W., & Ryan, R. M. (2003). The benefits of being present: Mindfulness and its role in psychological well-being. *Journal of Personality and Social Psychology, 84,* 822–848.

Chang, E. C., & D'Zurilla, T. J. (1996). Relations between problem orientation and optimism, pessimism, and trait affectivity: A construct validation study. *Behaviour Research and Therapy, 34,* 185–194.

Ciarrochi, J., Chan, A. Y. C., & Caputi, P. (2000). A critical evaluation of the emotional intelligence construct. *Personality and Individual Differences, 28,* 539–561.

Ciarrochi, J., Deane, F. P., & Anderson, S. (2002). Emotional intelligence moderates the relationship between stress and mental health. *Personality and Individual Differences, 32,* 197–209.

Ciarrochi, J., Forgas, J. P., & Mayer, J. D. (2001). *Emotional intelligence in everyday life: A scientific inquiry.* Philadelphia: Psychology Press/Taylor and Francis.

Ciarrochi, J., Scott, G., Deane, F. P., & Heaven, P. C. L. (2003). Relations between social and emotional competence and mental health: a construct validation study. *Personality and Individual Differences, 35,* 1947–1963.

Ciarrochi, J., & West, M. (2004). Relationships between dysfunctional beliefs and positive and negative indices of well-being: A critical evaluation of the Common Beliefs Survey-III. *Journal of Rational-Emotive and Cognitive Behavior Therapy, 22,* 171–188.

Clark, L. A., Watson, D., & Mineka, S. (1994). Temperament, personality, and the mood and anxiety disorders. *Journal of Abnormal Psychology, 103,* 103–116.

Cormier, L. S., & Cormier, W. H. (1998). *Interviewing strategies for helpers: Fundamental skills and cognitive behavioral interventions* (4th ed.). Pacific Grove, CA: Brooks/Cole.

Dahl, J., Wilson, K. G., & Nilsson, A. (2004). Acceptance and Commitment Therapy and the treatment of persons at risk of long-term disability resulting from stress and pain symptoms: A preliminary randomized trial. *Behavior Therapy, 35,* 785–802.

Davey, G. C., Jubb, M., & Cameron, C. (1996). Catastrophic worrying as a function of changes in problem-solving confidence. *Cognitive Therapy and Research, 20,* 333–344.

Diener, E., Suh, E. M., Lucas, R. E., & Smith, H. L. (1999). Subjective well-being: Three decades of progress. *Psychological Bulletin, 125,* 276–302.

Dugas, M. J., Freeston, M. H., & Ladouceur, R. (1997). Intolerance of uncertainty and problem orientation in worry. *Cognitive Therapy and Research, 21,* 593–606.

Dugas, M. J., Gagnon, F., Ladouceur, R., & Freeston, M. H. (1998). Generalized anxiety disorder: A preliminary test of a conceptual model. *Behaviour Research and Therapy, 36,* 215–226.

D'Zurilla, T. J., Chang, E. C., Nottingham, E. J., & Faccini, L. (1998). Social problem-solving deficits and hopelessness, depression, and suicidal risk in college students and psychiatric inpatients. *Journal of Clinical Psychology, 54,* 1091–1107.

Elliott, T. R., Herrick, S. M., MacNair, R. R., & Harkins, S. W. (1994). Personality correlates of self-appraised problem solving ability: Problem orientation and trait affectivity. *Journal of Personality Assessment, 63,* 489–505.

Elliott, T. R., & Marmarosh, C. L. (1994). Problem-solving appraisal, health complaints, and health-related expectancies. *Journal of Counseling and Development, 72,* 531–537.

Ellis, A. (2001). *Overcoming destructive beliefs, feelings, and behaviors: new directions for rational emotive behavior therapy.* Amherst, NY: Prometheus Books.

Feldner, M., Zvolensky, M., Eifert, G., & Spira, A. (2003). Emotional avoidance: An experimental test of individual differences and response suppression using biological challenge. *Behaviour Research and Therapy, 41,* 403–411.

Forgas, J. P. (1995). Mood and judgment: The Affect Infusion Model (AIM). *Psychological Bulletin, 117,* 39–66.

Freeston, M. H., Rheaume, J., Letarte, H., Dugas, M. J., & Ladouceur, R. (1994). Why do people worry? *Personality and Individual Differences, 17,* 791–802.

88 Mindfulness-Based Emotional Intelligence

Frenkel-Brunswik, E. (1949). Intolerance of ambiguity as an emotional and perceptual personality variable. *Journal of Personality, 18*, 108–143.

Hayes, S. C. (2004). Acceptance and Commitment Therapy, Relational Frame Theory, and the third wave of behavioral and cognitive therapies. *Behavior Therapy, 35*, 639–665.

Hayes, S. C., Barnes-Holmes, D., & Roche, B. (2001). *Relational frame theory: A post-Skinnerian account of human language and cognition.* New York: Kluwer.

Hayes, S. C., Brownstein, A. J., Haas, J. R., & Greenway, D. E. (1986). Instructions, multiple schedules, and extinction: Distinguishing rule-governed from schedule-controlled behavior. *Journal of the Experimental Analysis of Behavior, 46*, 137–147.

Hayes, S. C., Hayes, L. J., & Reese, H. W. (1988). Finding the philosophical core: A review of Stephen C. Pepper's world hypotheses. *Journal of Experimental Analysis of Behavior, 50*, 97–111.

Hayes, S. C., Strosahl, K. D., & Wilson, K. G. (1999). *Acceptance and Commitment Therapy: An experiential approach to behavior change.* New York: Guilford Press.

Hayes, S. C., Strosahl, K. D., & Wilson, K. G. (2002). Acceptance and Commitment Therapy: An experimental approach to behavior change. *Child and Family Behavior Therapy, 24*, 51–57.

Hayes, S. C., Strosahl, K. D., Wilson, K. G., Bissett, R. T., Pistorello, J., Polusny, M., et al. (2003). *The Acceptance and Action Questionnaire (AAQ) as a measure of experiential avoidance.* Manuscript under review.

Kabat-Zinn, J. (1990). *Full catastrophe living: Using the wisdom of your body and mind to face stress, pain, and illness.* New York: Dell Publishing.

Kapleau, P. (1989). *The three pillars of zen: Teaching, practice, and enlightenment.* New York: Anchor.

Kernis, M. H., Grannemann, B. D., & Barclay, L. C. (1989). Stability and level of self-esteem as predictors of anger arousal and hostility. *Journal of Personality and Social Psychology, 56*, 1013–1022.

Kernis, M. H., Paradise, A. W., Whitaker, D. J., Wheatman, S. R., & Goldman, B. N. (2000). Master of one's psychological domain? Not likely if one's self-esteem is unstable. *Personality and Social Psychology Bulletin, 26*, 1297–1305.

Laudan, L. (1981). A confutation of convergent realism. *Philosophy of Science, 48*, 19–49.

Linehan, M. M. (1993). *Cognitive-behavioral treatment of borderline personality disorder.* New York: Guilford Press.

Lyubomirsky, S. (2001). Why are some people happier than others? The role of cognitive and motivational processes in well-being. *American Psychologist, 56*, 239–249.

Mayer, J. D., Caruso, D. R., & Salovey, P. (1999). Emotional intelligence meets traditional standards for an intelligence. *Intelligence, 27*, 267–298.

Mayer, J. D., Salovey, P., & Caruso, D. R. (2002). *The Mayer-Salovey-Caruso Emotional Intelligence Test (MSCEIT): User's manual.* Toronto, Canada: Multi-Health Systems.

Meichenbaum, D. (1985). *Stress inoculation training.* New York: Pergamon Press.

Neuberg, S. L., & Newson, J. T. (1993). Personal need for structure: Individual differences in the desire for simpler structure. *Journal of Personality and Social Psychology, 65*, 113–131.

Nolen-Hoeksema, S. (1987). Sex differences in unipolar depression: Evidence and theory. *Psychological Bulletin, 101*, 259–282.

Nolen-Hoeksema, S., & Davis, C. G. (1999). "Thanks for sharing that": Ruminators and their social support networks. *Journal of Personality and Social Psychology, 77*, 801–814.

Nolen-Hoeksema, S., Larson, J., & Grayson, C. (1999). Explaining the gender difference in depressive symptoms. *Journal of Personality and Social Psychology, 77*, 1061–1072.

Nolen-Hoeksema, S., Parker, L. E., & Larson, J. (1994). Ruminative coping with depressed mood following loss. *Journal of Personality and Social Psychology, 67*, 92–104.

Ortony, A., Clore, G. L., & Collins, A. (1988). *The cognitive structure of emotion.* New York: Cambridge University Press.

Raskin, R., & Terry, H. (1988). A principal-components analysis of the Narcissistic Personality Inventory and further evidence of its construct validity. *Journal of Personality and Social Psychology, 54*, 890–902.

Rhodewalt, F. (2001). The social mind of the narcissist: Cognitive and motivational aspects of interpersonal self-construction. In J. P. Forgas & K. D. Williams (Eds.), *The social mind: Cognitive and motivational aspects of interpersonal behavior.* New York: Cambridge University Press.

Rhodewalt, F., & Eddings, S. K. (2002). Narcissus reflects: Memory distortion in response to ego-relevant feedback among high- and low-narcissistic men. *Journal of Research in Personality, 36*, 97–116.

Roger, D., & Jamieson, J. (1988). Individual differences in delayed heart-rate recovery following stress: The role of extraversion, neuroticism, and emotional control. *Personality and Individual Differences, 9*, 721–726.

Roger, D., & Najarian, B. (1989). The construction and validation of a new scale for measuring emotion control. *Personality and Individual Differences, 10*, 845–853.

Roger, D., & Najarian, B. (1998). The relationship between emotional rumination and cortisol secretion under stress. *Personality and Individual Differences, 24*, 531–538.

Rosenberg, M. (1965). *Society and the adolescent self-image.* Princeton, NJ: Princton University Press.

Rusting, C. L., & Nolen-Hoeksema, S. (1998). Regulating responses to anger: Effects of rumination and distraction on angry mood. *Journal of Personality and Social Psychology, 74*, 790–803.

Salovey, P., Mayer, J. D., Goldman, S., Turvey, C., & Palfai, T. (1995). Emotional attention, clarity, and repair: Exploring emotional intelligence using the Trait Meta-Mood Scale. In J. W. Pennebaker (Ed.), *Emotion, disclosure, and health* (pp. 125–154). Washington, DC: American Psychological Association.

Schmidt, F. L., & Hunter, J. E. (1998). The validity and utility of selection methods in personnel psychology: Practical and theoretical implications of 85 years of research findings. *Psychological Bulletin, 124*, 262–274.

Schutte, N. S., Malouff, J. M., Hall, L. E., Haggerty, D. J., Cooper, J. T., Golden, C. J., et al. (1998). Development and validation of a measure of emotional intelligence. *Personality and Individual Differences, 25*, 167–177.

Segal, Z. V., Williams, J. M. G., & Teasdale, J. D. (2002). *Mindfulness-based cognitive therapy for depression: A new approach to preventing relapse.* New York: Guilford Press.

Taylor, G. J. (2000). Recent developments in alexithymia theory and research. *Canadian Journal of Psychiatry, 45,* 134–142.

Taylor, G. J. (2001). Low emotional intelligence and mental illness. In J. Ciarrochi & J. P. Forgas (Eds.), *Emotional intelligence in everyday life: A scientific inquiry* (pp. 67–81). Philadelphia: Psychology Press/Taylor and Francis.

Taylor, G. J., & Bagby, R. M. (2000). An overview of the alexithymia construct. In R. Bar-On & J. D. A. Parker (Eds.), *The handbook of emotional intelligence: Theory, development, assessment, and application at home, school, and in the workplace* (pp. 40–67). San Francisco: Jossey-Bass.

Taylor, G. J., Bagby, R. M., & Luminet, O. (2000). Assessment of alexithymia: Self-report and observer-rated measures. In R. Bar-On & J. D. A. Parker (Eds.), *The handbook of emotional intelligence: Theory, development, assessment, and application at home, school, and in the workplace.* San Francisco: Jossey-Bass.

Thorpe, G. L., Walter, M. I., Kingery, L. R., & Nay, W. T. (2001). The Common Beliefs Survey-III and the Situational Self-Statement and Affective State Inventory: Test-rest reliability, internal consistency, and further psychometric considerations. *Journal of Rational-Emotive Therapy and Cognitive Behavior Therapy, 19,* 89–103.

Tokar, D. M., Fischer, A. R., & Subich, L. M. (1998). Personality and vocational behavior: A selective review of the literature, 1993-1997. *Journal of Vocational Behavior, 53,* 115–153.

Wegner, D. M. (1994). Ironic processes of mental control. *Psychological Review, 10,* 34–52.

Wegner, D. M., & Zanakos, S. (1994). Chronic thought suppression. *Journal of Personality, 62,* 615–640.

Wenzlaff, R. M., & Wegner, D. M. (2000). Thought suppression. *Annual Review of Psychology, 51,* 59–91.

Wilson, K. G., & Murrel, A. R. (2004). Values work in acceptance and commitment therapy: Setting a course for behavioral treatment. In S. C. Hayes, V. M. Follette, & M. M. Linehan (Eds.), *Mindfulness and acceptance: Expanding the cognitive-behavioral tradition* (pp. 120–151). New York: Guilford Press.

Wulfert, E., & Hayes, S. C. (1988). Transfer of a conditional ordering response through conditional equivalence classes. *Journal of the Experimental Analysis of Behavior, 50,* 125–144.

Zettle, R. D. (2003). Acceptance and Commitment Therapy (ACT) vs. systematic desensitization in treatment of mathematics anxiety. *Psychological Record, 53,* 197–215.

5

Social and Emotional Intelligence: Starting a Conversation about Their Similarities and Differences

Sun-Mee Kang
California State University, Northridge, USA

Jeanne D. Day
Naomi M. Meara
University of Notre Dame, USA

Summary

To facilitate conversation and collaborative research, we review historical developments and empirical findings from the literatures pertaining to emotional and social intelligence. Our review focuses on conceptual and measurement issues: internal consistency, criterion validity of the constructs, and comparison of their components with each other and components of academic intelligence. Additionally, we address challenges to interpreting research results occasioned by lack of theoretical coherence underlying empirical investigations and methods of measurement. We conclude that social and emotional intelligence are multidimensional, interdependent, and overlapping. It is suggested that future research might concentrate on such issues as the appropriate distinctions from academic intelligence (e.g., fluid vs. crystallized intelligence), differentiating components of constructs (e.g., knowledge of self vs. knowledge of others), and further development of measures and exploration of measurement issues.

5.1   INTRODUCTION

Social and emotional intelligence have a powerful intuitive appeal. That people vary in their ability to "understand others and act wisely in interpersonal relationships" (Thorndike, 1920, p. 228) is consistent with our experiences with others in social settings and with our observations of the social interactions of others. Similarly, that people vary in their ability "to perceive and express emotion, assimilate emotion in thought, understand and reason with emotion, and regulate emotion in the self and others" (Mayer, Salovey, & Caruso, 2000, p. 401; Mayer & Salovey, 1997) fits with the experiences and observations of many of us. Further, that people who behave in socially and emotionally intelligent ways seem to experience more success (e.g., in close relationships, in work settings) appears obvious. Indeed, the belief that social and emotional intelligence may be more important than academic intelligence, especially in one's realization of important life goals, has an equalizing aspect. That is, many laypeople and experts alike believe that social and emotional intelligence may be less genetically determined and, hence, more modifiable than academic intelligence (e.g., Matthews, Zeidner, & Roberts, 2002). That social, emotional, and academic intelligence are all labeled *intelligence*, implies that the abilities and skills involved are qualities of the person that can be revealed in multiple ways (e.g., exceptional knowledge, quickness) across a variety of settings and circumstances (e.g., on a test, during a social interaction) (Zeidner, Roberts, & Matthews, 2002) and, further, that these abilities and skills do not reflect *non-intellectual factors* such as interest, motivation, or personality (although see Bar-On, 1997, for a model of emotional intelligence that does include motivational factors and affective tendencies). That is, although smart individuals do stupid things (Sternberg, 2002), on balance, those who are more socially and emotionally (or academically) intelligent are not idiot savants (i.e., proficient in following rigidly a limited number of scripts).

Other remarkable similarities between the two constructs become apparent when Thorndike's (1920) definition of social intelligence (SI; understanding others and acting wisely in interpersonal relationships) and the Mayer et al. (2000) definition of emotional intelligence (EI; perceiving and expressing emotion, understanding and reasoning with emotion, and regulating emotion in self and others) are examined together. Each definition is broad and each includes both cognitive (e.g., understanding and perceiving) and behavioral (e.g., acting, regulating emotion in others) components. In fact, within each definition, the cognitive and behavioral components themselves each involve multiple and overlapping processes. For instance, perceiving (which appears more circumscribed than understanding) involves attending to and interpreting social and emotional cues. Similarly, regulating emotion in others (which seems more focused than "acting wisely") involves deciding on and implementing some strategy (e.g., calming talk), monitoring the success of that strategy, and, should the chosen strategy fail to meet one's goal, switching to a different strategy.

The breadth and inclusion of both cognitive and behavioral skills into the definitions of these two intelligences has led to difficulties in developing measures of these constructs and in establishing convergent, discriminant, and concurrent validity. Thus, although the breadth of the definitions and the inclusion of cognitive and behavioral dimensions in each are partly responsible for their appeal, these qualities also explain why these constructs remain so "empirically elusive" (Davies, Stankov, & Roberts, 1998; Sternberg, 2000). Below we review research on SI focusing first on conceptual and definitional issues and second on the measurement issues (especially convergent, discriminant, and criterion validity concerns) that follow from the conceptual and definitional ones. We then undertake a parallel review of the EI literature. We conclude with a recommendation that researchers of SI and EI converse with one another and suggestions about the exciting and informative research questions that could follow from such conversations.

5.2 SOCIAL INTELLIGENCE: CONCEPTUAL AND MEASUREMENT ISSUES

5.2.1 Conceptualizations of Social Intelligence

Several approaches have been used in attempts to define and conceptualize SI, like the psychometric approach and implicit-theory methodology, for example. Consequently, Thorndike's (1920) seemingly simple but elegant definition of SI has been parsed into several cognitive and behavioral factors or components (Chapin, 1942; Marlowe, 1986; O'Sullivan & Guilford, 1975; O'Sullivan, Guilford, & deMille, 1965; Walker & Foley, 1973). These component abilities include, but are not limited to:

1. social sensitivity, social insight, and social communication (with seven subordinate facets: role-taking, social inference, social comprehension, psychological insight, moral judgment, referential communication, and social problem-solving) (Greenspan, 1989);

2. prosocial attitude (i.e., both social interest and social self-efficacy), empathy skills, social skills, emotionality (emotional expressiveness and sensitivity to others' affective states), and social anxiety (Marlowe, 1986); and

3. understanding people, dealing well with people, being warm and caring, being open to new experiences and ideas, perspective taking ability, knowing social rules and norms, and social adaptability (Kosmitzki & John, 1993).

Notably, all of these components of SI were developed in the absence of an explicit theory, which likely contributed to the proliferation of components and corresponding measures. The measures, in turn, produced difficulties in establishing convergent and discriminant validity for SI.

5.2.2   Measurement Issues

Like laypeople, many researchers (e.g., Kosmitzki & John, 1993; Sternberg, Conway, Ketron, & Bernstein, 1981) believe that SI consists of several interrelated abilities that are probably correlated with, but also distinguishable from, academic intelligence. Historically, however, efforts to establish empirically the multidimensionality, yet coherence of SI, and its distinctiveness from academic intelligence, were largely unsuccessful (e.g., Gresvenor, 1927; Hoepfner & O'Sullivan, 1968; Keating, 1978; Pintner & Upshall, 1928; R. L. Thorndike & Stein, 1937). In fact, early studies showed that measures of SI (typically paper-and-pencil measures of cognitive aspects of SI) did not correlate highly among themselves but did correlate highly with measures of academic intelligence (Chapin, 1942; Gough, 1968; Gresvenor, 1927; Hoepfner & O'Sullivan, 1968; Hunt, 1927, 1928; Moss & Hunt, 1927; Pintner & Upshall, 1928; R. L. Thorndike & Stein, 1937). Thus, researchers concluded that: "The putative domain of social intelligence lacks empirical coherency" (Keating, 1978, pp. 221-222) and that social and academic intelligence might be conceptually (but not empirically) distinct (Ford & Tisak, 1983; Riggio, Messamer, & Throckmorton, 1991). The few studies that did document the distinctiveness of social and academic intelligence measured these two intelligences with different types of measures (e.g., traditional paper-and-pencil tests of academic intelligence that have right and wrong answers and self-report tests of SI that do not, strictly speaking, have right and wrong answers), thus confounding the traits of interest and the methods of measuring those traits (Ford & Tisak, 1983; Legree, 1995; Marlowe, 1986).

More recently, Day and her colleagues have further explored the multidimensionality and coherence of SI and its distinctiveness from academic intelligence using multitrait-multimethod designs and confirmatory factor analyses (CFAs; Jones & Day, 1997; Lee, Wong, Day, Maxwell, & Thorpe, 2000; Wong, Day, Maxwell, & Meara, 1995). Across these studies, multiple, different dimensions of SI were examined and contrasted with academic intelligence (defined and measured variously across the studies) including: social perception, social knowledge, social insight, social cognitive flexibility, social inference, and heterosexual social interaction (the latter is the only SI component in the list that involved observations of actual social interactions). The correlations among the SI constructs (e.g., social knowledge and social perception) ranged from .30 to .63. The correlations among the social and academic constructs ranged from .13 to .79. These patterns of correlations are consistent with prior conclusions: (a) that SI is multidimensional in nature (Keating, 1978; Kihlstrom & Cantor, 2000); and (b) that social and academic intelligence may be conceptually, but not empirically, distinct (at least not consistently and decisively distinct empirically).

At least one of these conclusions must be modified, however, based on additional data provided by the CFA models. In two of these investigations, which reported a total of three studies (Jones & Day, 1997; Wong et al. 1995), CFA models were constructed a priori in which: (a) pairs of SI constructs (and in one case a triad of SI constructs) were combined (to test whether SI was a single construct), (b) a social and an academic trait were combined with one another (to test whether social and academic intelligence could be discriminated), and (c) all social and academic intelligence measures were constrained to load on one factor. In only one model of six tested (Study 2 in Wong et al. 1995), did a CFA model that combined two SI constructs (specifically, social inference and social insight) fit the data better than a model that retained separate, but correlated, SI traits. In only one instance (of four tested) did a CFA model that combined an aspect of SI (social knowledge) and one component of academic intelligence (academic problem solving) fit the data (Jones & Day, 1997). These two constructs were, however, distinguishable in another study, when they were measured differently (Wong et al. 1995, Study 2). Nonetheless, none of the three models that combined all social and academic traits fit the data. Consistent with prior conclusions, these analyses suggest that SI is *multidimensional*. Contrary to prior conclusions, however, these analyses demonstrate that social and academic intelligence can be discriminated.

By some standards, for SI to be appropriately labeled an aspect of intelligence, measures of SI should correlate at least modestly with measures of academic intelligence (Carroll, 1993). In one study, however (Lee et al., 2000), Day and her colleagues demonstrated that social and academic intelligence might not be correlated. The purpose of the Lee et al. (2000) study was to determine whether lower-level crystallized and fluid academic intelligence factors could be combined into one higher-order academic intelligence construct and lower-level crystallized and fluid SI factors could be combined into one higher-order SI construct. In one model the two higher-order constructs were allowed to correlate; in the other the correlation between the higher-order social and academic intelligence constructs was set to zero. Both models fit the data. For academic intelligence, the path loadings from the higher-order trait to the lower-level crystallized and fluid academic intelligence traits were estimated at .60 or .52, depending on the model (i.e., whether the traits were correlated or not). For SI, the path loadings from the higher-order trait to the lower-level crystallized and fluid social intelligence traits were estimated at .50 or .37, depending on the model. Thus, some evidence of the coherence of SI was provided, given that a higher-order construct defined the lower-level ones. Some evidence was also provided that social and academic intelligence were related to one another. That is, in the model in which the two higher-order traits were allowed to correlate, the correlation was estimated at .37, which was statistically significant ($p < .05$). The model that set the correlation to zero did not, however, provide a significantly worse fit to the data than the model that allowed the higher-order social and academic constructs to correlate. A model with fewer paths to estimate is more parsimonious and is, therefore, the better model. These findings call into question, at least by some standards (e.g., Carroll, 1993), whether the construct labeled SI (as assessed in the Lee et al., 2000 study) can be rightfully identified as an intelligence at all.

5.2.3   Criterion Validity of Social Intelligence

Perhaps because researchers have mainly focused on establishing the convergent and discriminant validity of SI, only a handful of studies have examined whether SI tests actually relate to socially competent behavior. For example, (Ford & Tisak, 1983) found that measures of SI explained more variance in social-behavior effectiveness (assessed by judges' ratings on social behaviors in an interview) than academic intelligence tests (18% vs. 13%). This result challenged the earlier conclusion from Keating (1978)'s study that SI measures did not predict social competence (measured by the Social Maturity Index derived from the California Psychological Inventory by Gough, 1966). Notice that external criteria of SI were differently defined in these studies, which might account for the conflicting results. It also illustrates how difficult it is for researchers to operationally define social competence (Rose-Krasnor, 1997). Taken together, some evidence for criterion validity of SI measures exists, but this evidence is limited.

5.2.4   Summary

Early research on social and academic intelligence, as well as more recent work, are fairly consistent in showing that SI is multidimensional. These literatures are inconsistent, however, in documenting whether social and academic intelligence are distinct constructs. We believe that some of the strongest research (i.e., studies using multitrait-multimethod designs and CFAs) shows that social and academic intelligence are distinct. These conclusions must be tempered by acknowledgement that we lack a theory of SI that could provide a basis for explicating the similarities and differences between social and academic intelligence and, thus, a framework to develop more adequate measures of SI to test our intuitions. We also notice that few studies have examined whether SI tests actually relate to socially competent behavior. The evidence for the predictive validity of SI measures is limited.

5.3   EMOTIONAL INTELLIGENCE: CONCEPTUAL AND MEASUREMENT ISSUES

5.3.1   Conceptualizations of Emotional Intelligence

Although EI, like SI, is thought to include cognitive (e.g., perceiving emotion, understanding emotion) and behavioral components (e.g., expressing emotion, regulating emotions), fewer components of emotional than of social intelligence have been explicitly identified. Mayer and Salovey (1997), for example, identify only four, hierarchically organized, aspects of EI: Perception, Assimilation, Understanding, and Management. Additionally, Mayer et al. (2000) argue that these four competencies should be assessed, much as academic intelligence is assessed, with tests that have more and less correct answers. Inclusion of a limited number of competencies, a narrow focus on emotions, and reliance on ability tests that have right and wrong answers would likely facilitate the development of measures and the establishment of convergent, discriminant, and criterion validity of EI.

However, as noted by Mayer et al. (2000), some conceptualizations of EI are sufficiently broad to include non-ability factors such as personality and motivation. Bar-On (1997), for instance, conceptualizes EI as "an array of non-cognitive capabilities, competencies, and skills that influence one's ability to succeed in coping with environmental demands and pressures" (Bar-On, 1997, p. 14) and Goleman (1995) includes in his definition "self-control, zeal and persistence, and the ability to motivate oneself" (Goleman, 1995, , p. xii). These "mixed models" (Mayer et al. 2000, p. 401) have led researchers to create self-report measures of EI that overlap with measures of personality. Thus, two, apparently divergent, frameworks are operating—one that contrasts emotional and academic intelligence as abilities and employs tests with more or less right and wrong answers and one that focuses more on personality characteristics and employs self-report measures.

Self-report measures of EI are problematic for several reasons including: (1) they are susceptible to response biases, social desirability, and dissimulation (e.g., Roberts, Zeidner, & Matthews, 2001); (2) they seem to assess dimensions closely akin to well-established personality constructs rather than intelligence (Davies et al., 1998); and in at least one study (Derksen, Kramer, & Katzko, 2002), they had near zero correlations with academic intelligence. For these reasons, we will focus our review, below on the psychometric qualities of ability measures of EI (i.e., those measures for which a more or less agreed-upon correct answer exists).

5.3.2   Measurement Issues

As is the case with SI, researchers and laypeople alike believe that EI consists of several interrelated abilities (e.g., perception of emotions in self and others, regulation of emotion in self and others), which are likely correlated with, but also distinguishable from, abilities associated with academic intelligence. Early efforts to establish empirically the coherence of EI and its distinctiveness from academic intelligence were more successful than those for SI, possibly because emotion researchers focused narrowly on one aspect of EI, the perception of emotions in others (e.g., Mayer, DiPaolo, & Salovey, 1990; Mayer & Geher, 1996). This early work showed: (a) that perception of emotion across different stimuli (e.g., facial images, colors, abstract designs) cohered into a single construct, an EI construct that was positively correlated with empathy (Mayer et al., 1990) and (b) that perception of emotion in stories was positively correlated with empathy and self-reported SAT scores (Mayer & Geher, 1996).

Later research expanded ability tests of EI to include each of the four dimensions articulated by Mayer and Salovey (1997): Perception, Assimilation, Understanding, and Management (Caruso, Mayer, & Salovey, 2002; Mayer, Caruso, & Salovey, 1999; Mayer, Salovey, Caruso, & Sitarenios, 2003). Results for the initially developed measure (the Multifactor Emotional Intelligence Scale, or MEIS), although generally encouraging, were somewhat mixed. For example, the MEIS total score correlated positively with a measure of verbal intelligence ($r = .36$) and self-reported empathy ($r = .33$; see Mayer et al., 2000) but not with personality characteristics (Caruso et al., 2002). Exploratory factor analysis of the data, however, yielded a three (Perception, Understanding, and Managing), rather than the hypothesized four, factor solution (Mayer et al., 1999; although see Roberts et al., 2001 for support for a four factor solution) and some of the reliabilities of individual subscales of the MEIS were low (e.g., .31, .40) (Caruso et al., 2002; Roberts et al., 2001). Interestingly, correlations among the three EI factors were of similar magnitude to those obtained between SI constructs (between .33 and .49), and the correlations between EI factors and verbal intelligence were also of similar magnitude to those obtained in SI research (from .16 to .40; see Mayer et al., 2000). A similar pattern of intercorrelations from the SI literature was interpreted as indicating that SI is multidimensional. Another similarity (albeit based on limited data) between findings about EI and SI is that near-zero (and sometimes negative) correlations between EI factors as measured by the MEIS and the Raven's Progressive Matrices Test have been reported (Ciarrochi, Chan, & Caputi, 2000). In Section 5.4, we suggest that the crystallized/fluid distinction made in the academic intelligence literature might provide a means to understand some of the parallels between the social and emotional intelligence research traditions, as well as a means to resolve some of the discrepancies in these traditions.

5.3.3   Criterion Validity of Emotional Intelligence

To our knowledge, few studies report concurrent validity and even fewer predictive validity of EI. Correlations between overall scores on the MEIS and empathy are positive (e.g., $r = .33$ in Mayer et al., 2000; $r = .43$ in Ciarrochi et al., 2000). In addition, small but significant correlations between overall scores on the MEIS and other measures have been obtained for relationship quality ($r = .19$), life satisfaction ($r = .28$ in Ciarrochi et al., 2000; $r = .11$ in Mayer et al., 2000), and parental warmth ($r = .23$; Mayer et al., 2000; although this latter result was not replicated in Ciarrochi et al., 2000). Negative correlations between EI and tobacco and alcohol use (among adolescents) have also been found ($r = -.19$ and $-.16$, respectively) (Trinidad & Johnson, 2002). Currently, evidence for the concurrent and predictive validity of EI, like that of SI, is therefore limited.

5.3.4   Summary

As with the SI literature, research on emotional and academic intelligence provides mixed data on whether EI is a multidimensional domain of intelligence that is related to, and different (but not too different) from, academic intelligence.[1] The data from ability-based tests of EI (as opposed to self-report assessments) strongly suggest that EI is multidimensional and distinguishable from academic intelligence (as well as from established personality constructs). The data are less clear about its concurrent and predictive validity, and whether it is sufficiently related to academic intelligence to be called a form of intelligence.

5.4   DIRECTIONS FOR FUTURE RESEARCH

That social and emotional intelligence and their attendant research literatures share many similarities (e.g., their intuitive appeal as constructs, conceptual underpinnings, and measurement difficulties) is obvious, whereas the differences between the constructs seem subtle and more implicit. What appears less obvious—because to our knowledge it has not been done—is that careful examination of similarities and differences in conceptualizations and measurement of social and emotional intelligence and conversations about, and, perhaps, collaborative research on, those similarities and differences could advance understanding of both constructs and of their relationship to one another. Below, we suggest a few, but not exhaustive, topics of possible conversation and research.

5.4.1   Defining Social and Emotional Intelligence

If both social and emotional intelligence exist (an assumption which is open to investigation), they clearly overlap and probably have components that are interdependent. For example, perception of the emotional states of others (social/emotional perception) is an individual difference variable that is assessed in both research traditions (e.g., Salovey, Mayer, Caruso, & Lopes, 2003; Wong et al. 1995). Accurately perceiving the feelings of others is, presumably, a necessary, although not sufficient condition, for making sensitive social responses, which is why researchers in SI assess it. Yet, accurately perceiving the emotions of others may be more precisely conceptualized as a component of EI, albeit an aspect of EI that can inform judgments about how to respond in socially and emotionally intelligent ways. Similarly, social knowledge (e.g., knowledge of the norms and rules of one's culture or knowledge about the individuals involved) may be best conceptualized as a component of SI that can enhance one's awareness and understanding of the emotional responses of others when violations of those norms occur. Speculatively, perhaps if one perceives that an unusual or unexpected social or emotional response (either one's own or another's) has occurred in a given interpersonal situation, then one might reevaluate and add to, or otherwise modify, one's social or emotional knowledge. Even more speculatively, perhaps the more accurate the perception that the response was unusual (i.e., the higher one's EI), the more

---

[1]For other discussions of these topics and related issues, see Chapter 10 by Weis and Süß as well as Chapter 6 by Austin and Saklofske.

subtle and precise the modifications to one's social or emotional knowledge may be. If SI and EI are overlapping and interdependent, as we believe they are (and not competing constructs as others believe they are, e.g., Mayer & Geher, 1996; Mayer & Salovey, 1997), conversations about the similarities and differences between these two intelligences would help clarify and expand the conceptualization and measurement of each domain.

5.4.2   Crystallized and Fluid Social/Emotional Intelligence

Refinements in the explication and assessment of social and emotional intelligence might also be reached by appropriating distinctions from the academic intelligence literature (for instance, that between crystallized and fluid intelligence) (Matthews et al., 2002). Roberts et al. (2001) suggest that EI may primarily reflect acquired declarative and procedural knowledge (i.e., crystallized abilities). We would argue that SI also reflects acquired declarative and procedural knowledge about familiar social events (e.g., rules of social etiquette). However, we would also suggest that SI, like academic intelligence (Sternberg et al., 1981; Sternberg & Gastel, 1989) and possibly EI, may have fluid components that may be demonstrated by the ability to apply knowledge flexibly to solve novel problems (e.g., Jones & Day, 1997; Lee, Day, Meara, & Maxwell, 2002). Perhaps the hallmarks of socially and emotionally intelligent people include: (a) the availability, accessibility, and richness of social and emotional knowledge (e.g., Kang & Shaver, 2004) and (b) the ability to entertain multiple perspectives and hypotheses about unusual social/emotional behavior or behavior in unfamiliar social/emotional situations. Although extensive social, emotional, and academic knowledge may be a prerequisite for flexible application of that knowledge, possession of such knowledge does not guarantee its flexible use. That is, one could be very perceptive about one's own and others' emotional experiences and have a rich and detailed understanding about the situations that elicit such responses (i.e., be emotionally and socially knowledgeable) but fail to consider alternative explanations or alter one's behavioral strategies (i.e., be flexible). Similarly, one could be emotionally and socially knowledgeable and be more able to be flexible in either or both the social or emotional arenas. Thus, we suspect that the fluid/crystallized distinction made in the academic intelligence literature might be usefully applied in the SI and EI literatures. This last statement is not meant to imply that an individual with rich social knowledge and the ability to apply that knowledge flexibly will also have, and will apply, flexibly rich emotional or academic knowledge (although this possibility is worthy of investigation).

5.4.3   Knowledge of Self and of Others

Implicit in some discussions of SI and EI is an assumption that individuals with extensive self-knowledge (e.g., individuals who know how and why they would respond socially and/or emotionally in a given situation) probably have extensive knowledge of others. While we believe this assumption is probably correct, it is nevertheless conceivable that one could have extensive self-knowledge and little knowledge about anyone else. Further, if the fluid/crystallized distinction applies to SI and EI, then it is also possible that some individuals may be able to apply their knowledge flexibly with respect to themselves but not to others (or vice versa). The relationships among self-knowledge and its flexible application, and other-knowledge and its flexible application, merit conversations and, further research. Incidentally, implicit in research on social and academic intelligence is the assumption that individuals' knowledge of people in general (normative or typical social and emotional responses) will correlate with their knowledge of, for example, close friends. This too may merit discussion and research, although assessments of individuals' knowledge of their close friends would by necessity be individualized, would likely have to include participation of those friends in the research, and makes salient the very difficult issue of how best to score SI and EI tests (e.g., whether to use consensus, expert, or target scoring) given that such tests may not have clearly defined right or wrong answers (e.g., Roberts et al., 2001; Salovey et al., 2003).

A recent study (Kang & Shaver, 2004) is related to the some of the ideas expressed above. Kang and Shaver (2004) evaluated the assumption that individuals who have extensive emotional knowledge about themselves will also have greater empathy for, and perhaps will have higher-quality interpersonal relationships with, others. They developed and evaluated the construct validity of a self-report measure of emotional complexity (Range and Differentiation of Emotional Experience Scale, or RDEES) to evaluate whether emotional complexity, defined as experiencing a range of emotions and making subtle discriminations between similar emotions (such as sadness and depression), was related to empathic responding and better relationships. They found support for this claim and they present evidence that it was differentiation of emotions, more than the range of emotional experience, which predicted empathy and interpersonal adaptability.

We describe this particular study for three reasons. First, differentiation (of emotions or of social situations and social behaviors) might be important but largely unexamined components of both SI and EI. Second, differentiation can be assessed through a card-sorting activity (e.g., Kang & Shaver, 2004; Shaver, Schwartz, Kirson, & O'Connor, 1987), making it a viable candidate for ability assessments. That is, given cards with emotion words (or pictures of emotional expressions) and descriptions (or pictures) of social scenes, research participants with higher levels of differentiation may sort the cards into more categories in a particular card sort or into a larger number of different categories across multiple card sorts thus providing an ability measure of differentiation. And third, although in this paragraph we describe differentiation as an attribute of crystallized EI, we are uncertain about that characterization. We wonder if the ability to make subtle distinctions or differentiations is, in fact, an aspect of fluid intelligence. Thus, we feel even more strongly that discourse among researchers in social, emotional, and academic intelligence might prove fruitful.

5.5   CONCLUSIONS

Social and emotional intelligence share many similarities, both with one another and plausibly with academic intelligence. These intelligences also probably differ in important ways. We suggest that conversations among researchers in which those similarities and differences are carefully explored and explicated would advance theory and research in SI and EI. We provide a few ideas of topics that might serve to initiate those conversations.

We would like to conclude by outlining (in draft form) a study that could emerge from dialogue with others. The purpose of this study would be to establish the convergent and discriminant validity of fluid and crystallized abilities in each of three domains: academic, emotional, and social intelligence. Of course, other abilities, for example, processing speed, could be included in the design. For now, however, we will focus on crystallized and fluid abilities. A multitrait (i.e., fluid academic, crystallized academic, fluid emotional, crystallized emotional, and fluid social and crystallized social intelligence) multimethod (paper-and-pencil measures presented in writing, paper-and pencil measures presented in pictures, self-, and peer-report measures) design would be used. Various CFA models, some combining pairs of traits, others testing the equality of various correlations between traits, would be tested. Of course, decisions about how to define, for example, fluid ability (i.e., is differentiation the skill of most interest?), and which traits to assess (e.g., are emotion perception and knowledge of social rules and norms of most interest because they may interact?) would depend on the outcomes of the conversations. Different studies might emerge from conversations, but we believe that whatever research questions come to be seen as the most interesting, can only be answered with the same high-quality and methodologically rigorous approaches already evident in both research traditions.

REFERENCES

Bar-On, R. (1997). *BarOn Emotional Quotient Inventory (EQ–i): Technical manual.* Toronto, Canada: Multi-Health Systems.

Carroll, J. B. (1993). *Human cognitive abilities: A survey of factor-analytic studies.* New York: Cambridge University Press.

Caruso, D. R., Mayer, J. D., & Salovey, P. (2002). Relation of an ability measure of emotional intelligence to personality. *Journal of Personality Assessment, 79,* 306–320.

Chapin, F. S. (1942). Preliminary standardization of a social insight scale. *American Sociological Review, 7,* 214–225.

Ciarrochi, J., Chan, A. Y. C., & Caputi, P. (2000). A critical evaluation of the emotional intelligence construct. *Personality and Individual Differences, 28,* 539–561.

Davies, M., Stankov, L., & Roberts, R. D. (1998). Emotional intelligence: In search of an elusive construct. *Journal of Personality and Social Psychology, 75,* 989–1015.

Derksen, J., Kramer, I., & Katzko, M. (2002). Does a self-report measure for emotional intelligence assess something different than general intelligence? *Personality and Individual Differences, 32*, 37–48.

Ford, M. E., & Tisak, M. S. (1983). A further search for social intelligence. *Journal of Educational Psychology, 75*, 197–206.

Goleman, D. (1995). *Emotional intelligence: Why it can matter more than IQ.* New York: Bantam Books.

Gough, H. G. (1966). Appraisal of social maturity by means of the CPI. *Journal of Abnormal Psychology, 71*, 189–195.

Gough, H. G. (1968). *Manual for the Chapin Social Insight Test.* Palo Alto, CA: Consulting Psychologists Press.

Greenspan, S. I. (1989). Emotional intelligence. In K. Field, B. J. Cohler, & C. G. Wool (Eds.), *Learning and education: Psychoanalytic perspectives* (pp. 209–243). Madison, CT: International Universities Press.

Gresvenor, E. L. (1927). A study of the social intelligence of high school pupils. *American Physical Education Review, 32*, 649–657.

Hoepfner, R., & O'Sullivan, M. (1968). Social intelligence and IQ. *Educational and Psychological Measurement, 28*, 339–344.

Hunt, T. (1927). What social intelligence is and where to find it. *Industrial Psychology, 2*, 605–612.

Hunt, T. (1928). The measurement of social intelligence. *Journal of Applied Psychology, 12*, 317–334.

Jones, K., & Day, J. D. (1997). Discrimination of two aspects of cognitive social intelligence from academic intelligence. *Journal of Educational Psychology, 89*, 486–497.

Kang, S., & Shaver, P. R. (2004). Individual differences in emotional complexity: Their psychological implications. *Journal of Personality, 72*, 687–726.

Keating, D. P. (1978). A search for social intelligence. *Journal of Educational Psychology, 70*, 218–223.

Kihlstrom, J. F., & Cantor, N. (2000). Social intelligence. In R. J. Sternberg (Ed.), *Handbook of intelligence* (pp. 359–379). New York: Cambridge University Press.

Kosmitzki, C., & John, O. P. (1993). The implicit use of explicit conceptions of social intelligence. *Personality and Individual Differences, 15*, 11–23.

Lee, J.-E., Day, J. D., Meara, N. M., & Maxwell, S. E. (2002). Discrimination of social knowledge and its flexible application from creativity: A multitrait-multimethod approach. *Personality and Individual Differences, 32*, 913–928.

Lee, J.-E., Wong, C.-M. T., Day, J. D., Maxwell, S. E., & Thorpe, P. (2000). Social and academic intelligences: A multitrait-multimethod study of their crystallized and fluid characteristics. *Personality and Individual Differences, 29*, 539–553.

Legree, P. J. (1995). Evidence for an oblique social intelligence factor established with a Likert-based testing procedure. *Intelligence, 21*, 247–266.

Marlowe, H. A. (1986). Social intelligence: Evidence for multidimensionality and construct independence. *Journal of Educational Psychology, 78*, 52–58.

Matthews, G., Zeidner, M., & Roberts, R. D. (2002). *Emotional intelligence: Science and myth.* Cambridge, MA: MIT Press.

Mayer, J. D., Caruso, D. R., & Salovey, P. (1999). Emotional intelligence meets traditional standards for an intelligence. *Intelligence, 27,* 267–298.

Mayer, J. D., DiPaolo, M., & Salovey, P. (1990). Perceiving affective content in ambiguous visual stimuli: A component of emotional intelligence. *Journal of Personality Assessment, 54,* 772–781.

Mayer, J. D., & Geher, G. (1996). Emotional intelligence and the identification of emotion. *Intelligence, 22,* 89–113.

Mayer, J. D., & Salovey, P. (1997). What is emotional intelligence? In P. Salovey & D. J. Sluyter (Eds.), *Emotional development and emotional intelligence: Educational implications* (pp. 3–31). New York: Basic Books.

Mayer, J. D., Salovey, P., & Caruso, D. R. (2000). Models of emotional intelligence. In R. J. Sternberg (Ed.), *Handbook of intelligence* (pp. 396–420). New York: Cambridge University Press.

Mayer, J. D., Salovey, P., Caruso, D. R., & Sitarenios, G. (2003). Measuring emotional intelligence with the MSCEITV2.0. *Emotion, 3,* 97–105.

Moss, F. A., & Hunt, T. (1927). Are you socially intelligent? *Scientific American, 137,* 108–110.

O'Sullivan, M., & Guilford, J. P. (1975). Six factors of behavioral cognition: Understanding other people. *Journal of Educational Measurement, 12,* 255–271.

O'Sullivan, M., Guilford, J. P., & deMille, R. (1965). *The measurement of social intelligence* (Reports from the Psychological Laboratory No. 34). Los Angeles: University of Southern California.

Pintner, R., & Upshall, C. C. (1928). Some results of social intelligence tests. *School and Society, 27,* 369–370.

Riggio, R. E., Messamer, J., & Throckmorton, B. (1991). Social and academic intelligence: Conceptually distinct but overlapping constructs. *Personality and Individual Differences, 12,* 695–702.

Roberts, R. D., Zeidner, M., & Matthews, G. (2001). Does emotional intelligence meet traditional standards for an intelligence? Some new data and conclusions. *Emotion, 1,* 196–231.

Rose-Krasnor, L. (1997). The nature of social competence: A theoretical review. *Social Development, 6,* 111–133.

Salovey, P., Mayer, J. D., Caruso, D. R., & Lopes, P. N. (2003). Measuring emotional intelligence as a set of abilities with the Mayer-Salovey-Caruso emotional intelligence test. In S. Lopez & C. R. Snyder (Eds.), *Positive psychological assessment* (pp. 251–265). Washington, DC: American Psychological Association.

Shaver, P., Schwartz, J., Kirson, D., & O'Connor, C. (1987). Emotion knowledge: Further exploration of a prototype approach. *Journal of Personality and Social Psychology, 52,* 1061–1086.

Sternberg, R. J. (2000). *Handbook of intelligence.* New York: Cambridge University Press.

Sternberg, R. J. (2002). *When smart people behave stupidly.* New Haven, CT: Yale University Press.

Sternberg, R. J., Conway, B. E., Ketron, J. L., & Bernstein, M. (1981). People's conceptions of intelligence. *Journal of Personality and Social Psychology, 41,* 35–37.

Sternberg, R. J., & Gastel, J. (1989). Coping with novelty in human intelligence: An empirical investigation. *Intelligence, 13,* 187–197.

Thorndike, E. L. (1920). Intelligence and its use. *Harper's Magazine, 140,* 227–235.

Thorndike, R. L., & Stein, S. (1937). An evaluation of the attempts to measure social intelligence. *Psychological Bulletin, 34,* 275–285.

Trinidad, D. R., & Johnson, C. A. (2002). The association between emotional intelligence and early adolescent tobacco and alcohol use. *Personality and Individual Differences, 32,* 95–105.

Walker, R. E., & Foley, J. M. (1973). Social intelligence: Its history and measurement. *Psychological Reports, 33,* 839–864.

Wong, C.-M. T., Day, J. D., Maxwell, S. E., & Meara, N. M. (1995). A multitrait-multimethod study of academic and social intelligence in college students. *Journal of Educational Psychology, 87,* 117–133.

Zeidner, M., Roberts, R. D., & Matthews, G. (2002). Can emotional intelligence be schooled? A critical review. *Educational Psychologist, 37,* 215–231.

6

Far Too Many Intelligences? On the Communalities and Differences Between Social, Practical, and Emotional Intelligences

Elizabeth J. Austin
University of Edinburgh, Scotland
Donald H. Saklofske
University of Saskatchewan, Canada

Summary

This chapter considers three constructs which have been proposed as candidate intelligences: emotional intelligence (EI), practical intelligence (PI), and social intelligence (SI). The definition and measurement of each of these is discussed, including consideration of problems with current measures. We point out that two different and not necessarily equivalent approaches to measuring new intelligences have been developed. Ability measures emulate the problem-solving approach of conventional intelligence tests, whilst trait measures rely on self-reports. The conventional definition of an intelligence is then discussed in detail and the extent to which each of the candidate intelligences matches or fails to match this definition is considered. We conclude that applying the label *intelligence* to these constructs may be premature, although there is evidence that ability EI and SI have intelligence-like attributes. More research is needed both on defining these new constructs and in establishing the communalities and differences between them.

6.1   INTRODUCTION

In this chapter we discuss three constructs that may be regarded as candidate intelligences: emotional intelligence (EI), social intelligence (SI), and practical intelligence (PI). The definition and measurement of each construct is reviewed and the extent to which each actually meets the criterion for the "intelligence" designation is discussed. We also consider issues of how distinct these three intelligences are from one another.

In Section 6.2 some background information about each construct is given. Section 6.3 covers their measurement, and in particular considers the issue of performance versus self-report measures, which is currently an area of intense debate in EI research. Following a brief discussion of the extent of overlap of these constructs in Section 6.4, Section 6.5 sets out the definition of the term *intelligence* that we will adopt, taken directly from findings on psychometric intelligence; the extent to which each candidate intelligence matches this definition is then considered. The chapter ends with a general discussion and suggestions for future research in this area.

6.2   DEFINITION AND MEASUREMENT OF SOCIAL, PRACTICAL, AND EMOTIONAL INTELLIGENCE

6.2.1   Emotional Intelligence (EI)

Emotional intelligence provides a psychometric framework for the intuitive and appealing idea that people differ in their emotional skills and that these differences relate to real-life outcomes. For example, the superior interpersonal skills of high-EI individuals would be expected to lead to higher levels of career success, with EI having predictive power for this outcome over and above psychometric intelligence. EI has been defined in a variety of ways by different researchers. All EI models do, however, have overlapping core features comprising both intrapersonal (e.g., mood regulation, stress management) and interpersonal (e.g., emotion perception, social skills) components. EI has been characterized by some researchers as an ability (involving the cognitive processing of emotional information) which is therefore most appropriately measured by ability tests (e.g., Mayer, Caruso, & Salovey, 2000). An alternative approach assumes that EI represents a broad constellation of cognitive and non-cognitive components underlying emotions that can be measured by self-report questionnaire (e.g., Bar-On, 2000).

6.2.2   Social Intelligence (SI)

Social intelligence appears to have been first described as a performance construct by Thorndike in 1920. Together with abstract, verbal, practical, and/or mechanical intelligence, social intelligence was viewed as one of several interconnected but distinct intellectual abilities. Social intelligence was more specifically related to the capacity to understand, interact, and deal with people. The debate over the existence and relevance of social intelligence has been more or less active over the ensuing 80 years following Thorndike's pioneering statement. Matarazzo (1972) asserted that "we do not believe in such an entity... social intelligence is just general intelligence applied to social situations" (p. 209). However, the more recent multifactor intelligence theory proposed by Gardner (1993) has described three categories of intelligence: object-related, object-free, and person-related intelligences. Interpersonal and intrapersonal intelligence fall into the third category. Thus, both of the former focus on the capacity to understand and interact with others, whilst the latter relates to the construction of an accurate self perception that, in turn, can be used to effectively plan and direct a person's life. Also, in recent years, the social intelligence theme has been recast under such labels as social knowledge, social performance, social skills, and social competence (also see Chapter 10 by Weis & Süß). The latter description includes social intelligence and the acquisition of social skills, but also cognitive features related to social self-regulation, as well interpersonal personality traits (Schneider, Ackerman, & Kanfer, 1996). The measurement of social intelligence includes a mix of both performance-based and self-report scales that tap various cognitive and behavioral variables.

6.2.3   Practical Intelligence (PI)

Practical intelligence relates to the ability to deal with real-life problems, which are relatively unrelated to the more academic abilities assessed by IQ tests (Sternberg & Grigorenko, 2000). A more formal definition of the construct is: "Intelligence that serves to find a more optimal fit between the individual and the demands of the individual's environment, by adapting to the environment, changing (or shaping) the environment, or selecting a different environment" (Hedlund & Sternberg, 2000, p. 150). Advocates of PI argue that its association to problem solving in the real, as opposed to the academic, world means that it should act as a predictor of life success with incremental validity over psychometric intelligence. Studies of PI have involved the examination of both practical problem-solving skills and tacit knowledge. Tacit knowledge (TK), defined as knowledge which is relevant to a given situation, which is not formally acquired, and is procedural rather than declarative, has been identified as an important component of PI (Sternberg, Wagner, & Okagaki, 1993).

6.3   MEASUREMENT ISSUES

As mentioned above, instruments for the assessment of EI and SI using both self-report and performance methods have been devised. PI measures can be performance-based, for example requiring participants to deal with a simulated version of a workplace situation, but testing by self-report methods is also possible. Whilst self-report measures for new constructs can readily be devised using principles that have been established for assessing existing ones (e.g., personality), the construction of performance measures presents difficulties. Psychometric intelligence is a theoretically well-founded construct, which means that devising tests that have unambiguous right and wrong answers to assess any intelligence domain is a well-defined procedure; the existence of items with well-defined correct answers is regarded as an essential component of intelligence testing (Guttman & Levy, 1991; Most & Zeidner, 1995). For the candidate intelligences discussed in this chapter the problem of defining right answers is a more complex one, which we discuss in more detail in the passages that follow. In addition, the assessment of a construct by two very different measurement methods raises issues of whether the same construct is being measured. Naming the output from a self-report measure such as the EQ-i (Bar-On, 2000) and from a performance measure such as the Mayer-Salovey-Caruso Emotional Intelligence Test (MSCEIT; Mayer et al., 2000) as both measuring emotional intelligence rather pre-empts the issue (also see Chapter 2 by Neubauer & Freudenthaler). To resolve this discrepancy, Petrides and Furnham (2000, 2001) have proposed the labels trait (self-report) EI and ability (performance) EI; their work also draws attention to the issues of typical versus maximal performance which underlie the two measurement approaches (also see Chapter 9 by Pérez, Petrides, & Furnham). The same distinction could usefully be applied to measures of other new intelligences.

6.3.1   EI Measurement

A number of ability EI measures have been devised. Problems with such measures are related to difficulties in identifying the right answer to an EI problem, in the absence of a method for generating objective criteria to define the correct solution. The two main scoring systems which have been devised are expert scoring and consensus scoring (see Chapter 8 by Legree, Psotka, Tremble, & Bourne). The ability of EI experts to determine correct answers would appear to be problem-dependent. Thus, determining the correct answer to a facial expression recognition task appears relatively straightforward, whilst a problem involving complex social interactions presents greater difficulties. This problem is exacerbated by the fact that social behavior is determined by contextual and cultural factors, meaning that the concept of a right response is less well-defined (Matthews, Zeidner, & Roberts, 2002). It is also unclear whether EI researchers, who tend to be responsible for devising expert scoring criteria, actually qualify as emotional experts. Consensus scoring seeks to avoid these problems by defining the right answer as the response most frequently endorsed by a large normative group. Again, this scoring method appears vulnerable to ignoring situational and cultural effects, although use of different norms according to age, gender, and culture is possible. A second objection to this method is that it appears to be more applicable to simple emotional problems than to difficult ones. For example, again, facial expression recognition would appear to be appropriate for consensus scoring, but subtle problems of social interaction presumably need above-average EI abilities for their solution, so the group consensus here is likely to be actually incorrect (Matthews et al., 2002). In an extensive study of a performance EI measure, the Multifactor Emotional Intelligence Scales (MEIS; Mayer, Caruso, & Salovey, 1999), Roberts, Zeidner, and Matthews (2001), in addition to considering the general issues discussed above, identified specific problems: low sub-scale reliabilities, relatively low correlations between consensus and expert scores, and dependence of group differences on scoring method.

There are also problems associated with the assessment of EI by self-report. Thus, whilst questionnaire measures of EI are generally reliable and can be scored unambiguously, there are difficulties associated with consistent findings of medium to large correlations with personality measures. As an example, the aggregated results from a series of studies by the present authors (Austin, Saklofske, Huang, & McKenney, 2004; Saklofske, Austin, & Minski, 2003; Saklofske & Austin, 2004) with a combined N of 1422 give correlations of $-.29$ with Neuroticism (N), .44 with Extraversion (E), .25 with Openness (O), .41 with Agreeableness (A) and .26 with Conscientiousness (C). These results are consistent with the EI/personality correlations reported in a meta-analysis by Van Rooy and Viswesvaran (2004). In addition to this clear overlap between trait EI and personality, the idea that people are actually able to self-report on their emotional abilities has also been questioned (Bowman, Markham, & Roberts, 2002).

6.3.2   SI Measurement

As with EI, research on SI has employed both performance-based and self-report measures. While Legree (1995) presents arguments for the use of expert or consensus scoring for social intelligence measures, many of the current measures tapping SI appear to be based either on self-report or gleaned through informal measures that might draw from observation, interview or even extant records. A recent study by Weis and Süß (see Chapter 10) examined the potential relationship between self-report measures of social cognitive and behavioral skills, several performance measures of SI, and hypothetically related personality traits. They concluded that there was no support for the convergent construct validity of self-report and performance-based SI measures.

In the clinical context, specific subtests from the Wechsler intelligence scales have often been considered to tap social intelligence. One common example is the Picture Arrangement subtests found on the child and adult versions of this test. However, there is little evidence to support this contention, leading Kamphaus (1998) to argue that "a Picture Arrangement subtest score should not be interpreted as a measure of social judgment" (p. 54). The measurement approach recommended by practitioners who subscribe to Gardner's (1993) views of Multiple Intelligences include a pot pourri of data collection methods ranging from portfolio, observation, work samples, and self-report descriptions. While this approach has gained considerable acceptance in educational settings, it does not meet the criteria for sound psychometrically grounded measurement. The difficulty here is that the answer to the measurement question rests in the definition of the construct to be measured or assessed. Unfortunately, to date, consensual definitions of SI have not been forthcoming in the literature.

6.3.3   PI Measurement

A number of PI and TK tests have been developed (Sternberg & Grigorenko, 2000). Whilst the scoring procedure for practical problem solving tests is generally well defined, TK test scoring is subject to the same problems as performance EI scoring. A typical TK test involves choosing between or ranking alternative courses of action when confronted with a work-related situation (e.g., Wagner & Sternberg, 1985), leading to a requirement of defining the right choices. One method used to achieve this is again expert scoring, with correct answers being defined by high performers in the domain of interest. This scoring method would appear to be less problematic than for EI, as there are reasonably objective criteria, for identifying experts. An alternative approach to scoring is to examine response differences between expert and less expert groups.

6.4   OVERLAPS AND DIFFERENCES BETWEEN SI, PI, AND EI

It is clear from the definitions of these constructs that there is some degree of overlap between them, although in there is currently a dearth of studies in which all three (or any pair) have been directly compared. The study of Davies, Stankov, and Roberts (1998) found no significant correlations between EI and SI measures. By contrast, the work of Weis and Süß (Chapter 10, this volume) shows EI, SI and TK measures loading in theoretically interpretable ways on social understanding, social memory and social knowledge factors. These communalities clearly require further investigation. The issue of ability and trait measures discussed above is also relevant, for example if a performance-based definition, as originally envisaged by Thorndike, of SI is adopted, SI would be expected to show stronger correlations with ability EI than with trait EI.

Although overlap is expected, the definitions of EI, PI, and SI do suggest the existence of some differences between them, which we now discuss in more detail. EI is explicitly defined as having both inter- and intrapersonal components; the existence of these two strands, allowing incorporation of individual differences in, for example, mood regulation and stress management, make it appear a richer construct than SI or PI, since the latter do not explicitly cover any type of internal regulatory processes. SI is defined primarily in terms of inter-personal skills and knowledge of social rules and conventions, so SI would appear to have some overlap with the interpersonal aspects of EI. Some distance between SI and EI is, however, suggested by results on different links to conflict behavior, with SI being found to relate positively to aggressive behavior as well as to peaceful conflict resolution, whereas empathy, an important EI component in many models, is associated more strongly with non-aggressive resolution strategies (Björkqvist, Österman, & Kaukiainen, 2000). The descriptions of PI and SI differ from EI in not being conceptualized as being specifically emotional. Moreover, PI does not even explicitly relate to inter-personal skill; there may, however, be an implicit component of PI, that is, it represents one of the ways of acquiring tacit knowledge, specifically, by socializing well in order to be optimally placed to learn skills from other individuals.

6.5   DO SI, PI, AND EI COUNT AS INTELLIGENCES?

6.5.1   Criteria for a Construct To Be "an Intelligence"

Extensive study of human ability differences has lead to a consensus on the structure of psychometric intelligence (Carroll, 1993). The accepted model of psychometric intelligence has a hierarchical structure, with general ability g at the top stratum, group factors at the second stratum, and specific factors at the third stratum. For a new intelligence to qualify as a candidate, it should (ideally) fit into this structure, possess a similar degree of predictive validity to that found for other forms of psychometric intelligence, and also show links to underlying biological and cognitive processes. In addition, the candidate intelligence should be well defined, in the sense that it can be operationalized as a cognitive ability, that is, a clear link between an intelligence and the kind of problems it is used to solve can be established. It is also expected that the problem-solving should be linked to purely cognitive processes such as verbal fluency, pattern completion, and so forth. Within the traditional formulation of psychometric intelligence, modes of problem-solving linked to dispositional or cultural factors are excluded, with this exclusion being linked to the idea that intelligence test problems should have unique right answers. In the following sections the current status of psychometric intelligence is discussed in more detail with reference to these criteria, and SI, PI, and EI are compared with psychometric intelligence in these respects.

Correlations with other intelligence measures and with non-intelligence measures: Convergent and discriminant validity.   The existence of positive manifold—that is, positive correlations amongst both group factors and specific factors—underpins the hierarchical model of intelligence discussed above. New intelligences are therefore expected to fit this model by correlating positively with existing ones; such correlations should be large enough to be meaningful, whilst not being so large that the new intelligence is indistinguishable from an existing one. If SI, PI, and EI are to fit in the existing hierarchy, one possibility is that each construct would be at the second stratum; that is, as group factors, with, for example, EI subcomponents forming specific factors. Alternatively, these constructs might fit at the third stratum; for EI Matthews et al. (2002) discuss the evidence that it can be regarded as a sub-component of crystallized ability, whilst for PI Gottfredson (2003) argues that the specificity of current measures place them also in the third stratum. Psychometric intelligence also meets discriminant validity criteria; the modest size of correlations between intelligence measures and personality traits (Ackerman & Heggestad, 1997) shows that intelligence and personality address distinct aspects of the psychological differences between individuals; again there would appear to be a requirement for SI, PI, and EI to show similar distinctness.

Criterion and predictive validity.   Psychometric intelligence has good predictive validity for life outcomes in areas where these associations would be expected on theoretical grounds, in particular educational and career success (Gottfredson, 1997; Neisser et al., 1996; Schmidt & Hunter, 1998). SI, PI, and EI would be expected to show similar predictive ability for appropriate theoretically linked outcomes. There are also issues of incremental validity, that is, new intelligences should give enhanced predictive power over old ones. As an example of an incremental validity exercise, regression models using psychometric intelligence and EI separately and combined as predictors of career success, and so forth, could be compared. Each variable alone would be expected to have some predictive ability; a key test of the usefulness of EI is whether it adds significantly to the predictive power of psychometric intelligence. This question can be addressed by comparing R^2 measures for models with psychometric intelligence alone and psychometric intelligence and EI as predictors. Consistent findings of no significant improvement in predictive ability with a range of outcomes would suggest that the new intelligence is not measuring anything different from the old one.

Biological associations and associations with lower-level cognitive tasks. Psychometric intelligence is known to be highly heritable (Plomin & Petrill, 1997), suggesting that there is a biological contribution to intelligence differences. Evidence pointing in the same direction linking intelligence to speed of information processing comes from findings on associations between psychometric intelligence and faster performance on reaction time and inspection time tasks, and event related potential differences between low- and high-g individuals, although the mechanisms for these associations are not well understood (Deary, 2000). Similar genetic and biological associations should be sought for new candidate intelligence measures; to date no systematic attempts at uncovering the biological and lower-level cognitive mechanisms underlying EI, SI and PI have been reported.

6.5.2   EI as an Intelligence

For ability EI, there is accumulating evidence of reasonably sized positive correlations with conventional psychometric intelligence measures (Mayer et al., 1999; Roberts et al., 2001). Associations appear to be stronger for crystallized than for fluid ability measures, an observation suggesting that EI may overlap more with acculturated than with fluid abilities (Bowman et al., 2002). Mayer et al. (1999) argue that performance EI can be operationalized as a set of abilities in a manner analogous to psychometric intelligence, although it should be noted that, as discussed above, there is some controversy and disagreement about the methods of scoring emotional performance problems (Matthews et al., 2002). By contrast, trait EI measures show small or zero correlations with psychometric intelligence (e.g., Derksen, Kramer, & Katzko, 2002).

Turning to issues of discriminant validity, ability EI measures show small or zero correlations with personality (Roberts et al., 2001; Mayer et al., 2000). By contrast, trait EI measures show medium to large correlations with personality, and the extent to which trait EI is distinct from personality is a topic of current debate in the literature. Some part of the correlation patterns observed for trait and ability EI may be due to common method variance. There is also the possibility that trait EI may relate to ability EI in the same way that self-reported intelligence relates to intelligence objectively assessed by IQ tests. Here the finding is that self-reported intelligence correlates at around .30 with IQ (e.g., Furnham, 2001). These findings indicate that people can report on their own ability level to some imperfect extent, notwithstanding the response biases inevitable in self-assessing this most socially desirable characteristic. Similar considerations may well apply to EI; whilst respondents will presumably believe high EI to be desirable, they may be capable of making some kind of realistic assessment of how emotionally intelligent they actually are.

In terms of the predictive validity of EI, positive associations with happiness, life satisfaction, and social network size and quality and negative associations with depression, depression-proneness, and loneliness have been found (Austin et al., 2004; Ciarrochi, Chan, & Bajgar, 2001; Dawda & Hart, 2000; Saklofske et al., 2003; Schutte et al., 1998). A summary of the small number of studies which have addressed this issue (Matthews et al., 2002), however, suggests that the incremental predictive validity of ability EI with psychometric intelligence controlled for, and of trait EI with personality controlled for, are both small.

Tables 6.1 and 6.2 summarize some results from our own research in which the incremental validity of trait EI was assessed using regression modelling. The group of variables happiness, life satisfaction, loneliness and social networks would all be expected to relate to EI (negatively in the case of loneliness, otherwise positively) because of the superior inter-personal skills of high-EI individuals. A negative relationship between depression-proneness and EI would be anticipated because of intrapersonal EI skills such as mood management. The final set of variables, all related to health behaviors would also be expected to show associations with EI, with high-EI individuals tending to take better care of their health, although the arguments for this are less direct and assign a coping style-like role to EI. As an example, inter-personal EI skills would be expected to facilitate resistance to peer pressure to consume excessive amounts of alcohol (Trinidad & Johnson, 2002), whilst at the same time making high-EI individuals more receptive to guidance on alcohol consumption from health professionals and others. In addition, intrapersonal EI skills such as mood regulation might be expected to reduce the need to use al-

Table 6.1   Correlations of EI With Theoretically-Linked Outcomes

	Study 1	Study 2	Study 3
Happiness	.45***		
Life Satisfaction	.39***	.30***	.30***
Loneliness (family)	−.29***		
Loneliness (social)	−.33***		
Loneliness (romantic)	−.19***		
Depression proneness	−.38***		
Social network size		.36***	
Social network quality		.17**	
Alcohol consumption		−.19*	−.07
Exercise			.12*
Self-reported health		−.02	.01
Number of doctor's visits		−.03	.10
Alternative health treatment use			.11*
Healthy diet			.17**

Notes. Study 1 (Saklofske et al., 2003) $N = 354$, Study 2 (Austin, Saklofske, & Egan, 2005) $N = 704$, Study 3 (Saklofske & Austin, 2004) $N = 364$.
$^* p < .05$, $^{**} p < .01$, $^{***} p < .001$.

cohol as a means of mood management. The correlations in Table 6.1 confirm some associations are indeed found between EI and positive health behaviors, as well as associations in the predicted direction with the social variables and depression. These correlations are, however, difficult to interpret. Personality traits also correlate significantly with the Table 6.1 outcomes, which suggests that the correlations may partly be accounted for by the common associations amongst EI, personality and outcomes. Regression modelling can be used to test these ideas, by identifying the most salient predictors for each outcome. In addition, the incremental validity of EI can be assessed by comparing models with personality traits as predictors with and without the additional inclusion of EI; the change in R^2 between the two models provides an incremental validity measure. Our general finding has been that there are cases where EI has some degree of incremental predictive validity over personality, but the increases in R^2 are not large.

Table 6.2 shows the result of using regression modelling to identify the significant predictors of each outcome. It can be seen that EI does appear as a predictor in several models and in particular is the best predictor of social network size and of taking exercise. The result for social network size is of particular interest since this provides a good match to the theoretical idea that high-EI individuals should have more and better quality relationships with friends, colleagues, and family. By contrast, self-reported social network quality is determined by personality, appearing to fit the general tendency of individuals who are high on Neuroticism to report dissatisfaction with all aspects of their lives. The mechanism by which EI relates to exercise behavior is less obvious but, as with the example of alcohol consumption discussed above,

Table 6.2   Significant Regression Predictors

	Study 1	ΔR^2	Study 2	ΔR^2	Study 3	ΔR^2
Happiness	E(+)N(−)A(+)EI(+)	1.3				
Life Satisfaction	N(−)EI(+)E(+)	1.8	N(−)	2.9	N(−)E(+)EI(+)	3.2
Loneliness (family)	N(+)A(−)EI(−)O(−)	1.4				
Loneliness (social)	N(+)E(−)EI(−)	1.3				
Loneliness (romantic)	N(+)EI(−)	1.2				
Depression proneness	N(+)E(−)O(+)EI(−)	1.0				
Social network size			EI(+)	5.0		
Social network quality			N(−)	0.1		
Alcohol consumption			E(+)	3.9	E(+)	0.5
Exercise					EI(+)	0.2
Self-reported health			N(−)A(+)	3.1	E(+)N(−)	0.3
Number of doctor's visits			C(+)	1.2		
Alternative health treatment use					O(+)	0.6
Healthy diet					A(+)C(+)	0.9

Note. $\Delta R^2 = R^2$ change (%).

could relate to both interpersonal (positive social aspects of sporting activities) and intrapersonal (using exercise for mood regulation) facets of EI. For each outcome the change in R^2 between models using the five personality trait scores as predictors and models using EI in addition to personality is shown (see columns labelled ΔR^2). It can be seen that all these values are small, with the largest being 5% and several below 1%, suggesting that the incremental validity of trait EI over personality does give cause for concern. For exercise behavior two structural equation models were compared. A model in which EI mediates the effects of personality on exercise behavior is shown in Figure 6.1. This was compared with a regression model in which C, E, and EI contribute independently to exercise behavior, but with the correlation between E and C being retained. Comparison of the fit of the two models supported the mediating model ($\chi^2(2)$ was 3.7 for the mediating model and 57.0 for the regression model with respective mean standardized off-diagonal residual covariance matrix elements of 0.024, 0.12).

Possible explanations for the mediating role of EI are discussed above, essentially mediation might be expected if EI plays a similar role to coping style,

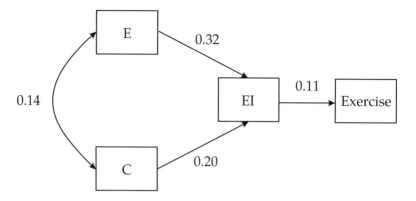

Figure 6.1 Model showing EI acting as a mediator of the relationship between personality and exercise.

which is often found to mediate personality/behavior associations (Deary et al., 1996). There are also studies showing that trait EI scores differ in the predicted direction between a range of criterion groups (Bar-On, 1997; Schmidt & Hunter, 1998). For example, therapists score significantly higher than therapy clients or prisoners, and more successful members of certain occupational groups have been found to have higher EI scores than their less successful counterparts. Trait EI has also been found to be a predictor of academic success in first-year university students (Parker, Summerfeldt, Hogan, & Majeski, 2004). This finding can be interpreted in terms of the usefulness of inter- and intrapersonal skills in dealing with the novel university environment, a point that administrators, for example, might find eminently useful, suggesting both that EI might be used alongside personality and ability tests when selecting university applicants and that emotional skills enhancement programs might form part of student support services.

Unlike PI and SI, there has been some progress in linking EI (or alexithymia, which is related to low EI; Parker, Taylor, & Bagby, 2001) to performance on tasks which assess individual differences in the processing of emotional information (Austin, 2004; Bates, 1999; Ciarrochi et al., 2001; Parker, Taylor, & Bagby, 1993a, 1993b; Petrides & Furnham, 2003). The trait approach to EI measurement raises the issue of whether people can self-report on their emotional skills without actually demonstrating them in the same way as it is known they can on their personality traits. In particular, does a person's response to an item such as "I find it easy to read people's facial expressions" bear any relation to their actual ability to read facial expressions during social interactions with others. From a more fundamental viewpoint, it seems plausible to suggest that individual differences in EI might in part be underpinned by individual differences in the speed of processing of emotional information.

The idea of a possibly biologically based information processing component to EI links to the information processing approach to psychometric intelligence discussed in Section 6.5.1. The existence of individual differences in emotion

Table 6.3   Correlations Amongst Computer Tasks And The NART

	NART	Happy-IT	Sad-IT	Symbol-IT
Happy-IT	−.09 (72)			
Sad-IT	.07 (72)	.42*** (92)		
Symbol-IT	.06 (72)	.48*** (92)	.46*** (92)	
Ekman-60	−.06 (67)	.40*** (87)	.33** (87)	.18 (87)

Notes. NART = National Adult Reading Test (total correct), Happy IT = happy face inspection time score (total correct), Sad IT = sad face inspection time score (total correct), Symbol IT = symbol inspection time score (total correct). N for each correlation is given in brackets.
** $p < .01$, *** $p < .001$.

processing speed and potential relationships with EI has not yet been widely investigated. The main objective of the study described in this section (Austin, 2004) was to examine the associations between scores on a trait EI measure and performance on speeded (inspection time [IT]) and unspeeded tasks involving the recognition of facial expressions of emotion. A second objective was to investigate the extent to which the speed of emotional information processing relates to the speed of processing of non-emotional information. In this study, 92 participants completed a trait EI scale and three IT tasks in which discriminations were performed between (a) happy and neutral faces, (b) sad and neutral faces, and (c) two emotionally-neutral symbols. Participants also completed a personality questionnaire and were assessed on the NART (Nelson & Willison, 1991), a measure of crystallized ability, and on an unspeeded facial expression recognition task.

Table 6.3 shows the correlations amongst the computer tasks and the NART. It can be seen that there are large significant correlations amongst scores on the three IT tasks. Both emotional inspection time tasks are also significantly correlated with the unspeeded facial expression recognition task (Ekman-60; Young, Perrett, Calder, Sprengelmeyer, & Ekman, 2002), whereas the symbol inspection time task is not. NART scores are not correlated with any of the computer tasks and personality traits were also found to be uncorrelated with emotional task performance. Overall EI and intrapersonal EI sub-factors were found to be uncorrelated with performance on any of the tasks but an interpersonal EI sub-factor assessing the ability to read the emotions of others was significantly correlated with performance on the two IT tasks involving emotional stimuli ($r = .22$ for happy faces, .25 for sad faces, both $p < .05$). The correlation between interpersonal EI and Ekman faces task performance was similar in size, although failing to reach significance with a slightly smaller sample size for this task ($r = .22$, $p = .055$). Since performance on the symbol IT task can be regarded as a measure of general processing speed, the effect of partialling-out symbol task performance on the correlation between the two emotional IT tasks was examined. This relationship remained significant ($r = .28$, $p < .05$), suggesting a contribution to the correlation related to the specific emotional content of the two tasks. Correlations between the Ekman-60 task and the two emotional IT tasks also remained significant ($r = .40$, $p < .001$ for happy faces, $r = .28$, $p < .05$ for sad faces). Taken together, the correlations suggest that a common processing speed factor accounts in part for performance on the IT tasks. In addition, an underlying emotion-processing factor appears to contribute to emotional IT performance. The patterning of correlations with trait EI provides support for its validity, in that self-reports of interpersonal emotion perception ability are related to (interpersonal) emotion task performance, whilst self-reports of intrapersonal aspects of emotion management are unrelated to performance on these tasks. There is also evidence for discriminant validity from personality, in that personality, unlike EI, was found to be unrelated to performance on emotion-related tasks. Associations between trait EI and emotional information processing ability have also been reported by Bates (1999) and Petrides and Furnham (2003). From the findings discussed above, it seems reasonable to conclude that ability EI has many of the required features of an intelligence in terms of its general pattern of correlations with other measures. Trait EI does not fit the definition of an intelligence, but is weakly related to the ability to process emotion-related information. There is clearly scope for improvement of both ability and trait measures. For ability EI measures the issue of scoring, discussed earlier, needs to be addressed, whilst the development of trait EI measures which are more distinct from personality than current instruments would be highly desirable.

6.5.3   SI as an Intelligence

Whilst much of the earlier work on social intelligence produced confusing and contradictory results, leading many researchers to conclude that the construct was not worth studying, some recent work using established psychometric and modeling techniques, including confirmatory factor analysis (CFA) suggests a possible revival. A study by Lee, Wong, Day, Maxwell, and Thorpe (2000) provides evidence that SI divides into the domains of social-cognitive (understanding people, knowing social rules) and social-behavioral (being good at dealing with people). This study also provides evidence supporting both the existence of fluid and crystallized SI and of SI fitting into the intelligence hierarchy, with SI measures showing reasonable sized correlations with academic intelligence. A study by Legree (1995) similarly derived a separate social intelligence factor with CFA indicating a hierarchical factor structure with SI loading on g along with verbal, speed, quantitative and technical factors. These results suggest that like ability EI, SI, appropriately defined and measured, has intelligence-like attributes (see Chapter 10).

The ongoing debate during much of the 20th century over the relevance and need for a description of social intelligence to both complement but also extend other descriptions of intelligence has not yet achieved any kind of consensus. Certainly social knowledge, understanding, and application are already reflected in many of the subtests assessing crystallized abilities found on the Wechsler scales (e.g., Comprehension, Picture Arrangement). Once the concept of SI includes social self-regulation and personality traits, it might appear to be better described within a framework of contemporary social cognitive models (Matthews, Schwean, Campbell, Saklofske, & Mohamed, 2000) and measured possibly as both an ability and trait, following current practices in the assessment of EI. Whether social intelligence is akin to the specific kinds of intrapersonal and interpersonal intelligences described by Gardner, a reflection of various cognitive abilities underlying social themes, a link or bridge between personality and intelligence, or more properly viewed as a part of personality seen from both a trait and social cognitive perspective, remains to be seen. Current research efforts need to be directed at both isolating a SI factor (whether a major or group factor) and also demonstrating its relevance to the description of individual differences.

6.5.4   PI as an Intelligence

Whilst a number of specific, situation-based tests of practical problem solving and tacit knowledge have been constructed for particular groups (e.g., managers, the military), no general-purpose PI test is currently available. This may appear a difficult objective given the domain-specificity of PI, but within a framework where TK acquisition abilities are postulated to underlie PI, a general-purpose TK skills instrument would appear to be feasible. In order for PI to be fully assessed for its fit with the intelligence hierarchy, it is necessary to measure individual differences in the implied underlying cognitive ability that allows individuals to acquire domain-specific PI skills. At present there is no test battery available that would enable a general PI factor of this nature and PI subcomponents to be extracted and examined for predictive validity and correlations with other intelligence measures (Gottfredson, 2003).

In terms of establishing correlations of existing PI measures with psychometric intelligence, the findings to date present problematic features. PI and TK test performance have been reported to have negligible or even negative correlations with psychometric intelligence (Sternberg & Grigorenko, 2000), which would preclude the inclusion of PI in the intelligence positive manifold. Evidence of criterion/predictive validity has been found with PI being, for example, positively associated with a range of career success measures in academic psychologists and business managers (Wagner & Sternberg, 1985). A detailed survey of the published PI literature (Gottfredson, 2003) has, however, questioned results on PI obtained to date. The issues raised by Gottfredson, some of which are also pointed out by Bowman et al. (2002), include the use of small samples, inconsistent findings, restriction of ability range in the groups studied, the lack of a general-purpose PI instrument, and difficulties in generalization from the results obtained on the narrow range of occupational groups studied. She also suggests that the gulf between academic and practical intelligence is not as wide as has been suggested with, for example, many conventional IQ tests having tacit knowledge aspects, and academic ability having predictive power for the ability to solve real-life practical problems. Gottfredson's review also raises an interesting issue related to the discriminant validity of PI from personality that merits attention. Tests designed to assess the tacit knowledge required to succeed in a particular career may well also tap into traits linked to pursuing one's own interests and creating a good impression with superiors; in this context studies of associations between TK tests and traits such as Machiavellianism (Christie & Geis, 1970) and impression management (Paulhus, 1984) would be of interest.

Given the relatively sparse data on PI currently available and the intense debate over its interpretation (Gottfredson, 2003; Sternberg, 2003) the question of whether PI does fit into the intelligence manifold is perhaps best regarded as open whilst further results are awaited. PI nonetheless appears to be potentially useful for predicting real-world success, and merits further study and the gathering of more data for this reason, as well as in order to establish its associations with other intelligence measures.

6.6 DISCUSSION

6.6.1 Are EI, SI, and PI "Intelligences"?

For all three constructs it is perhaps unfortunate that the label *intelligence* has been applied to them in advance of supporting evidence being obtained. From the literature reviewed here it appears that ability EI shows a correlation pattern that should allow it to be fitted into the psychometric intelligence manifold, with trait EI being located closer to the personality domain. There is some similar evidence for SI as an intelligence, but establishing the position for PI seems to require more work, as indeed is also required to clarify the status of EI and SI.

The application of the *intelligence* label to new constructs also points to some areas where individual difference researchers may perhaps be thinking too simplistically. Firstly, are we obliged to call everything that predicts real-life success an intelligence? The best counter-example here is the personality trait of Conscientiousness, which is a predictor of career and academic success (e.g., Hurtz & Donovan, 2000; Paunonen & Ashton, 2001) but is clearly a personality trait, not an intelligence. Secondly, the idea of defining either "intelligences" or personality traits as globally adaptive once we move away from the solid ground of psychometric intelligence is hard to defend. Situational factors can clearly play a role in what is adaptive and what is not. For example, the EI subcomponent of empathy could be adaptive in some situations (understanding a partner's or friend's feelings and acting upon that knowledge to enhance the relationship) and maladaptive in others (pursuing career success in a competitive environment where too much understanding of and concern for the feelings of others may impede one's own progress).

6.6.2 How Do These "Intelligences" Interrelate?

Whilst EI, PI, and SI clearly have some degree of overlap, it is hard to draw definite conclusions on how extensive this might be, given the current lack of comparative studies. There is an urgent need for large-scale studies in which all three are assessed together and tested against each other as predictors of real-life outcomes. Such studies should where possible include both trait and performance measures. Hedlund and Sternberg (2000) have made the interesting suggestion that EI, PI, and SI can all be integrated within a tacit knowledge framework. It seems problematic to justify this position experimentally based on the present findings on TK, given (a) the lack of a general-purpose measure of TK and (b) the lack of work on correlations between measures of EI, SI, and PI. Nonetheless, this argument is theoretically appealing, in that emotional and social abilities can be hypothesized to be acquired by the tacit learning route in an analogous manner to that proposed for practical skills. In this formulation the intra- and interpersonal aspects of EI would be regarded as comprising tacit knowledge about managing oneself and managing others respectively (Matthews et al., 2002).

6.6.3   Do These Constructs Have a Biological Underpinning?

Work on the biological basis of PI and SI is currently non-existent. Some progress is starting to be made with EI. Further work is needed on its underlying biological basis by further study of the relationships between both trait and ability EI scores and performance on lower-level emotion-processing tasks. This information processing approach has proved very fruitful in the study of psychometric intelligence and should be equally helpful in the study and validation of EI (and by extension PI and SI). One caution here is that initially the tasks should be selected from those for which the right answers are unambiguous, to avoid the scoring problems which have on occasion been found with ability EI measures (Matthews et al., 2002). For all three constructs, behavior genetic studies would also be of great interest; if any or all of them are established to be significantly heritable, this would in itself provide both evidence for underlying biological mechanisms and act as a starting point in the search for relevant genes. One promising initial finding on the biological basis of EI comes from a study (Bar-On, Tranel, Denburg, & Bechara, 2003), which has linked brain lesions that impair emotional signaling with both poor decision-making and low EI scores.

6.6.4   Measurement Issues

The trait/ability distinction is a potential issue for all three constructs but has been most fully developed for EI, to which we confine the discussion in this subsection. The distinction between trait and ability measures should be maintained, thereby avoiding fallacy of giving two different things the same name ("jingle", Block, 1995; Thorndike, 1904). The study of the relationships between the two forms of EI promises to be fruitful; it is clearly of interest to establish the extent to which people can self-report on their own emotional skills The relationships found between trait EI and emotional task performance described above show that trait EI can act as a measure of emotional processing abilities, notwithstanding its overlaps with personality. An important argument for continuing to work on the development of trait EI measures is that testing by questionnaire is more straightforward and less expensive than the use of performance tests. Questionnaires can be mailed out to large samples and completed by respondents under unsupervised conditions, a major advantage compared to the usual supervised administration of performance tests. As discussed above, it is to be hoped that further work on questionnaire EI measures will produce scales which show less overlap with personality than the current generation of EI scales.

6.7   CONCLUSIONS

Much work remains to be done on establishing the nature, validity, and usefulness of EI, PI, and SI and it is likely that they will remain problematic for the foreseeable future. This is partly due to the gaps in research pointed out above, but also because they are all, to some extent, conceptualized as being on the cognition/emotion boundary. Such bridging constructs are not easy to fit into the individual differences perspective, which has tended to assign cognitive phenomena to intelligence and issues of dealing with emotions to personality. This is an over-simplified view, in that cognition and emotion clearly do overlap, as shown, for example, by evidence supporting Damasio's (1994) somatic marker hypothesis, which links impairments of decision-making with impaired emotional signalling. Part of the challenge of these new intelligences is that they suggest a change in our thinking about the links between cognition and emotion and also about what we mean by intelligent behavior. The question of whether the addition of EI, PI, and SI to the psychometric canon gives us too many intelligences cannot be resolved at present. More work on these constructs singly and in comparison with each other will be required to test their validity, usefulness and independence from one another.

REFERENCES

Ackerman, P. L., & Heggestad, E. D. (1997). Intelligence, personality, and interests: Evidence for overlapping traits. *Psychological Bulletin, 121,* 219–245.

Austin, E. J. (2004). An investigation of the relationships between trait emotional intelligence and emotional task performance. *Personality and Individual Differences, 36,* 1855–1864.

Austin, E. J., Saklofske, D. H., & Egan, V. (2005). Personality, well-being and health correlates of trait emotional intelligence. *Personality and Individual Differences, 38,* 547–558.

Austin, E. J., Saklofske, D. H., Huang, S. H. S., & McKenney, D. (2004). Measurement of trait emotional intelligence: Testing and cross-validating a modified version of Schutte et al.'s (1998) measure. *Personality and Individual Differences, 36,* 555–562.

Bar-On, R. (1997). *BarOn Emotional Quotient Inventory (EQ–i): Technical manual.* Toronto, Canada: Multi-Health Systems.

Bar-On, R. (2000). Emotional and social intelligence: Insights from the Emotional Quotient inventory. In R. Bar-On & J. D. A. Parker (Eds.), *The handbook of emotional intelligence: Theory, development, assessment, and application at home, school, and in the workplace* (pp. 363–388). San Francisco: Jossey-Bass.

Bar-On, R., Tranel, D., Denburg, N. L., & Bechara, A. (2003). Exploring the neurological substrate of emotional and social intelligence. *Brain, 126,* 1790–1800.

Bates, T. (1999, July). *Domain-specific information-processing speed model of emotional intelligence (IQ e).* Paper presented at the 9th Biennial Meeting of the International Society for the Study of Individual Differences, Vancouver, Canada.

Björkqvist, K., Österman, K., & Kaukiainen, A. (2000). Social intelligence – empathy = aggression? *Aggression and Violent Behavior, 5,* 191–200.

Block, J. (1995). A contrarian view of the five-factor approach to personality description. *Psychological Bulletin, 117,* 187–215.

Bowman, D. B., Markham, P. M., & Roberts, R. D. (2002). Expanding the frontiers of human cognitive abilities: so much more than (plain) g! *Learning and Individual Differences, 13,* 127–158.

Carroll, J. B. (1993). *Human cognitive abilities: A survey of factor-analytic studies.* New York: Cambridge University Press.

Christie, R., & Geis, F. L. (1970). *Studies in Machiavellianism.* New York: Academic Press.

Ciarrochi, J., Chan, A. Y. C., & Bajgar, J. (2001). Measuring emotional intelligence in adolescents. *Personality and Individual Differences, 31,* 1105–1119.

Damasio, A. R. (1994). *Descartes' error: Emotion, reason, and the human brain.* New York: Grosset/Putnam.

Davies, M., Stankov, L., & Roberts, R. D. (1998). Emotional intelligence: In search of an elusive construct. *Journal of Personality and Social Psychology, 75,* 989–1015.

Dawda, D., & Hart, S. D. (2000). Assessing emotional intelligence: Reliability and validity of the Bar-On Emotional Quotient inventory (EQ-i) in university students. *Personality and Individual Differences, 28,* 797–812.

Deary, I. J. (2000). *Looking down on human intelligence.* Oxford, UK: Oxford University Press.

Deary, I. J., Blenkin, H., Agius, R. M., Endler, N. S., Zealley, H., & Wood, R. (1996). Models of job-related stress and personal achievement among consultant doctors. *British Journal of Psychology, 87,* 3–29.

Derksen, J., Kramer, I., & Katzko, M. (2002). Does a self-report measure for emotional intelligence assess something different than general intelligence? *Personality and Individual Differences, 32,* 37–48.

Furnham, A. (2001). Self-estimates of intelligence: Culture and gender differences in self and other estimates of both general (g) and multiple intelligences. *Personality and Individual Differences, 31,* 1381–1405.

Gardner, H. (1993). *Frames of mind: The theory of multiple intelligences* (2nd ed.). New York: Basic Books.

Gottfredson, L. S. (1997). Why g matters: The complexity of everyday life. *Intelligence, 24,* 79–132.

Gottfredson, L. S. (2003). Dissecting practical intelligence theory: Its claims and evidence. *Intelligence, 31*, 343–397.

Guttman, L., & Levy, S. (1991). Two structural laws for intelligence tests. *Intelligence, 15*, 79–103.

Hedlund, J., & Sternberg, R. J. (2000). Too many intelligences? Integrating social, emotional and practical intelligence. In R. Bar-On & J. D. A. Parker (Eds.), *The handbook of emotional intelligence: Theory, development, assessment, and application at home, school, and in the workplace* (pp. 136–167). San Francisco: Jossey-Bass.

Hurtz, G. M., & Donovan, J. J. (2000). Personality and job performance: The Big Five revisited. *Journal of Applied Psychology, 85*, 869–879.

Kamphaus, R. W. (1998). Intelligence test interpretation: Acting in the absence of evidence. In A. Prifitera & D. H. Saklofske (Eds.), *WISC–III clinical use and interpretation* (pp. 40–57). San Diego, CA: Academic Press.

Lee, J.-E., Wong, C.-M. T., Day, J. D., Maxwell, S. E., & Thorpe, P. (2000). Social and academic intelligences: A multitrait-multimethod study of their crystallized and fluid characteristics. *Personality and Individual Differences, 29*, 539–553.

Legree, P. J. (1995). Evidence for an oblique social intelligence factor established with a Likert-based testing procedure. *Intelligence, 21*, 247–266.

Matarazzo, J. D. (1972). *Wechsler's measurement and appraisal of adult intelligence* (5th ed.). New York: Oxford University Press.

Matthews, G., Schwean, V. L., Campbell, S. E., Saklofske, D. H., & Mohamed, A. A. R. (2000). Personality, self-regulation and adaptation: A cognitive-social framework. In M. Boekaerts, P. R. Printrich, & M. Zeidner (Eds.), *Handbook of self-regulation* (pp. 171–207). New York: Academic Press.

Matthews, G., Zeidner, M., & Roberts, R. D. (2002). *Emotional intelligence: Science and myth.* Cambridge, MA: MIT Press.

Mayer, J. D., Caruso, D. R., & Salovey, P. (1999). Emotional intelligence meets traditional standards for an intelligence. *Intelligence, 27*, 267–298.

Mayer, J. D., Caruso, D. R., & Salovey, P. (2000). Selecting a measure of emotional intelligence: The case for ability testing. In R. Bar-On & J. D. A. Parker (Eds.), *The handbook of emotional intelligence: Theory, development, assessment, and application at home, school, and in the workplace* (pp. 320–342). San Francisco: Jossey-Bass.

Most, B., & Zeidner, M. (1995). Constructing personality and intelligence test instruments: Methods and issues. In D. Saklofske & M. Zeidner (Eds.), *International handbook of personality and intelligence* (pp. 475–503). New York: Plenum.

Neisser, U., Boodoo, G., Bouchard, T. J., Jr., Boykin, A. W., Brody, N., Ceci, S. J., et al. (1996). Intelligence: Knowns and unknowns. *American Psychologist, 51*, 77–101.

Nelson, H. E., & Willison, J. (1991). *National adult reading test* (2nd ed.). Windsor, UK: NFER Nelson.

Parker, J. D. A., Summerfeldt, L. J., Hogan, M. J., & Majeski, S. A. (2004). Emotional intelligence and academic success: Examining the transition from high school to university. *Personality and Individual Differences, 36*, 163–172.

Parker, J. D. A., Taylor, G. J., & Bagby, R. M. (1993a). Alexithymia and the processing of emotional stimuli: An experimental study. *New Trends in Experimental Clinical Psychiatry, 9*, 9–14.

Parker, J. D. A., Taylor, G. J., & Bagby, R. M. (1993b). Alexithymia and the recognition of facial expressions of emotion. *Psychotherapy and Psychosomatics, 59,* 197–202.

Parker, J. D. A., Taylor, G. J., & Bagby, R. M. (2001). The relationship between emotional intelligence and alexithymia. *Personality and Individual Differences, 30,* 107–115.

Paulhus, D. L. (1984). Two-component models of socially-desirable responding. *Journal of Personality and Social Psychology, 46,* 598–609.

Paunonen, S. V., & Ashton, M. C. (2001). Big five predictors of academic achievement. *Journal of Research in Personality, 35,* 78–90.

Petrides, K. V., & Furnham, A. (2000). On the dimensional structure of emotional intelligence. *Personality and Individual Differences, 29,* 313–320.

Petrides, K. V., & Furnham, A. (2001). Trait emotional intelligence: Psychometric investigation with reference to established trait taxonomies. *European Journal of Personality, 15,* 425–448.

Petrides, K. V., & Furnham, A. (2003). Trait emotional intelligence: Behavioural validation in two studies of emotion recognition and reactivity to mood induction. *European Journal of Personality, 17,* 39–57.

Plomin, R., & Petrill, S. (1997). Genetics and intelligence: What's new. *Intelligence, 24,* 53–77.

Roberts, R. D., Zeidner, M., & Matthews, G. (2001). Does emotional intelligence meet traditional standards for an intelligence? Some new data and conclusions. *Emotion, 1,* 196–231.

Saklofske, D. H., & Austin, E. J. (2004). [Emotional intelligence, personality and health behaviours in Canadian students]. Unpublished data.

Saklofske, D. H., Austin, E. J., & Minski, P. S. (2003). Factor structure and validity of a trait emotional intelligence measure. *Personality and Individual Differences, 34,* 707–721.

Schmidt, F. L., & Hunter, J. E. (1998). The validity and utility of selection methods in personnel psychology: Practical and theoretical implications of 85 years of research findings. *Psychological Bulletin, 124,* 262–274.

Schneider, R. J., Ackerman, P. L., & Kanfer, R. (1996). To "act wisely in human relations": Exploring the dimensions of social competence. *Personality and Individual Differences, 4,* 469–481.

Schutte, N. S., Malouff, J. M., Hall, L. E., Haggerty, D. J., Cooper, J. T., Golden, C. J., et al. (1998). Development and validation of a measure of emotional intelligence. *Personality and Individual Differences, 25,* 167–177.

Sternberg, R. J. (2003). Our research program validating the triarchic theory of successful intelligence: Reply to Gottfredson. *Intelligence, 31,* 399–413.

Sternberg, R. J., & Grigorenko, E. L. (2000). Practical intelligence and its developments. In R. Bar-On & J. D. A. Parker (Eds.), *The handbook of emotional intelligence: Theory, development, assessment, and application at home, school, and in the workplace* (pp. 215–243). San Francisco: Jossey-Bass.

Sternberg, R. J., Wagner, R. K., & Okagaki, L. (1993). Practical intelligence: The nature and role of tacit knowledge in work and at school. In J. M. Puckett & H. W. Reese (Eds.), *Mechanisms of everyday cognition* (pp. 205–227). Hillsdale, NJ: Lawrence Erlbaum.

Thorndike, E. L. (1904). *An introduction to the theory of mental and social measurements.* New York: Teachers College, Columbia University.

Thorndike, E. L. (1920). Intelligence and its use. *Harper's Magazine, 140,* 227–235.

Trinidad, D. R., & Johnson, C. A. (2002). The association between emotional intelligence and early adolescent tobacco and alcohol use. *Personality and Individual Differences, 32,* 95–105.

Van Rooy, D. L., & Viswesvaran, C. (2004). Emotional intelligence: A meta-analytic investigation of predictive validity and nomological net. *Journal of Vocational Behavior, 65,* 71–95.

Wagner, R. K., & Sternberg, R. J. (1985). Practical intelligence in real world pursuits. *Journal of Personality and Social Psychology, 49,* 436–458.

Young, A. W., Perrett, D., Calder, A. J., Sprengelmeyer, R., & Ekman, P. (2002). *Facial expressions of emotion—Stimuli and tests (FEEST).* Bury St. Edmunds, UK: Thames Valley Test Company.

Part II

Measures of Emotional Intelligence

7

Measures of Emotional Intelligence: Practice and Standards

Oliver Wilhelm

Humboldt University of Berlin, Germany

Summary

In this chapter emotional intelligence (EI) is discussed from a psychometric perspective with a focus on ability measures. Prior research is used to demonstrate that in EI research, like in other psychological fields, measures addressing the same construct but being based on performance or self-report show little to no convergence. It is argued that performance based measures are better suited as indicators of EI. The Mayer-Salovey-Caruso Emotional Intelligence Test (MSCEIT) as one such measure is presented and its validity is discussed. Whether or not ability measures of EI can be considered to be intelligence tasks is considered from several perspectives. This critique of EI measures tries to outline research questions warranting more attention in the future. The proposed recommendations include (a) trying to develop tasks with a strong background in Emotion Psychology, (b) using a broader variety of tasks in multivariate studies, and (c) using more appropriate criteria in validating EI.

7.1 INTRODUCTION

When new constructs of individual differences are introduced into psychology scientists are supposed and expected to react fairly skeptically, critically, and conservatively. When new measures are associated with new constructs things get even tougher. There might be two causes for these defensive routine reactions. First, viewed historically, lay persons did not contribute valuable constructs and measurement instruments to individual differences research, and although it was psychologists investigating the idea of an emotional intelligence (EI) first (Mayer, DiPaolo, & Salovey, 1990), it was popularized—even within psychology—by lay persons (Goleman, 1995, 1998). Second, psychologists feel the need to legitimize why they make such a big fuss about *their* measures of dispositions of persons (i.e., what makes their personality measures any different from the ad hoc questionnaires in Cosmopolitan magazine). These routine reactions make good sense in order to avoid false positives when it comes to establishing new constructs and new measures—on the other side there is the threat of being overly cautious and rejecting new ideas and new measures even though they might be worth being further investigated, developed, and used in practical settings. Being overly conservative might cause an unacceptable high rate of false negatives. Slightly simplifying historical events (see Matthews, Zeidner, & Roberts, 2002, for an adequate description) EI intruded the quiet waters of individual differences research, testing, and assessment in the early 1990s (Mayer et al., 1990; Mayer & Salovey, 1993; Salovey & Mayer, 1990) and sparked strong public interest (Goleman, 1995, 1998) in the construct and its measurement subsequently. This public interest can be considered to be indicative of the demand that is more or less satisfied through measurement instruments developed within the scientific community. Some researchers are investigating the construct to the best of their knowledge and abilities while others turn both thumbs down and direct the construct and associated measures to psychology's unmarked grave of poor ideas.

This chapter will first focus on an important distinction between various instruments proposed for the measurement of EI: the assessment of typical versus maximal behavior. A brief evaluation of EI measures of typical behavior is followed by a more extensive discussion of measures of maximal behavior. The latter begins with a description of the Mayer-Salovey-Caruso Emotional Intelligence Test (MSCEIT V.2; Mayer, Salovey, Caruso, and Sitarenios, 2002; Mayer, Salovey, Caruso, & Sitarenios, 2003), continues with requirements to classify a measure as an intelligence test, and concludes with a critique and some recommendations for future research.

7.2   TYPICAL AND MAXIMAL BEHAVIOR

A distinction between typical and maximal behavior was first drawn by Cronbach (1949). The distinction between measures of typical and maximal behavior is strongly associated with the content of a measure. Typical behavior is usually assessed with self-reports of preferences and valences. Sometimes life data are used to measure typical behavior. Maximal behavior is associated with measuring abilities, achievement, skills, and declarative knowledge. Situations in which maximal behavior is recorded are usually characterized by

(a) the assessed person being aware of the performance appraisal, (b) the assessed person being willing and able to demonstrate maximal performance, and (c) the standards for evaluating performance being adequate for assessment (Sackett, Zedeck, & Fogli, 1988).

The difference between performance based and self-report measures has several aspects. Performance based measurement procedures rely on maximal behavior, they are external appraisals of performances, they have minimal response bias, they are effortful and lengthy to administer and they are supposed to measure an "ability". On the other side, self-report based measures rely on reported typical behavior, they are internal appraisals of preferences, response bias can be substantial—specifically in high stakes testing, they are easy and quick to administer and they are supposed to measure personality-like constructs. Measures of typical behavior are used predominantly in personality psychology and measures of maximal behavior in individual differences in proficiencies, abilities, and achievement.

It is important to note that the distinction in typical and maximal performance leaves open how close to their maximal behavior people operate when behaving typically. Similarly, putting more effort into maximal behavior is not always possible or instrumental (Kahneman, 1973). Efforts to bridge the gap between constructs of maximal and typical behavior can be attempted from both sides. It is possible to assess personality constructs with measures of maximal behavior, and it is possible to assess abilities with measures of typical behavior (Riemann & Abels, 1994). There are several examples where the latter approach has been taken and it is possible to profit from considering these approaches when dealing with emotional intelligence.

First, in aging research there is a frequent use of self-reported memory complaints (Hertzog, Park, Morrell, & Martin, 2000) and these self-reports compete with objective measures of memory performance. Second, in clinical neuropsychology self-report measures have been developed that demonstrate a loss of insight into objectively measured performance decrements on measures of maximal behavior (McGlynn & Schacter, 1989; Seidenberg, Haltiner, Taylor, Hermann, & Wyler, 1994). Third, in cognitive psychology there are several self-report measures to assess attention slips and memory failures (Broadbent, Cooper, Fitzgerald, & Parkes, 1982; Herrmann, 1982; Reason, 1993) and these measures can be related to measures of maximal behavior of working memory, short-term memory, and attention (Oberauer, Süß, Schulze, Wilhelm, & Wittmann, 2000). Finally, in educational psychology, differential psychology, and social psychology there have been several self-report measures trying to capture typical academic and intellectual engagement (Cacioppo & Petty, 1982; Epstein, Pacini, Denes-Raj, & Heier, 1996; Goff & Ackerman, 1992; McCrae, 1990, 1996; Wilhelm, Schulze, Schmiedek, & Süß, 2003) and these questionnaires can be related to established intelligence tests.

In all of these areas researchers have not been successful in establishing substantial or high correlations. In fact, only for the last domain there are small to moderate relations between measures from both sides of the gap (i.e., between typical intellectual engagement and intelligence measures). It has been argued in the past that traditional measures of maximal behavior are usually administered in controlled settings and that the laboratory context of the measurement keeps these tests from being useful predictors of relevant criteria (Dennis, Sternberg, & Beatty, 2000). Indeed, if one thinks about everyday activities the number and duration of situations in which humans behave to the best of their abilities might be quite limited. However, when it comes to prediction the power of measures of maximal behavior is soundly established and of substantial magnitude (Ones, Viswesvaran, & Dilchert, 2004).

Available evidence suggests that for EI the pattern of results found for comparable constructs summarized above is replicated—disregarding problems on the conceptual and empirical end for measures of both typical and maximal behavior. The pattern of results suggests that despite a considerable conceptual overlap of what constitutes EI, in the context of typical and maximal behavior there is little to no relation between measures from both ends (see e.g., O'Connor & Little, 2003). These zero correlations leave little room for alternative interpretations other than that both forms of measures assess distinct characteristics. Attributing the absence of a correlation to the relevance of method artifacts is not satisfactory if the goal is to establish a new construct that is associated with new measures (see Chapter 9 by Pérez, Petrides, & Furnham). In terms of multitrait-multimethod validation substantial correlations across methods and within a trait (monotrait-heteromethod) are required, and if measures of typical and maximal behavior are considered as different methods, these correlations are not of sufficient magnitude. On the other side, heterotrait-monomethod correlations should be low or zero, and they are typically not in the case of constructs assessed with self-reported EI measures. Ability measures of EI correlate modestly and meaningfully with other abilities. Similar results have been found in the domain of social intelligence (see Chapter 10 by Weis & Süß).

If measures of typical and maximal EI are unrelated they should not have the same label. EI apparently is intended to be an ability construct. Hence, self-report measures of EI should not be given the label intelligence. Workaround labels like "trait EI" do not resolve the problem because "ability"-based EI is considered to be a trait too.

7.3   SELF-REPORTED AND SELF-RATED EMOTIONAL INTELLIGENCE

The attempts to measure emotional intelligence are clearly twofold (Mayer, Caruso, & Salovey, 2000). On the one side there are traditional self-reports of typical behavior, and on the other side there are measures conceptually related to traditional ability measures. The latter will be labelled "ability models" here although it is not yet established whether or not these measures unequivocally qualify as ability measures. This issue will be addressed below in Section 7.5. Given that both forms of EI measurement are basically unrelated and given that the term *intelligence* is associated with the use of measures provoking maximal behavior, self-report measures of EI should not include the term *intelligence*.

More profound than this terminological problem is the status of corresponding self-report measures. Such measures have been developed based on various definitions of what constitutes emotionally intelligent behavior. Bar-On (1997, 2000) distinguishes some 15 components of successful emotional functioning. These 15 components are organized within 5 broader interrelated dimensions including intrapersonal EI, interpersonal EI, adaptability EI, stress management EI, and general mood EI. The test corresponding to this model is called the BarOn Emotional Quotient Inventory EQ-i (Bar-On, 1997). However, the proposed as well as alternative structures could not be supported empirically (Palmer, Manocha, Gignac, & Stough, 2003; Petrides & Furnham, 2000, 2001). Similarly, the Schutte et al. Emotional Intelligence Inventory (Schutte et al., 1998) and its extensions (Saklofske, Austin, & Minski, 2003) has been extensively used but no final decision about its internal structure can be made at this time. Amongst other available measures the Trait Emotional Intelligence Questionnaire (TEIQue) seems to be the most promising candidate in terms of available evidence and effort in validating the measure (see Chapter 9 by Pérez et al.). The TEIQue is a measure with 144 items assigned to ten scales: adaptability, assertiveness, emotion perception, emotion expression, emotion regulation, empathy, low impulsivity, relationship skills, social competence, and stress management.

One problem with the TEIQue and similar measures is that the items are mostly taken from existent measures such as Emotional Empathy (Mehrabian & Epstein, 1970), the Toronto Alexithymia Scale (Bagby, Parker, & Taylor, 1994a, 1994), and other self-report measures of emotional intelligence. Technically then the TEIQue is mostly an assembly of existent items and the constructs assessed by the questionnaire therefore can hardly be new. A second problem for the TEIQue, as well as for similar measures, is that no satisfying measurement model on the item level for the total test or individual scales has been established so far. A third problem for all self-report measures of EI is that redundancy with competing and established constructs emerging from self-report measures has not been adequately assessed as yet. The last point is very important. Within individual differences research abundant efforts have been devoted to establish the dimensionality of traditional self-reports. The five-factor model (Costa & McCrae, 1992) is the most prominent of these efforts and within this model several lower-order facets have been proposed and investigated for each of the factors. Additionally, there is a broad variety of other self-report dimensions that have been investigated in the past. When new constructs based on self-reports are established, unequivocal evidence that individual differences on the new measure cannot be reduced on individual differences as assessed with available self-report measures is required. After controlling for a broad battery of competing self-report dimensions, measures of the new construct should still be meaningfully and substantially related with each other. Additionally, the new measure should incrementally predict interesting criteria over and above competing self-report dimensions and other established predictors. To date there seems to be no scientific evidence that support the unidimensionality, incremental validity, and utility of self-reported EI.

Therefore, the self-report measures for EI proposed so far should not be labelled EI. Available evidence does not prove that these measures assess something new. Considering these measures as indicators of a new construct—say emotional self-efficacy—requires more sophisticated embedding into related and established nomological nets.

Self-ratings of abilities fall in the "no-man's-land" between measures of typical and maximal behavior (Stankov, 1999). It is not unusual to find items that represent self-ratings of abilities in measures that are supposed to assess some self-report dimension. Items like "I am good in expressing my moods and feelings" are not very far from structured attempts to measure self-ratings of emotional intelligence. Such items do not properly reflect preferences for typically behaving emotionally intelligently but rather express insight into the relative standing on the ability to adequately express moods and feelings. For some abilities it is easier than for others to provide appropriate self-ratings. The more appropriate introspection and knowledge about abilities are, the higher the relation between the ability and self-ratings. It is important to note though that in traditional areas of intelligence the correlations between self-ratings and actual abilities usually are somewhere between .20 and .50 (Ackerman, Beier, & Bowen, 2002). Although there is some convergent and discriminant validity in the relations between various self-ratings of ability and knowledge and actual measurement of these traits, these numbers are surprisingly low because human lives are filled with feedback about how well they perform in a variety of fields. The correlation between self-rated EI and ability EI is not likely to be any higher. Based on correlations well below .50 it is certainly not appropriate to use self-ratings as proxies for ability EI. Additionally, it is unclear what self-ratings of emotional intelligence actually reflect. Preferences, valences, abilities, a bias to overestimate or underestimate actual abilities, and other personality constructs are the most salient candidates to account for self-ratings of abilities. In order to establish a new construct and new measurement procedures, self-ratings are of very limited use, both as criteria and predictors. Hence, the reminder of this chapter will be devoted to so-called ability EI.

7.4   THE MSCEIT: DESCRIPTION, STRUCTURE, AND VALIDITY

The Mayer-Salovey-Caruso Emotional Intelligence Test (MSCEIT) is a shortened and improved version of the Multi-Factor Emotional Intelligence Scales (MEIS; Mayer et al., 2002; Mayer, Caruso, & Salovey, 1999). The major goals in developing the MSCEIT were to abbreviate the very lengthy MEIS and to improve the psychometric properties of individual scales and items. The MSCEIT is highlighted in this discussion because it represents the most recent and up-to-date development of the research group surrounding Mayer, Salovey, and

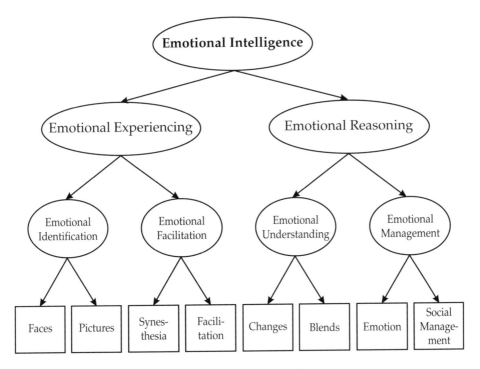

Figure 7.1   Subscales of the MSCEIT and its proposed structure.

Caruso, and it is the most widely used and best developed ability measure of emotional intelligence.

There are eight subscales of the MSCEIT (see the squares in Figure 7.1). These eight subscales combine in four pairs to represent four branches of emotional intelligence. The four branches combine to form two area-levels. These two area-levels in turn combine to make the MSCEIT total score. The MSCEIT thus represents a higher-order model of emotional intelligence. There are three levels in the model that are assigned ability status. Emotional intelligence at the top of the hierarchy, the two area-level scores of emotional experiencing and emotional reasoning, and the four branch-level scores of perceiving emotions, using emotions, understanding emotions, and managing emotions. Figure 7.1 additionally represents a fourth level—the specific tests as indicators of the MSCEIT.

Interpretation of test results is proposed down to the branch-level scores and can include interpretation of task-level scores in rare individual cases. Following the higher-order model there is a total of seven abilities that are measured by the MSCEIT. The interpretation of the four branches on the lowest level is:

Perceiving emotions: Participants with high scores are able to accurately identify and recognize their own and others' emotions. These participants are also able to express feelings accurately and they are sensitive to faked and false emotional expression.

Using emotions: Participants with high scores are able to generate emotions to support problem solving. Those participants are also able to direct their attention to relevant changes, take several perspectives in considering emotions, and facilitate thinking by using different kinds of moods.

Understanding emotions: Participants with high scores understand causes and changes of emotions, both abstractly and in terms of relations. Those participants are also able to adequately recognize similarities amongst emotions of varying intensities and to reason about the dynamics of feelings in an interpersonal context.

Managing emotions: Participants with high values are successful in using their emotional awareness in drawing optimal decisions while assigning adequate importance to their emotions. Those participants manage to stay open to feelings, to engage and disengage when necessary and appropriate, and they are good in meta-evaluating their moods in terms of typicality, acceptability, and relevance.

The first two of these abilities can be aggregated into the ability of emotional experiencing. This ability is supposed to reflect accurately perceiving, responding to, and manipulating emotional information. The second pair of abilities combines to form emotional reasoning. This ability is expected to reflect understanding and managing emotions and how accurately a person understands the meaning of emotions and how those emotions can be managed in oneself and in relevant others.

On top of the proposed hierarchy is general emotional intelligence (Mayer & Salovey, 1997; Mayer, Salovey, & Caruso, 2000). It is computed as the mean of emotional experiencing and emotional reasoning. It is interpreted as the ability to perceive emotions, to use emotions so as to assist thought, to understand emotions, and to successfully regulate emotions.

There are many good descriptions of the tasks included in the MSCEIT (Mayer et al., 2002) and its predecessor—the MEIS (see also Chapter 2 by Neubauer & Freudenthaler). The scoring of the MSCEIT follows the same scheme for all subtests. The frequency distribution of the response options for a subscale is used to weight the response of an individual on that test. For example, in the "Faces" task individuals rate how much happiness a photograph of a face expresses and select one of the five options, ranging from no happiness to extreme happiness. Assume that for a certain photograph the five options in ascending order of happiness are endorsed by 10%, 20%, 40%, 20%, and 10% of participants, respectively. An individual endorsing response option 3 would thus be credited with a score of .40 while an individual endorsing response option 5 would only be credited with a score of .10. The same procedure is repeated for all responses and the scores on individual items of a subtest are averaged to express performance for this subtest. The rationale for such a scoring procedure is that for many important domains of human abilities and knowledge no universally accepted unequivocal standards of correctness are available (see Chapter 8 by Legree, Psotka, Tremble, & Bourne). Consensus-based scoring is widely and successfully used in Situational Judgment Tests (McDaniel, Morgeson, Finnegan, Campion, & Braverman, 2001) and can be justified in domains of tacit or procedural knowledge. For the MSCEIT an empirical comparison between scores computed by application of a general consensus method—based on participants from the standardization group—and an expert consensus method—based on 21 experts from the International Society for Research on Emotions—reveals very high correlations of scores. The validity of the MEIS and the MSCEIT is under intense investigation and firm conclusions would certainly be premature. Rather than exhaustively presenting available evidence, the focus here will be on an eclectic summary of available prototypic investigations; specific attention will be devoted to (a) the MSCEIT as the momentary state of the art measure of EI and (b) some desiderata and standards for future research.

The structure of the MSCEIT in the data collected so far seems by and large to be robust. However, a structural model assuming four correlated factors can only be estimated if the covariance between the Identification and Facilitation factors and the covariance between the Understanding and Management factors are constrained to be equal to one another (Mayer et al., 2003). In exploratory factor analysis the proposed distinctions between factors are supported mostly. However, the loadings of tasks vary widely in both confirmatory and exploratory factor analysis, implying that factors are dominated by individual tasks. For example, the task "Synesthesia" has a much higher loading on the Facilitation factor than the second task "Facilitation" that is assigned to this factor. Consequently, the factors lack broadness in content. Content validity of the MSCEIT has not been demonstrated thoroughly so far. There is also a problematic mismatch between factor labels and tasks of the MSCEIT. For example, Branch 1 is labelled by the test authors "Perception and Expression of Emotion" but seemingly only perception of emotion is assessed.

Predictive validity of the MSCEIT has been assessed by correlating the scores with a variety of criteria. Correlations with fluid intelligence are generally small and correlations of some tasks with crystallized intelligence are substantially higher. MacCann, Roberts, Matthews, and Zeidner (2004) report correlations of individual EI tasks with broad visualization (Gv) tasks in the range of .20. A recent meta-analysis provides evidence that the MEIS—unlike self-report measures of EI—is associated with general mental ability ($\rho = .33$; $SD\rho = .093$) (Van Rooy & Viswesvaran, 2004). In various samples correlations between the MSCEIT and self-reports of empathy were found ranging from .17 to .52. Correlations with other self-report scales are mostly small although significant in several cases. Ciarrochi, Chan, and Caputi (2000) report a correlation of .31 with self-esteem. Correlations with Life Satisfaction vary widely but coefficients for larger studies are around .20 (Mayer et al., 2002). Emotional intelligence is substantially negatively associated with peer-nominated aggression and positively associated with prosocial behavior (Mayer et al., 2002). EI in general and Emotional Experiencing in particular are associated negatively with illegal drug use, alcohol use, and deviant behavior and these correlations are due to the male subgroup exclusively (Brackett, Mayer, & Warner, 2004). Correlations between the four branches and the total score of the MSCEIT and self-report measures of EI do not exceed .28 and are mostly substantially smaller (Brackett & Mayer, 2003). In this study the MSCEIT was predictive of social deviance, even after controlling for the Big-five and verbal SAT scores. Despite this evidence a variety of controversies and problems remain and these issues will be discussed in the following sections.

7.5   IS "ABILITY" EI AN INTELLIGENCE?

The term *intelligence* in the construct label EI has caused considerable discussion. What are the reasons to subsume a new construct under the rubric of intelligence? First, measuring intelligence is a shortcut for success in applied settings (Ones et al., 2004). Intelligence is the single best predictor psychology has invented. Intelligence tests are widely used and integrating a new construct into such a context might facilitate acquiring some of the fame and credibility of an established construct.

Besides such marketing considerations it can also be argued that measures of emotional intelligence require effortful information processing and people are more or less apt at this processing. If information processing is less effortful *ceteris paribus* there will be poorer performance. The Levels of Emotional Awareness Scale (LEAS; Lane, Quinlan, Schwartz, Walker, & Zeitlin, 1990) is a cognitive-developmental measure of emotion that distinguishes between five levels of increasing complexity, thus distinguishing between easier and more sophisticated information processing. The five levels of complexity are bodily sensations, action tendencies, single emotions, blends of emotions, and combinations of blends (Lane & Schwartz, 1987). Participants are presented with twenty vignettes and write their responses to the two questions "How would you feel?" and "How would the other person feel?". The LEAS has been carefully developed and validated (Ciarrochi, Scott, Deane, & Heaven, 2003; Lane et al., 1998) and—due to its explicit consideration of information processing—represents an interesting and possibly better way of assessing emotional intelligence than measures relying on consensus or expert scoring. At present, the notion of information processing is not explicitly discussed for the MSCEIT. Developing alternative and additional measures that apply the model of five levels of emotional complexity to assess the generality of emotional awareness would be interesting. The role of aspects of information processing is even more strongly pronounced in several experimental measures of emotion like the Emotional Stroop Test for example (Coffey, Berenbaum, & Kerns, 2003; Matthews et al., 2002). It is presently unclear, however, how these measures of emotional information processing relate to other ability measures of emotional intelligence and how coherent such measures are. A third reason to label EI an intelligence might be that unlike self-report measures, EI measures, like other ability measures, can be scored by agreement with some external correctness standard (Guttman, 1965). Such a standard usually classifies individual responses as right or wrong. Sometimes partial credit is given introducing degrees of correctness into assessment. These correctness standards apply to ability tests only. In most attitude measures, for example, participants are asked to provide us with information about how favorable their evaluation of some object is. In assessing personality traits participants are usually asked to provide us with information about how typical a behavior, thought, and the like is for them. In ability tests responses are compared to some explicit rule and classified as more or less correct. There are various evaluation standards that can be used in classifying response behavior in ability tests (Nevo, 1993). Performance can be assessed as number of correct responses, as latency per correct response, as variety of responses generated, or as agreement with authority. In assessing emotional intelligence the standards that have been used predominantly so far in assessing response behavior of an individual are target scoring, general consensus scoring, and expert consensus scoring—all varieties of the "authority" type of performance assessment. The response norms used in EI measures can be conceptualized as correctness standards. Although not desirable, it is common that various measures of a specific construct apply a single correctness standard. For example, reasoning tasks usually apply logical standards, mental speed tasks apply standards of work rate, and measures of emotional and practical intelligence most frequently apply consensus standards.

A fourth reason that is put forward in supporting a classification of EI measures as intelligence tasks is their relation with other intelligence measures. Starting from the positive manifold found amongst tests classified as intelligence measures, it is argued that if measures of EI represent an intelligence they must be correlated with other measures of intelligence. However, there are other indicators associated with intelligence that scientists would not be willing to classify as intelligence tests. For example, parents' education might be correlated with offspring intelligence and it would be very unusual to use parental education as an indicator of offspring intelligence. From a perspective endorsing a general factor and a positive manifold emanating from it the correlation between any two established intelligence tests is primarily or exclusively a function of their correlation with the general factor. Still, positive manifold is not itself the cause of observed relations amongst intelligence measures. Intelligence measures are correlated positively with each other because they tap the same underlying abilities. It has been argued repeatedly that measures of emotional intelligence should be correlated with general intelligence (Mayer, Salovey, Caruso, & Sitarenios, 2001; Roberts, Zeidner, & Matthews, 2001; Zeidner, Matthews, & Roberts, 2001). The reason such a correlation is expected is that it is a well replicated finding that there is a positive manifold between all measures that have been labelled intelligence tests. Hence, if emotional intelligence qualifies as an aspect of general intelligence there should be a positive correlation between indicators of emotional and "traditional" intelligence.

There are extensions and elaborations of this argument that go beyond a mere statistical necessity. Specific measures of emotional intelligence were expected and found to be correlated with some aspects of intelligence but not others (MacCann et al., 2004). Psychologically, there is no problem in specific measures of emotional intelligence being unrelated with specific or general aspects of intelligence. If there is no overlap in the causes of individual differences there is no need that two measures be correlated. In most cases, however, there will be some overlap. For example, some reasoning ability is involved in measures that are subsumed under the "Understanding" branch of the MSCEIT. Similarly, some measures do have demands on visual processing and hence they might be related to broad visualization. Other measures of emotional intelligence require basic knowledge and hence they might be associated with crystallized intelligence. On the other side, some of the relations that have been found might represent artifacts. If, for example, a measure of emotional intelligence heavily relies on extensive verbal descriptions in the vignette, reading comprehension might be a necessary but not sufficient condition to actually get to the part dealing with the emotional content of an item. As a result, there might be an artifactual relation between performance on such an EI measure and reading comprehension, verbal intelligence or even general intelligence.

On the other hand, it has been argued that it supports the validity of performance measures of EI if they are unrelated to personality scales. Although high correlations would certainly be a cause for concern, moderate correlations could very well be meaningful. If, for example, openness to aesthetics, a facet of openness to new experiences, is correlated with performance on the "Designs" task from the MSCEIT, such a relationship could reflect aesthetic engagement of participants as expressed in their preference for behaviors that include an openness towards aesthetics. By mere exposition time, or by intellectual elaboration, persons with high openness for aesthetics might be better at performing on tasks like "Designs" because they are more familiar with the stimuli and have a more elaborated knowledge base of what various designs could actually express. There are other similar personality constructs that could be meaningfully correlated with performance on measures of emotional intelligence. Thus, ability models of emotional intelligence cannot simply be validated convergently by showing positive relationships with other ability measures and discriminantly by showing zero relationships with personality measures. What constitutes convergent and discriminant evidence is a psychological question in need of substantiation in every case.

The decision of whether or not tasks such as the ones from the MSCEIT should be labelled as intelligence tests has several conceptual aspects. Intelligence itself is so imprecisely defined that it is impossible to draw a clear line that allows for assigning the status of an intelligence test or withdrawing such a status. Assigning the status of cognitive ability measures to tasks as the ones used in the MSCEIT seems to be an option. A cognitive ability measure should certainly possess some features. For example, performance on a measure of cognitive ability should decrease if less time is available for working on the problems. Performance on cognitive ability measures—except measures of knowledge—should *ceteris paribus* also decrease if less effortful processing is warranted from participants; that is, if participants are asked to perform on a typical level performance should be worse than when they are asked to perform at a maximal level. Similarly, instructions to fake good performance (i.e., to demonstrate better performance) will usually not work with an ability measure. If participants get a chance to work a second time on the same problems of a traditional intelligence test, they will improve substantially. A profound understanding of the ability involved in a cognitive ability measure implies to have some good ideas about how to manipulate the difficulty of problems. These and similar possibilities have not been thoroughly tested with measures of EI so far. With respect to retesting, Caruso, Mayer, and Salovey (2002) report a decrease of performance in the retest for nine of the twelve measures of the MEIS, the remaining three tests showing no change in performance level. Currently available evidence does not allow firm conclusions about whether or not EI measures from ability models qualify as cognitive ability measures.

7.6   CRITIQUE AND RECOMMENDATIONS

To be totally explicit, past experience in individual differences research, current evidence in research on EI, and the hope for a prosperous future for the construct all indicate that EI should not be investigated on the level of self-reports or self-ratings. Simply annotating the term *emotional intelligence* with some arbitrary addition will not do the job of clearly expressing that self-reported and performance appraised measures labelled emotional intelligence are conceptually fundamentally different and empirically by and large independent from each other. Furthermore, self-report measures are easy to develop and collect. Hence, there are many self-report measures and there is a large body of research exploring as well as testing the structure of individual differences on such self-reports. Every attempt to establish a new construct that is assessed solely or exclusively by relying on self-reports must establish the distinctiveness of these measures from established measures. With a broadly defined construct like emotional intelligence it will also be necessary to investigate the internal structure of the proposed indicators and to thoroughly check whether or not there is enough coherence amongst the various indicators to be summarized under one label. A collection of indicators from which one best fits to self-reported extraversion and another one to self-reported agreeableness is not satisfying. It is desirable to demonstrate at least some level of independence from the methods used for investigation. For example, a relation between corresponding life-data and self-report data is desirable. Substantial convergence of self-reports and peer-reports on the same participants is another example of demonstrating some method independent trait variance. Finally, in order to be worth pursuing it is eventually necessary that the new measure demonstrates some incremental validity of non-trivial magnitude. All of these steps are essential in establishing a construct of EI conceptualized as typical behavior. It would remain, however, that a construct of this sort should be labelled differently from the construct assessed by ability measures of EI. A term like *typical emotional engagement* might be a good label for such a prospective and elusive construct.

On the ability side the MEIS and the MSCEIT represent the broadest assessment of EI. The MEIS and the MSCEIT are the EI measures that have been subject to most of the validation efforts undertaken so far and they have gained the largest proportion of attention in research and application. The critique and recommended research strategy presented below thus focuses on the MEIS and the MSCEIT—alternative measures should meet a similar set of requirements and challenges.

7.6.1   Scoring

For EI as an ability it is theoretically assumed that all participants from the intended application population possess this ability in varying degrees, and that this ability has some stability over time. The required psychometric properties of measurement instruments for EI should follow established standards. In proceeding through these psychometric requirements it is important to bear in mind that the psychometric evaluation of a measurement instrument is usually started after the assignment of numbers to specific responses. The process of this assignment—the scoring of a measure—is in need of justification itself (see Chapter 8 by Legree et al., for a detailed description of consensus based scoring). Consensus based scoring is one procedure used to assign numbers to responses. It can be defended for use with measures assessing tacit or procedural knowledge (Chapter 8 by Legree et al.), but it does not seem as if proponents of EI have adopted the idea that EI assesses such implicit knowledge. Interestingly, consensus based scoring is used in two other domains of psychology. Situational Judgment Tests (SJT) describe a methodology to assess job relevant implicit knowledge using consensus based scoring (McDaniel et al., 2001; McDaniel & Nguyen, 2001) and Practical Intelligence (PI) is a recently proposed highly controversial construct (Gottfredson, 2003; Sternberg, 2003) that is intended to measure success in real-life contexts (Wagner, 1987). A critical question prevalent in research on PI and SJT is whether or not PI can be assessed without relying on tests using consensus based scoring. The same question can be asked for EI: is there a coherent construct of EI and does the collected evidence on the validity of the construct and associated measures transfer to other measures of EI that do not rely on consensus based scoring? There is currently not sufficient evidence to answer this question.

A more technical but possibly critical difficulty is that various procedures of consensus based scoring do not sufficiently converge (MacCann et al., 2004). The question thus arises, which scoring procedure is the most appropriate one. Relying on psychometric results to pick the procedure that produces the most reliable or consistent scores is not an adequate solution. The procedure selected to score ability measures must be rationally appropriate too. The procedures compared by MacCann et al. are not very different on the rational end. There are thus competing and not converging scoring procedures for tests like the MEIS and the MSCEIT. Satisfactory convergence between expert and consensus scoring is not yet sufficient to justify the MSCEIT scoring.

7.6.2   Available Validity Studies

Within the domain of psychometric measures, be they self-report or ability measures, correlational evidence can be pretty hard to assess. This is mostly due to a somehow arbitrary interpretation of associations. This problem is not new. Whenever a new intelligence test is constructed it is validated by correlating it with established measures. It is usually assumed that the correlations should be high but not perfect. If the correlations were perfect, there would be no point in establishing a new measure. If the correlation is high, there is some room for the new measure to be better than existent measures. However, high but not perfect correlations in no way imply that scenario. It could as well be the case that the new measure is psychometrically deficient and if it would be better the correlations with existent measures would be perfect. The situation is similar with measures of EI. If, for example, it is found that a new self-report measure of EI is correlated .70 with a measure of happiness and −.50 with a measure of neuroticism, is this indicating the validity of the measure? It could be argued that this provides strong evidence for the convergent validity of the self-reported EI questionnaire. However, it could also be argued that this result leaves little to no place for uniqueness of measures of self-reported EI and that apparently the construct is completely redundant with established constructs. Similarly, small to moderate correlations between a measure of emotional abilities and an established ability measure, say verbal intelligence, can be said to demonstrate discriminant validity—the EI measure is likely to measure something not captured by verbal intelligence measures. On the other hand, it could be argued that the small to medium correlation expresses an artifact of the test medium and that participants with high verbal intelligence are advantaged when taking measures of EI. Finally, it can be argued that the small correlation expresses some shared variance that can be attributed to general intelligence. Given that there are several explanations for the same result, the interpretation is necessarily arbitrary. If the truth be told: this scenario is not very different from the situation that exists for any specific intelligence test and its relations with other established ability measures. However, for most decent intelligence measures there is additional and replicated evidence demonstrating their embeddedness in a nomological net, their incremental utility in practical settings, their theoretically predicted redundancy with other, similar and dissimilar forms of tests, and much more. Although the majority of the studies on traditional intelligence tests are merely conceptual replications of each other there are many studies left that exclude alternative explanations for correlative results, thereby strengthening the interpretation and validity of the results.

7.6.3 Unavailable Validity Studies

Although there is a range of validity evidence that has been collected so far there is a surprising gap when it comes to exploring the relationship between the MEIS or the MSCEIT and related tasks. For example, the work on EI has rarely used indicators of performance measures of social intelligence as correlates. Similarly, there has been little research including experimental paradigms, for example, standard procedures used in face recognition research or the Emotional Stroop task. Closely related approaches to the investigation of individual differences in emotion related abilities—like the LEAS described above—have also been rarely used as correlates. An eclectic effort including many more than the standard MSCEIT tasks and representing a much broader variety of emotional tasks, including distinct scoring procedures, would provide us with a lot of invaluable information for further development of the investigated fields. With respect to construct validity it is crucial to learn more about how emotional intelligence is embedded in the nomological net of related constructs and measures. Besides established human cognitive ability constructs (Carroll, 1993) it is also relevant to discuss EI and its relation to social intelligence, empathic accuracy, PI, interpersonal abilities, intrapersonal abilities, and emotional awareness. Unfortunately, most of the above mentioned constructs are of dubious value.

7.6.4 Alternative Models

Not enough emphasis is given to possible alternative models of the data. Figure 7.2 shows just three of such alternative models in Panels A, B, and C (see Schulze, 2005, for a discussion of various model architectures).

The models in Figure 7.2 describe structures that are pretty similar to the one adopted in the MSCEIT. However, there are also important discrepancies. Some of the models do without a general factor (see Panels A and B). In other words, assuming the models provide a decent fit to empirical data, adequate explanations of the covariances between tasks can be established without postulating something like a general emotional intelligence factor. The structure of individual differences on available EI measures is not well established. Eclectic research applying a great bandwidth of available measures is warranted and necessary in order to compare various structural models of emotional intelligence with each other.

Continuing to stress this point the number of abilities that are supposed to be assessed with the MSCEIT is very high. Based on only eight tasks, participants receive feedback on seven abilities. This is the case because the scores of each test are used three times. The first time in computing values for the four branches, the second time when these four branches are combined into the two area scores, and the third time when the two area scores are combined into the MSCEIT total value. Doing poorly on a specific task will thus hurt you three times. The redundancy of this use of information is not sufficiently explicated to the participants and implications from the higher-order structure

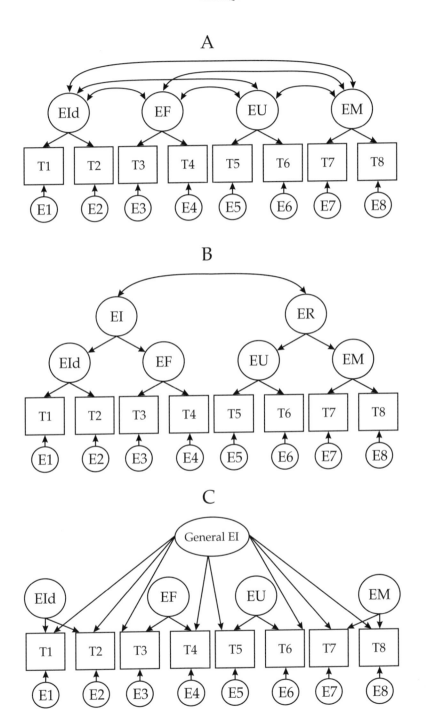

Figure 7.2   Alternative models for the MSCEIT.

of the model supposedly underlying the MSCEIT are not sufficiently considered. In order to avoid repeatedly analyzing the same information for the same data the variance of the indicators could be fractionated into variance due to general EI and lower-order factors.

7.6.5   Number of Tasks per Factor and Generality of Factors

In the MSCEIT, not enough tasks are used to assess the branches of emotional intelligence. For the branch level scores only two task types are used per ability. The interpretation of the factors goes far beyond the contents actually included in the test. A much broader variety of task types should be used before postulating abilities. For example, there are decades of research demonstrating over and over again that matrices tasks are decent measures of a construct labelled fluid intelligence. There is thus abundant evidence to use the task as an indicator of such a construct. Of course, it is a characteristic of good psychological measurement to rely on more than a single task type. On the other hand, each indicator used should qualify as a decent measure of the construct. It can easily be tested whether or not a specific indicator is fitting within a measurement model of an ability. What is required are four or more indicators that are all purported to measure the same ability. With only three indicators a measurement model would be just identified—no adequate test of such a model would thus be possible. With only two tasks it is necessary to extend the model to include additional factors and variables in order to be meaningful. The status of the four branches of the MSCEIT cannot be tested adequately. More tasks for each of the proposed constructs are required.

7.6.6   Alternative Tasks (Number and Variety)

There is considerable arbitrariness when deriving a task from a construct description. Technically, the definitions of most individual differences constructs allow for an unlimited number of tasks to be derived from the construct description. Much specificity of ability indicators is considered to be irrelevant in measuring the ability we are interested in. The person administrating the test, the test medium, the specific stimuli used in a measure (for example, which faces are displayed in the Faces task) are all considered to be irrelevant for the measured construct. Variations in the task instructions and in the response scales used should have no substantial influence on what is measured with a specific test. The description of EI abilities allows for many more variations. For example, the perception of emotions can be assessed with music, prose, with videos of facial expression, with artificial stimuli, and so forth. Without variations in the form of measurement care must be taken to not overgeneralize the results from tests. For the MEIS and the MSCEIT substantially more and more diverse indicators are warranted before concluding that the four branch model is a sufficient and appropriate model of EI. In other words, the MSCEIT provides a very general interpretation of emotional intelligence but uses very specific tasks.

7.6.7   Test Construction

Test construction should proceed as deductive derivation from theory whenever possible. The measurement intention for EI measures should be inspired by experimental and neuropsychological research whenever possible. A critical and important issue is to create and maintain a strong relationship between psychometric research on measures for individual differences and general theories of emotion. The use of a measure should be justified by what it measures. After a precise description of the measurement intention and operationalization psychometric criteria are important but the test content is crucial. Although the tasks of the MEIS and the MSCEIT seem to be good indicators for the proposed branches little is known about alternatives and—for the tests themselves—nothing about the emotion background. It is desirable to create and maintain stronger links between individual indicators and the constructs they are supposed to measure.

7.7   CONCLUSIONS

Despite the need to consider the points raised above it is important to note that the MSCEIT represents the most ambitious and, to date, most appropriate approach to the broad assessment of emotion related capabilities. There are many challenges, both methodologically and psychologically. While the field is at an early stage in debating the validity and utility of the concept and proposed measures it is necessary to be very careful in applications of the measures proposed so far. Taken together, the proponents of performance based measures of EI have done a decent job. While it is too early for reification of a simple model the field has made considerable progress in the last decade. Besides the adverse impacts of premature use of measures and inflation of the concept as a whole, public attention to EI has had a major beneficial effect too: it has directed scientific efforts into an important and neglected area of human abilities.

On the other side, the enthusiastic uptake of the initial proposals of the construct EI has blurred sight for the state-of-the-art procedures used when investigating new ideas. One threatening consequence from this enthusiasm is that measures and interventions based on EI are underway and used in practice before crucial questions have been answered empirically. In fact, we might not even be able to spell out the right questions yet.

To conclude optimistically with some research prospects, one promising approach that is motivated and inspired by neuropsychological and experimental work on face recognition will be highlighted. Good face perception and face recognition allow humans to infer information about age, sex, mood, and identity of a person. Consequently, face recognition can be considered to be a limiting factor for some aspects of EI. Individual differences for these aspects of EI can thus be attributed to individual differences in face recognition. There is decent physiological evidence that there are two distinct components of face recognition. The first of these components has to do with the encoding of faces. Successful and unsuccessful learning of unfamiliar faces are associated with neurophysiological differences (Schweinberger, Pfütze, & Sommer, 1995; Sommer, Komoss, & Schweinberger, 1997). The second component has to do with the retrieval of familiar and unfamiliar faces. The so-called early repetition effect is different for personally familiar persons, famous persons and celebrities, and unfamiliar persons (Herzmann, Schweinberger, Sommer, & Jentzsch, 2004). The promise of this and similar research is that there is convincing evidence for individual differences that can be attributed to the encoding and retrieval of faces (Pfütze, Sommer, & Schweinberger, 2002). It is thought provoking to think about options in this area. How about developing measures that assess perception and recognition of changes in facial expression, or measures that address just noticeable differences in facial expression?

REFERENCES

Ackerman, P. L., Beier, M. E., & Bowen, K. R. (2002). What we really know about our abilities and our knowledge. *Personality and Individual Differences, 33,* 587–605.

Bagby, R. M., Parker, J. D. A., & Taylor, G. J. (1994a). The Twenty-Item Toronto Alexithymia Scale–II: Convergent, discriminant, and concurrent validity. *Journal of Psychosomatic Research, 38,* 33–40.

Bagby, R. M., Parker, J. D. A., & Taylor, G. J. (1994b). The Twenty-Item Toronto Alexithymia Scale–I: Item selection and cross-validation of the factor structure. *Journal of Psychosomatic Research, 38,* 23–32.

Bar-On, R. (1997). *BarOn Emotional Quotient Inventory (EQ–i): Technical manual.* Toronto, Canada: Multi-Health Systems.

Bar-On, R. (2000). Emotional and social intelligence: Insights from the emotional quotient inventory. In R. Bar-On & J. D. A. Parker (Eds.), *The handbook of emotional intelligence: Theory, development, assessment, and application at home, school, and in the workplace* (pp. 363–388). San Francisco, CA: Jossey-Bass.

Brackett, M. A., & Mayer, J. D. (2003). Convergent, discriminant, and incremental validity of competing measures of emotional intelligence. *Personality and Social Psychology Bulletin, 29,* 1147–1158.

Brackett, M. A., Mayer, J. D., & Warner, R. M. (2004). Emotional intelligence and its relation to everyday behaviour. *Personality and Individual Differences, 36,* 1387–1402.

Broadbent, D. E., Cooper, P. J., Fitzgerald, P. F., & Parkes, K. R. (1982). The Cognitive Failures Questionnaire (CFQ) and its correlates. *British Journal of Clinical Psychology, 21,* 1–16.

Cacioppo, J. T., & Petty, R. E. (1982). The need for cognition. *Journal of Personality and Social Psychology, 42,* 116–131.

Carroll, J. B. (1993). *Human cognitive abilities: A survey of factor-analytic studies.* New York: Cambridge University Press.

Caruso, D. R., Mayer, J. D., & Salovey, P. (2002). Relation of an ability measure of emotional intelligence to personality. *Journal of Personality Assessment, 79*, 306–320.

Ciarrochi, J., Chan, A., & Caputi, P. (2000). A critical evaluation of the emotional intelligence construct. *Personality and Individual Differences, 28*, 539–561.

Ciarrochi, J., Scott, G., Deane, F. P., & Heaven, P. C. L. (2003). Relations between social and emotional competence and mental health: a construct validation study. *Personality and Individual Differences, 35*, 1947–1963.

Coffey, E., Berenbaum, H., & Kerns, J. G. (2003). The dimensions of emotional intelligence, alexithymia, and mood awareness: Associations with personality and performance on an emotional stroop task. *Cognition & Emotion, 17*, 671–679.

Costa, P. T., Jr., & McCrae, R. R. (1992). *Revised NEO personality and five factor inventory professional manual*. Odessa, FL: Psychological Assessment Resources.

Cronbach, L. J. (1949). *Essentials of psychological testing*. New York: Harper & Row.

Dennis, M. J., Sternberg, R. J., & Beatty, P. (2000). The construction of "user-friendly" tests of cognitive functioning: A synthesis of maximal– and typical–performance measurement philosophies. *Intelligence, 28*, 193–211.

Epstein, S., Pacini, R., Denes-Raj, V., & Heier, H. (1996). Individual differences in intuitive–experiential and analytical–rational thinking styles. *Journal of Personality and Social Psychology, 71*, 390–405.

Goff, M., & Ackerman, P. L. (1992). Personality–intelligence relations: Assessment of typical intellectual engagement. *Journal of Educational Psychology, 84*, 537–552.

Goleman, D. (1995). *Emotional intelligence: Why it can matter more than IQ*. New York: Bantam Books.

Goleman, D. (1998). *Working with emotional intelligence*. New York: Bantam.

Gottfredson, L. S. (2003). Dissecting practical intelligence theory: Its claims and evidence. *Intelligence, 31*, 343–397.

Guttman, L. (1965). A faceted definition of intelligence. *Scripta Hierosolymitana, 14*, 166–181.

Herrmann, D. J. (1982). Know thy memory: The use of questionnaires to assess and study memory. *Psychological Bulletin, 92*, 434–452.

Hertzog, C., Park, D. C., Morrell, R. W., & Martin, M. (2000). Ask and ye shall receive: Behavioral specificity in the accuracy of subjective memory complaints. *Applied Cognitive Psychology, 14*, 257–275.

Herzmann, G., Schweinberger, S. R., Sommer, W., & Jentzsch, I. (2004). What's special about personally familiar faces? A multimodal approach. *Psychophysiology, 41*, 688–701.

Kahneman, D. (1973). *Attention and effort*. Hillsdale, NJ: Prentice-Hall.

Lane, R., Quinlan, D., Schwartz, G. E., Walker, P., & Zeitlin, S. (1990). The levels of emotional awareness scale: A cognitive–developmental measure of emotion. *Journal of Personality Assessment, 55*, 124–134.

Lane, R., Reiman, E., Axelrod, B., Yun, L.-S., Holmes, A. H., & Schwartz, G. E. (1998). Neural correlates of levels of emotional awareness: Evidence of an interaction between emotion and attention in the anterior cingulate cortex. *Journal of Cognitive Neuroscience, 10*, 225–235.

Lane, R., & Schwartz, G. E. (1987). Levels of emotional awareness: A cognitive-developmental theory and its application to psychopathology. *American Journal of Psychiatry, 144*, 133–143.

MacCann, C., Roberts, R. D., Matthews, G., & Zeidner, M. (2004). Consensus scoring and empirical option weighting of performance–based emotional intelligence (EI) tests. *Personality and Individual Differences, 36*, 645–662.

Matthews, G., Zeidner, M., & Roberts, R. D. (2002). *Emotional intelligence: Science and myth*. Cambridge, MA: MIT Press.

Mayer, J. D., Caruso, D. R., & Salovey, P. (1999). Emotional intelligence meets traditional standards for an intelligence. *Intelligence, 27*, 267–298.

Mayer, J. D., Caruso, D. R., & Salovey, P. (2000). Selecting a measure of emotional intelligence: The case for ability testing. In R. Bar-On & J. D. A. Parker (Eds.), *The handbook of emotional intelligence: Theory, development, assessment, and application at home, school, and in the workplace* (pp. 320–342). San Francisco: Jossey-Bass.

Mayer, J. D., DiPaolo, M., & Salovey, P. (1990). Perceiving affective content in ambiguous visual stimuli: A component of emotional intelligence. *Journal of Personality Assessment, 54*, 772–781.

Mayer, J. D., & Salovey, P. (1993). The intelligence of emotional intelligence. *Intelligence, 17*, 433–442.

Mayer, J. D., & Salovey, P. (1997). What is emotional intelligence? In P. Salovey & D. J. Sluyter (Eds.), *Emotional development and emotional intelligence: Educational implications* (pp. 3–31). New York: Basic Books.

Mayer, J. D., Salovey, P., & Caruso, D. R. (2000). Models of emotional intelligence. In R. J. Sternberg (Ed.), *The handbook of intelligence* (pp. 396–420). New York: Cambridge University Press.

Mayer, J. D., Salovey, P., & Caruso, D. R. (2002). *The Mayer, Salovey, and Caruso Emotional Intelligence Test: Technical manual*. Toronto: Multi-Health Systems.

Mayer, J. D., Salovey, P., Caruso, D. R., & Sitarenios, G. (2001). Emotional intelligence as a standard intelligence. *Emotion, 1*, 232–242.

Mayer, J. D., Salovey, P., Caruso, D. R., & Sitarenios, G. (2003). Measuring emotional intelligence with the MSCEIT V2.0. *Emotion, 3*, 97–105.

McCrae, R. R. (1990). Traits and trait names: How well is openness represented in natural languages. *European Journal of Personality, 4*, 119–129.

McCrae, R. R. (1996). Social consequences of experiential openness. *Psychological Bulletin, 120*, 333–337.

McDaniel, M. A., Morgeson, F. P., Finnegan, E. B., Campion, M. A., & Braverman, E. P. (2001). Use of situational judgment tests to predict job performance: A clarification of the literature. *Journal of Applied Psychology, 86*, 730–740.

McDaniel, M. A., & Nguyen, N. T. (2001). Situational judgment tests: A review of practice and constructs assessed. *International Journal of Selection & Assessment, 9*, 103–113.

McGlynn, S. M., & Schacter, D. L. (1989). Unawareness of deficits in neuropsychological syndromes. *Journal of Clinical and Experimental Neuropsychology, 11*, 143–205.

Mehrabian, A., & Epstein, S. (1970). A measure of emotional empathy. *Journal of Personality, 40*, 525–543.

Nevo, B. (1993). In search of a correctness typology for intelligence. *New Ideas in Psychology, 11*, 391–397.

Oberauer, K., Süß, H.-M., Schulze, R., Wilhelm, O., & Wittmann, W. W. (2000). Working memory capacity—Facets of a cognitive ability construct. *Personality and Individual Differences, 29*, 1017–1045.

O'Connor, R. M., & Little, I. S. (2003). Revisiting the predictive validity of emotional intelligence: self–report versus ability–based measures. *Personality and Individual Differences, 35*, 1893–1902.

Ones, D. S., Viswesvaran, C., & Dilchert, S. (2004). Cognitive ability in selection decisions. In O. Wilhelm & R. W. Engle (Eds.), *Handbook of understanding and measuring intelligence* (pp. 431–463). London: Sage.

Palmer, B. R., Manocha, R., Gignac, G., & Stough, C. (2003). Examining the factor structure of the Bar-On Emotional Quotient Inventory with an Australian general population sample. *Personality and Individual Differences, 35*, 1191–1210.

Petrides, K. V., & Furnham, A. (2000). On the dimensional structure of emotional intelligence. *Personality and Individual Differences, 29*, 313–320.

Petrides, K. V., & Furnham, A. (2001). Trait emotional intelligence: Psychometric investigation with reference to established trait taxonomies. *European Journal of Personality, 15*, 425–448.

Pfütze, E.-M., Sommer, W., & Schweinberger, S. R. (2002). Age–related slowing in face and name recognition: Evidence from event–related brain potentials. *Psychology and Aging, 17*, 140–160.

Reason, J. T. (1993). Self–report questionnaires in cognitive psychology: Have they delivered the goods? In A. D. Baddeley & L. Weiskrantz (Eds.), *Attention: Selection, awareness, and control* (pp. 152–170). Oxford: Clarendon Press.

Riemann, R., & Abels, D. (1994). Personality abilities: Construct validation. In B. de Raad, W. K. B. Hofstee, & G. L. M. van Heck (Eds.), *Personality psychology in europe* (Vol. 5, pp. 201–215). Tilburg: Tilburg University Press.

Roberts, R. D., Zeidner, M., & Matthews, G. (2001). Does emotional intelligence meet traditional standards for an intelligence? Some new data and conclusions. *Emotion, 1*, 196–231.

Sackett, P. R., Zedeck, S., & Fogli, L. (1988). Relations between measures of typical and maximal job performance. *Journal of Applied Psychology, 73*, 482–486.

Saklofske, D. H., Austin, E. J., & Minski, P. S. (2003). Self–reported emotional intelligence: Factor structure and evidence for construct validity. *Personality and Individual Differences, 34*, 707–721.

Salovey, P., & Mayer, J. D. (1990). Emotional intelligence. *Imagination, Cognition and Personality, 9*, 185–211.

Schulze, R. (2005). Modeling structures of intelligence. In O. Wilhelm & R. W. Engle (Eds.), *Handbook of understanding and measuring intelligence* (pp. 241–263). London: Sage.

Schutte, N. S., Malouff, J. M., Hall, L. E., Haggerty, D. J., Cooper, J. T., Golden, C. J., et al. (1998). Development and validation of a measure of emotional intelligence. *Personality and Individual Differences, 25*, 167–177.

Schweinberger, S. R., Pfütze, E.-M., & Sommer, W. (1995). Repetition priming and associative priming of face recognition: Evidence from event–related potentials. *Journal of Experimental Psychology: Learning, Memory, and Cognition, 21,* 722–736.

Seidenberg, M., Haltiner, A., Taylor, M. A., Hermann, B. B., & Wyler, A. (1994). Development and validation of a multiple ability self–report questionnaire. *Journal of Clinical and Experimental Neuropsychology, 14,* 93–104.

Sommer, W., Komoss, E., & Schweinberger, S. R. (1997). Differential localization of brain systems subserving memory for names and faces in normal subjects with event–related potentials. *Electroencephalography and Clinical Neurophysiology, 102,* 192–199.

Stankov, L. (1999). Mining on the "no man's land" between intelligence and personality. In P. L. Ackerman, P. C. Kyllonen, & R. D. Roberts (Eds.), *Learning and individual differences: Process, trait, and content determinants* (pp. 315–337). Washington, DC: American Psychological Association.

Sternberg, R. J. (2003). Our research program validating the triarchic theory of successful intelligence: Reply to Gottfredson. *Intelligence, 31,* 399–413.

Van Rooy, D. L., & Viswesvaran, C. (2004). Emotional intelligence: A meta-analytic investigation of predictive validity and nomological net. *Journal of Vocational Behavior, 65,* 71–95.

Wagner, R. K. (1987). Tacit knowledge in everyday intelligent behavior. *Journal of Personality and Social Psychology, 52,* 1236–1247.

Wilhelm, O., Schulze, R., Schmiedek, F., & Süß, H.-M. (2003). Interindividuelle Unterschiede im typischen intellektuellen Engagement [Individual differences in typical intellectual engagement]. *Diagnostica, 49,* 49–60.

Zeidner, M., Matthews, G., & Roberts, R. D. (2001). Slow down, you move too fast: Emotional intelligence remains an "elusive" intelligence. *Emotion, 1,* 265–275.

8

Using Consensus Based Measurement to Assess Emotional Intelligence

Peter J. Legree
Joseph Psotka
Trueman Tremble
U.S. Army Research Institute for the Behavioral and Social Sciences, USA

Dennis R. Bourne
American Psychological Association, USA

More than a century ago, the Russian novelist Leo Tolstoy wrote:
"Happy families are all alike; every unhappy family is unhappy in its own way."

Summary

Situational judgment tests (SJTs) have been developed in the fields of Industrial/Organizational and Cognitive Psychology to predict performance and to evaluate theories of cognition. Production of these scales has usually required the opinions of subject matter experts to produce scoring keys or criterion data to compute empirically based standards. A simpler, elegant procedure is considered that allows examinee responses to be scored as deviations from the consensus defined by the response distributions of the examinee sample. This approach is termed *Consensus Based Measurement* and has been applied to validate scales in domains, such as Emotional Intelligence, that lack certified experts and well-specified, objective knowledge. Data are summarized demonstrating substantial convergence between SJT scores computed using expert and examinee based scoring standards for which substantial expert and examinee data are available. The convergence indicates that examinee response distributions may be used to score SJTs when expert responses are not available. Validity data for SJTs that are scored with this approach are summarized.

8.1   INTRODUCTION

Over the past decade, scenario-based scales have been developed to measure knowledge and expertise in performance domains such as leadership and driver safety, as well as to assess emotional, social, and general intelligence (Legree, 1995, Legree, Heffner, Psotka, Martin, & Medsker, 2003, Legree, Martin, & Psotka, 2000, Mayer, Salovey, Caruso, & Sitarenios, 2003, McDaniel, Morgeson, Finnegan, Campion, & Braverman, 2001).

While most applications have utilized expert groups to develop scoring standards (see Hedlund et al., 2003), other attempts have constructed scoring keys based on data collected from large groups of respondents who were knowledgeable concerning the subject domain but could not be qualified as experts (Legree, 1995; Legree et al., 2000, 2003). The scoring keys from these groups of non-experts were believed to have closely approximated the scoring standards that would have been obtained from experts. In these earlier papers, the use of non-expert groups to develop scoring standards was termed *Consensual Scoring* or more broadly, *Consensus Based Measurement (CBM)*. CBM provides a maximal performance based method to assess knowledge-related constructs and is relevant to conceptualizations of emotional intelligence (EI) that propose a related set of knowledge, skills, and abilities (see Chapter 2 by Neubauer & Freudenthaler).

The promise of CBM rests in the fact that it expands the spectrum of knowledge addressed in psychological research to include domains for which neither *bona fide* experts can be identified, nor objective factual knowledge located. CBM is relevant to measuring EI, the common theme running throughout the current volume, because it is an example of a domain that is still lacking in the availability of experts and objective knowledge. In fact, the theoretical development of EI is still broadly viewed as in a stage of formative development. This fact notwithstanding, CBM has been used to score well-developed performance-based EI scales, including the Multi-factor Emotional Intelligence Scale (MEIS; Mayer, Caruso, & Salovey, 1999) and the Mayer-Salovey-Caruso Emotional Intelligence Test (MSCEIT; Mayer et al., 2003). However, the notion that non-experts can be used to develop the expert knowledge required to score these instruments may be unappealing to test developers, who are not yet familiar with the strengths and limitations of this approach, and those commentators who have questioned its assumptions (e.g., Roberts, Zeidner, & Matthews, 2001; Schaie, 2001; Zeidner, Matthews, & Roberts, 2001). Thus, a chapter describing CBM and its development in disparate areas of applied psychology (along with a summary of relevant data and theory) could help some favorable consensus to develop. We will present a case for using CBM for ill-specified knowledge domains, such as EI, and for other domains, where experts might not be available, because of some unique advantages associated with consensual scoring.

8.2   TEST CONSTRUCTION FOR POORLY SPECIFIED KNOWLEDGE DOMAINS

Many psychological knowledge tests are based on a job (or task or cognitive) analysis that associates knowledge and performance domains. Based on available data, this approach has proven its worth in many pragmatic areas of assessment and counseling (see Anastasi & Urbina, 1997). Implicit in this approach, are expectations that formal and tacit knowledge underlies much performance, and that observed behavior supports inferences connecting behavior with those knowledge attainments. Construction of knowledge scales traditionally has drawn either on an available formal corpus of accumulated knowledge (such as books written by experts; or pedagogical materials developed over decades of instruction and analysis) or on an available pool of institutionally recognized experts.

However, much knowledge is intuitive and tacit, and might be called mere opinion, so there may be no formal knowledge sources, or even experts who can provide appropriate standards. In many areas, such as art, music, politics, government, and economics, experts may have, or seem to have, markedly different views, rationales, and evidentiary sources than the stratified populations of interest to researchers. CBM offers unique, analytic powers in these situations.

8.2.1   Limitations of Traditional Scale Construction

While CBM may have some noteworthy limitations, we would like to point out that traditional item construction, based on de facto expertise, also has its limitations. Item construction in formal, well-defined knowledge domains can easily incorporate general knowledge and expertise, and item revision is often based on the use of item statistics or factor analytic techniques, to maximize scale characteristics such as reliability and validity. Because predictor and criterion reliability limit scale validity, the maximization of test reliability is of critical importance, and test construction decisions are frequently based on requirements to improve scale reliability. To maximize reliability, item statistics and especially low item correlations with total test score have been commonly used to identify questionable items for revision or deletion. From an item response theory perspective, concerns with analogous goals results in the characterization of items as inefficient in providing information and requiring modification. Scales, and especially predictor scales, are produced using a subset of the items selected to differentiate high and low performing examinees. Resultant tests are usually accurate, reliable, and frequently valid, against some external criterion.

For many academic and industrial purposes, this traditional approach has been adequate for the development of knowledge measures that are both valid and useful for personnel management and training decisions. Much mathematical knowledge, for example, is well developed and linked to performance, and it is relatively simple to identify the correct answer for a range of questions requiring the understanding of basic concepts. Likewise, words and expressions have specific meanings and connotations, as detailed in dictionaries. Vocabulary knowledge is frequently assessed with items corresponding to these dictionary definitions and is sometimes used to estimate general intelligence. Initial item construction is possible largely because of the presence of expert knowledge usually reflecting the availability of an information corpus and sometimes the opinions of experts. Even simple arithmetic and algebra problems require expertise, although it is widely available. The impact of the use of item statistics is to construct consistency within the measure, and create a stronger relationship between performance and the likelihood to respond correctly on all items. Seen from the perspective of CBM, this procedure in effect creates a consensus among the standardization group. From this perspective, all scales are consensually constructed, and consensus based scoring is a variant on a long established theme.

8.2.2 When Consensus Goes Awry

Obviously, items may occasionally be created for which consensus understandings are not correct or for which different groups have markedly different understandings: What is the capital of Israel (Tel Aviv/Jerusalem)? Should the US have invaded Iraq (Yes/No)? Where is the US federal government located (White House/Capital Building/Supreme Court/Executive Buildings)? These are all items for which different groups may have different understandings, or for which different understandings may have varying validity. A reasonable response to the presence of these occasional disagreements is not to reject CBM, but to understand the basis of these disagreements and thereby identify implications relating to the development and assessment of knowledge and opinion. Furthermore, the possibility that the knowledge underlying many questions might be deduced by analyzing the opinions of large numbers of non-experts is intriguing.

8.2.3 Knowledge Domains without Experts

It seems incontrovertible that knowledge domains may exist without the presence of an expert knowledge source, either in the form of an information corpus or verifiable experts. Consider that before the efforts of Noah Webster (1758–1843), assessing English language vocabulary knowledge of American colonists would have been problematic from the standpoint of scoring responses. Lacking a convenient information source for word knowledge (i.e., the dictionary), an 18th century vocabulary test developer might have felt compelled to determine, through expert opinions, acceptable definitions for American terms, such as "hickory", and for common terms that might have multiple meanings, such as "bed". Whether expert opinions would judge a flower garden reference as an acceptable definition for "bed" is an open question, but the direction of the judgment would impact individual scores.

But what population would constitute appropriate subject matter experts for the common English vocabulary knowledge of Webster's time? The use of highly regarded 18th century, United Kingdom English professors as subject matter experts might seem reasonable and would have foreshadowed approaches commonly used in Industrial/Organizational Psychology to develop and score situational judgment tests (SJTs), but these opinions might have been skewed in an academic direction. It may be interesting that Noah Webster, who was also an important patriot dedicated to the democratic ideals of the American Revolution, incorporated definitions for uniquely North American terms such as "hickory" and "skunk". He also simplified spelling in a manner more consistent with Benjamin Franklin's preferences, substituting "center" for "centre" and "music" for "musick" (see http://www.m-w.com/). Royal English professors at Oxford and Cambridge universities would seem unlikely candidates to accept these innovations, and this expected resistance would have produced questionable results if they were used as subject matter experts. It would be more reasonable (and Jeffersonian!) to survey a representative sample of English speaking American colonists/citizens and develop guidelines to identify acceptable responses for vocabulary definition items. In short, if we had to develop a vocabulary test today, without the benefit of dictionaries, using a democratic sampling of a broad spectrum of educated adults to act as experts would seem a reasonable approach.

This reasoning illustrates how knowledge domains may exist that are lodged in opinion and have no objective standard for verification other than societal views, opinions, and interpretations. Yet these knowledge domains may provide important information concerning one's abilities; after all, vocabulary knowledge has traditionally been very highly loaded on psychometric g (Carroll, 1993). For such knowledge domains, it may be mandatory to use standards based on a social knowledge perspective to evaluate individual responses. The concept that much knowledge is experientially based and linked to opinion is rooted in the writings of philosophers, such as Plato and John Stuart Mill. And, the concept that the opinions of common people may reflect higher standards is at the heart of democratic institutions.

The assessment of knowledge corresponding to "soft", emerging domains such as emotional and social intelligence, where the codification and formalization of knowledge is only beginning, cries out for the use of these new technologies. These ill-defined domains are often of considerable consequence: knowledge and expertise related to driving safety, leadership, and social functioning can and does substantially impact on an individual's quality of life. It is important to this discussion that these knowledge domains are analogous to the situation that our 18th century vocabulary test developer would have ex-

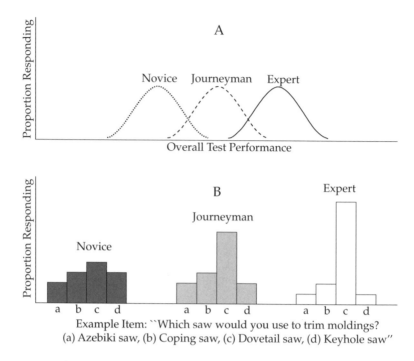

Example Item: ``Which saw would you use to trim moldings?
(a) Azebiki saw, (b) Coping saw, (c) Dovetail saw, (d) Keyhole saw''

Figure 8.1   Performance on a conventional test at the scale and item level across three levels of expertise. Panel A: Overall scale performance distributions for a multiple-choice test. Panel B: Theoretical response distributions for a multiple-choice item where "c" is the correct answer.

perienced, because for these domains, well-developed knowledge corpora are not available and, equally important, identifying appropriate groups of subject matter experts is problematic. Scales developed to assess these domains might evaluate the consistency of an individual's cognitive structures with a scoring standard corresponding to a group consensus and therefore would be methodologically similar.

8.3   KNOWLEDGE, RESPONSE DISTRIBUTIONS, AND LEVELS OF EXPERTISE

Our conceptualizations regarding CBM evolved from expectations about how item response distributions might change as a function of the expertise of various respondent samples. Knowledge is customarily viewed as growing as levels of expertise increase in a specific domain. Therefore, if a sample of apprentices were tracked over time, and repeatedly surveyed with standard knowledge items as novices (or initiates), journeymen, and experts, the response distributions shown in Panel A (Figure 8.1) might describe their growth in expertise.

These distributions in Panel A illustrate both individual differences as well as increasing knowledge. For any test item, more respondents would choose the correct response as expertise increased, as is illustrated in Panel B.

However, suppose a sample of students studying EI were surveyed with items that required examinees to endorse statements on a Likert scale. For example, examinees might be requested to rate their agreement with the statement: "EI may be defined as the individual's fund of knowledge about the social world"; similar statements have been proposed to define social intelligence (see Cantor & Kihlstrom, 1987), but not EI. For this type of question, the item response distributions associated with increased levels of expertise might vary in both central tendency and in variance. A change in central tendency might occur as students learn that some EI conceptualizations carry implications for social knowledge. Changes in the central tendency of these types of response distributions are illustrated in Figure 8.2 (Panel A).

A reduction in variance might also occur as students become more refined in their understandings of EI, recognizing that while EI conceptualizations focus on emotion constructs (see Chapter 2 by Neubauer & Freudenthaler), they also carry implications for social knowledge. Panel B in Figure 8.2 illustrates a reduction in variance of response distributions associated with increased accuracy.

Both these trends have general relevance to understanding the growth and refinement of knowledge through reflection, experience, and formal education. By definition, naïve individuals have poorly formed conceptual structures for understanding relationships or events, and their responses may not be sensible, sometimes indicating ignorance of even basic relationships and sometimes overstating their importance. But with increasing degrees of sophistication, individuals will become increasingly aware and accurate in their understanding of relationships and events. It is worth considering that, to the extent poor performance on a knowledge test can be viewed as reflecting error, non-expert responses will be more variable than those of experts, as well as possibly having a different central tendency.

This conceptualization suggests that as error is reduced examinees will tend to agree with each other to a greater extent as expertise increases for both conventional and scenario-based test items. The central tendency of expert response distributions for individual, scenario-based items should be roughly equal to the central tendency of non-expert (e.g., journeymen) response distributions when the growth of knowledge over expertise is associated primarily with changes in variance (Figure 8.2, Panel B). This observation also applies to conventional multiple-choice items (Figure 8.1, Panel B), but it is of little practical value because writing sensible, multiple-choice items requires that the correct response be known a priori. Scenario-based items do not always require that the correct response be specified or even known.

However, it is equally possible for increasing expertise to show changes in central tendency as well as variance. This model is intermediate and is represented in Panel C in Figure 8.2. At this time we have little meaningful to say about what kinds of items should show changes over levels of expertise in

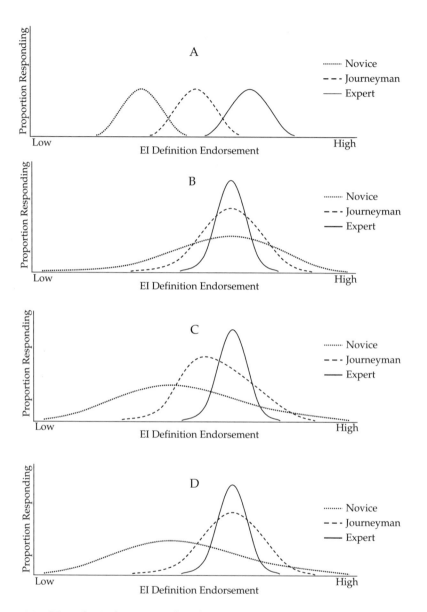

Figure 8.2   Hypothetical response distributions across three levels of expertise corresponding to a Likert-based item requiring endorsement of the statement: "EI may be defined as the individual's fund of knowledge about the social world". Panel A: Item distributions associated with changing central tendency and equal variance. Panel B: Item distributions associated with equal central tendency and differing variance. Panel C: Expected item distributions with differing central tendency and differing variance. Panel D: Observed item distributions for scenario-based items.

variance, central tendency, or both, with changing expertise, but simply point out the logical possibility and consider that a research agenda on CBM should investigate these relationships.

One powerful implication of successful CBM scales and inventories is a vindication and affirmation of broadly democratic processes that overturn the tyranny of autocratic expertise. Examining the hypothetical distributions of many novices (or initiates) against those of a handful of experts should reveal broader, flatter distributions that can more easily adapt and change with changing world knowledge. If one assumes that the correlation between novices' and experts' knowledge in these instruments is mediated by the intersection of their correlations with some broader truth,[1] it may well turn out that diverse groups of novices may have a more accurate reflection of truth than experts; at least, this is a worthy hypothesis to investigate for limiting conditions. Some implications of these relationships are drawn below.

8.4   SITUATIONAL JUDGMENT TESTS AS MEASURES OF EMOTIONAL INTELLIGENCE

We recognized that SJTs are ideal for studying changes in item response distributions over expertise, in both central tendency and variance as described above. We describe SJTs broadly as scales that:

1. Either implicitly or explicitly describe a scenario in order to simulate or depict an event, situation, or process. The scenarios may represent problems requiring solutions, the maintenance of success, or the interpretation of events. Understanding these depictions may require the application of knowledge gained either experientially or formally.

2. Provide a list of alternatives associated with each scenario. The alternatives may describe actions or interpretations, or provide the examinee the opportunity to respond in an open-ended manner to describe his/her opinion and knowledge.

3. Obligate examinees to either evaluate the alternatives associated with the scenarios (e.g., rating the appropriateness of the alternatives) or to generate new alternatives and analyses in the case of an open-ended response.

Performance on SJTs is quantified by analyzing the examinee evaluations. An SJT may contain many scenarios with scenarios treated as items or describe a single scenario with alternatives treated as items. How these evaluations are scored against some standard, and how these standards are developed, is the topic of concern in the passages that follow.

The scoring standards for most existent SJTs are developed by having subject matter experts evaluate or rate the alternatives for each scenario (see McDaniel et al., 2001). These data are then used to construct the expert scoring

---

[1]That is, $R(K_n, K_e) = R(K_n, K_t) \cap R(K_e, K_t)$.

Table 8.1   **Some Approaches Used to Consensually Score SJTs**

Method	Application	Citation
Percent Agreement/Endorsement: Likert data are collected and the response frequencies are used to weight each option.	Emotional Intelligence	Mayer et al. (2003)
Simple Distance: Likert data are used to compute item means over examinees. Distances are computed as the absolute difference between the individual and the mean rating for each item. Examinee performance is quantified as mean item distance.	Driving Knowledge	Legree et al. (2003)
Standardized Distance: Similar to the Simple Distance method, but ratings are first transformed to standardize within individual. The approach controls for the tendency of some respondents to use only a sub-segment of the scale.	Social Intelligence & Psychometric g	Legree (1995) Legree et al. (2000)
Squared Difference: Similar to Simple Distance, but item values are computed as the square of the difference. Provides additional weight to larger differences.	Tacit Knowledge	Sternberg et al. (2000)
Correlation: The value of the correlation of an individual's ratings with the mean ratings quantifies performance.	Leadership	Psotka, Streeter, Landauer, Lochbaum, and Robinson (2004)

standards, for example by computing mean expert ratings for each alternative. To evaluate examinee responses in comparison to the expert-based standards, a percent-correct agreement, a deviation measure, or a correlation of an examinee's set of ratings with the scoring standard is computed. Consistent with the use of a variety of procedures to evaluate performance on SJTs with expert-based scoring standards, various procedures might be used to consensually score SJTs. Information describing these possible methods is contained in Table 8.1.

While these approaches have implicitly adopted a classical test theory perspective, it is sensible that item response theory analyses might be undertaken given sufficient data. An SJT developed to evaluate tacit driving knowledge is presented in Table 8.2 to illustrate this approach.

The driving knowledge test leveraged a model of driving performance recognizing that drivers may moderate risk by altering their speed in response to the presence of road hazards (Legree et al., 2003). This SJT was scored by

Table 8.2 Safe Speed Knowledge Test

Assume someone is driving a safe car in light traffic under optimal/perfect conditions. Given the following considerations, please *estimate* how much that individual (driver) should or shouldn't slow down and change speed to ensure safety.

CONDITIONS:	−20 MPH Slow Down	−10 MPH	0 MPH Same Speed
1. Snow and heavy traffic	OOOOOOOOOOOOOOOOOOOOOOOOOOOO		
2. Clear weather and light traffic	OOOOOOOOOOOOOOOOOOOOOOOOOOOO		
3. Snow and no traffic	OOOOOOOOOOOOOOOOOOOOOOOOOOOO		
4. Dry roads at midnight	OOOOOOOOOOOOOOOOOOOOOOOOOOOO		
5. Stressed driver due to problems at work	OOOOOOOOOOOOOOOOOOOOOOOOOOOO		
6. Moderately heavy traffic	OOOOOOOOOOOOOOOOOOOOOOOOOOOO		
7. Gravel and light traffic	OOOOOOOOOOOOOOOOOOOOOOOOOOOO		
8. Clear roads and somewhat breezy	OOOOOOOOOOOOOOOOOOOOOOOOOOOO		
9. Light rain and curvy roads	OOOOOOOOOOOOOOOOOOOOOOOOOOOO		
10. Angry and light rain	OOOOOOOOOOOOOOOOOOOOOOOOOOOO		
11. Light traffic and hilly terrain	OOOOOOOOOOOOOOOOOOOOOOOOOOOO		
12. Slightly worn tires	OOOOOOOOOOOOOOOOOOOOOOOOOOOO		
13. Upset with family over finances/money	OOOOOOOOOOOOOOOOOOOOOOOOOOOO		
14. Sick with a head cold	OOOOOOOOOOOOOOOOOOOOOOOOOOOO		
	−20 MPH Slow Down	−10 MPH	0 MPH Same Speed

computing distance scores between examinee responses and the scoring standard for each of the 14 items.

Most SJT's have been produced for application within organizations. These scales usually present job-related problem scenarios and instruct examinees to choose among possible solution actions. In contrast, scales on the MEIS and the MSCEIT, and arguably Conditional Reasoning Tests (see James, 1998) present information and instruct examinees to choose among possible interpretations. Thus, the scales on the MEIS and the MSCEIT may be considered more abstract than standard SJT measures because they explore intermediate cognitive processes underlying EI, as opposed to simply simulating observable decisions.

It is relevant to the current volume that SJTs might be developed in other nontraditional manners to elucidate additional aspects of EI (or any other construct). For example, an SJT might be constructed that presents information and then estimates the time required for examinees to evaluate simple statements, or non-verbal stimuli, in a manner analogous to reaction or inspection time tasks (see Detterman, Caruso, Mayer, Legree, & Conners, 1992). Such an SJT would measure latency associated with EI cognitions and would be consistent with conceptualizations regarding psychometric speed and chronometry (see Carroll, 1993; Jensen, 1998).

8.5   CBM: EMPIRICAL FINDINGS

8.5.1   Supervisory and Social Intelligence SJT Data

In earlier work with SJTs (Legree, 1995; Legree & Grafton, 1995), we evaluated our conceptualization of knowledge development by comparing expert based scoring standards that reflected the opinions of a small number of subject matter experts (i.e., mean expert ratings) and the mean ratings for the items as computed across examinees. That supervisor SJT described 49 scenarios and listed a total of 198 alternatives, with between 3 and 5 alternatives per scenario. Each scenario described an interpersonal problem and presented alternatives as possible solutions to the problem. The scale was administered to examinees and experts who rated the appropriateness of the actions described in the alternatives for each scenario. We computed mean examinee ratings for each of the 198 alternatives and observed a high correlation between the expert-based scoring standard and the mean examinee item ratings (i.e., $r = .72$, $N = 198$, $p < .001$) and estimated a very high correlation (.95) by correcting the observed correlation for attenuation of the reliability of each set of observations (i.e., the mean expert and examinee ratings).

Initially, we had expected that examinee means would provide only a rough approximation of the expert-scoring standard. We had hoped this approximation would be evidenced by a moderate correlation between the means that would range between .40 and .60. We had planned to use a recursive procedure to sequentially identify groups of individuals with increasing levels of knowledge and then apply this approach to score scales for which expert opinions were not available. Information from the more select groups of individuals would then be used to develop increasingly valid scoring standards for the Supervisory SJT that would more closely approximate the expert standards. These standards would then be referred to as *consensus based standards* and the process as CBM.

Based on the observed and corrected correlations between the examinee and expert means, .72 and .95, the use of recursive procedures to refine the scoring pattern defined by the entire group of examinees was judged as not necessary. We also computed examinee scores using two different standards based on the expert and examinee means and then correlated the two sets of scores; this correlation was .88, ($N = 198$, $p < .001$).

These correlations indicated that the mean ratings of examinees might provide an alternate-scoring standard for the SJT, and this realization raised issues concerning the appropriateness of the two standards. We concluded that the examinee-based standard was preferable because these values were more reliable than the experts' standard, due to the large number of individuals ($N = 193$). We then applied this method to score two additional social intelligence scales for which expert opinions were not available. A confirmatory factor analysis of these three scales and a standard ability battery (the Armed Service Vocational Aptitude Battery), demonstrated the existence of a separate g-loaded factor corresponding to our social intelligence model (Legree, 1995).

8.5.2   Applications to Assess g and Driver Safety

While the social intelligence model was confirmed, we recognized that the value of CBM needed to be buttressed in other domains by validating consensus based scores against conceptually relevant and important criteria, and by showing correspondence between scores based on examinee and expert opinions. In additional research, we explored the power of CBM by developing and validating two types of scales: six Unobtrusive Knowledge Tests (UKTs), constructed to measure general cognitive ability, and two Tacit Driving Knowledge Tests, developed in order to assess knowledge related to driver safety. Most of these measures (there was one exception) required individuals to respond to items using Likert scales; for example, estimating the frequency of words and terms used in oral communication or the extent to which drivers should moderate speed when confronted with driving hazards. Construction of these scales leveraged conceptualizations of incidental learning and tacit knowledge to predict and understand human performance. This type of knowledge and associated expertise is usually acquired slowly and incrementally as a result of experience and reflection upon those experiences (Sternberg et al., 2000). For these scales, neither an objective knowledge base nor experts could be identified to develop scoring standards. Thus, performance on these scales could only be evaluated using consensus based scoring algorithms.

The UKT battery was administered to a highly selected military sample comprised of Air Force recruits. Factor scores extracted from this experimental battery correlated .54 with factor scores extracted from a conventional test battery (i.e., psychometric g); and a .80 correlation estimate was obtained by correcting for range restriction (Legree et al., 2000). Five of the six experimental scales also correlated significantly with psychometric g. This parameter estimate of .80 is typical of correlations obtained among IQ test batteries (see Carroll, 1993). A confirmatory factor analysis of the corrected correlation matrix estimated a .97 path coefficient between the two latent factors corresponding to the Unobtrusive Knowledge and Conventional Test Batteries. Thus, we intentionally produced and scored a very highly g-loaded test battery without using subject matter experts or objective knowledge, instead using CBM.

The tacit driving knowledge tests were administered to Army soldiers, for whom automobile crash involvement data were also collected. Compared to most performance domains, crash involvement is unusual because it has only very minor relationships with knowledge, skill, and ability measures, including general intelligence, based on meta-analyses (Arthur, Barrett, & Alexander, 1991; Veling, 1982). However, as reported in Table 8.3, both of the tacit driving knowledge tests correlated significantly with crash involvement criteria, $-.11$ to $-.20$ (Legree et al., 2003).

Table 8.3   Safe Speed Knowledge Item Response Distributions and Factor Loadings

Test Items	M	SD	% Speed[a]	Factor Loadings		
				Emotional Knowledge	Uncom-plicated	Precipi-tation
Upset with family finances	8.39	5.30	16	**.73**	−.01	.04
Sick with a head cold	8.50	5.08	13	**.73**	−.09	−.05
Slightly worn tires	7.62	4.92	3	**.55**	.05	−.02
Stressed over work	7.61	4.90	18	**.46**	.06	.17
Light traffic & hilly	6.17	4.28	20	**.44**	.17	.05
Clear & light traffic	1.50	3.19	78	−.02	**.92**	−.11
Clear & breezy	2.77	3.52	49	−.02	**.68**	.14
Dry & midnight	4.52	3.79	28	.20	**.62**	.02
Light rain & curves	10.40	4.07	1	.06	−.08	**.59**
Angry & light rain	10.59	4.43	3	.23	−.12	**.44**
Snow & no traffic	11.17	4.11	2	.02	.01	**.49**
Snow & heavy traffic	14.81	4.01	0	−.07	.13	**.40**
Mod. heavy traffic[b]	7.70	4.17	8			
Gravel and light traffic[b]	7.77	4.02	7			

	Criteria Correlations			Factor Correlations		
	Fault Rate	Fault Status[c]	g			
Emotional	−.19‡	−.20‡	.10*	1.00	.19	.50
Dry Weather	−.10*	−.16†	.31‡		1.00	.25
Precipitation	−.16‡	−.16†	.11†			1.00

Note. $N = 387$. [a]Percent of respondents reporting that speed should not be reduced. [b]Variables excluded from analysis because of cross-loadings. [c]Fault status reflected an N of 211.
* $p < .10$. † $p < .05$. ‡ $p < .01$.

While these values may appear modest, they exceed coefficients typically obtained for stable characteristics and they carry implications for improving driver safety. Thus, the values we obtained demonstrate the utility of using consensus based scoring to assess tacit knowledge for this arguably atypical performance domain.

The Safe Speed Knowledge test, presented in Table 8.2, was one of two scales developed to assess tacit driving knowledge. Confirming the importance of constructs related to EI, when the Safe Speed items were factored, one of the three factors was defined by emotionally and internally relevant items (refer to Table 8.3). Although this factor had a very minimal g loading, it was most predictive of the at-fault crash criteria. These data show safer drivers are more aware of the importance of moderating speed when under emotional (or internal) stress.

Of course individuals could have been nominated as experts to develop the scoring standards associated with the domains referenced by the UKT and tacit driving knowledge tests, but, it is our belief, all expert accreditations or knowledge corpora linked to these domains are suspect for their intended purposes. Nominated experts, having no more real expertise than the examinees in this study, would differ qualitatively, and not quantitatively, from the examinees who completed the scales. Knowledge of word frequency during oral communication and safe driving speed are exemplars of domains associated with experience that lack bona fide experts.

The implicit association task, which is the only experimental test that did not use a Likert response scale, is even more unique. The implicit association task assessed an examinee's ability to understand binary patterns (see Psotka, 1977), and each item required examinees to continue a series of X's and O's (e.g., XOXOXO?). No scoring standard could be invoked because the patterns used as stimuli were not chosen in accordance with pre-specified rules or relationships that would dictate the correct answer. As a result, these items could only be consensually scored. Nevertheless, performance on this task correlated with psychometric g.

8.5.3   Additional Datasets Supporting Expert and Examinee Comparisons

The above data demonstrate the efficacy of CBM, for producing predictive validity, and so for useful scoring standards. There is little doubt that CBM can be used to score tests developed for these unusual soft knowledge domains that lack formal sources of knowledge, which either may be very highly g-loaded, or have very minimal g loadings. Our conceptualization also predicted a very high correlation between expert and consensus based scoring standards, as well as the scores based on those two standards. For example, in our initial evaluation of the model the Supervisor SJT, the expert and consensus scoring standards correlated .72 and scores based on these standards correlated .88. Because experts are often hard to find and expensive once found, much research with expert-based measures has low reliability. We are aware of three other data sets that used expert based standards derived from a large number of experts and are thus likely to have the needed level of reliability. There are likely to be additional datasets that could support these types of analyses, but examinee data are rarely used to approximate expert judgments.

Non-Commissioned Officer (NCO) SJT.   The largest of these data sets corresponds to the Non-commissioned Officer (NCO) SJT developed to evaluate supervisory skills for senior enlisted soldiers. The NCO SJT described 71 problem scenarios and listed 362 actions. To evaluate CBM, response protocols were scored using both expert ($N = 88$) and consensus ($N = 1891$) based standards (Heffner & Porr, 2000, W. B. Porr, personal communication, July 2003). Overall performance scores correlated .95 and scoring standards correlated .89.

Emotional intelligence data.   The MSCEIT (Mayer et al., 2003, see also Chapters 2 and 7 of the current volume), which is arguably the best-developed performance EI battery, provides both expert and consensus based scores. The expert group corresponded to 21 members of the International Society for Research on Emotions, and the consensus scores corresponded to 2112 examinees, all of whom completed the scale. The correlation between the scores based on the two sets of standards was .98 and the score standards correlated .91. These researchers also reported inter-rater kappa coefficients for the experts and for two samples of the non-expert examinees: expert kappas were consistently higher than the examinee kappas ($\kappa = .43$ versus $\kappa = .31/\kappa = .38$, $p < .01/p < .05$) as suggested by a model of decreasing variance with increasing expertise, while central tendency remains constant.

Tacit knowledge for military leadership data.   The third database corresponds to the Tacit Knowledge for Military Leadership (TKML) scale (Hedlund et al., 2003; Psotka et al., 2004). The TKML was designed to measure the practical, action-oriented knowledge that Army leaders typically acquire from experience. The TKML was developed with the idea that an ordered hierarchy of expertise in Military Leadership can be created by using the scores of Lieutenant Colonels as a standard and comparing them with U.S. Military Academy (West Point) Cadets, and U.S. Army Lieutenants, Captains, and Majors. The scale was administered to groups of soldiers including: 355 Cadets, 125 Lieutenants, 117 Captains, 98 Majors, and 50 Lieutenant Colonels. The Lieutenant Colonels comprised the expert group, and this group contains the highest ranking soldiers and those who have served longest in the military (with an average of 18 years service). Comparisons of the consensus based cadet (355 cadets) and expert (50 Lieutenant Colonels) scoring standards and scores provide very consistent results with the earlier data. The two sets of score standards correlated .96, and the cadet scores computed using those standards correlated $r = 1$ (i.e., above .995). Similar results were found by analyzing the data for the intermediate (lieutenant, captain, and major) groups.

While obtaining high correlations between the expert-based and consensus based standards helps validate the approach, values approaching $r = 1$ were unexpected. In addition, the use of recursive procedures to refine consensus based standards was not required for the scales we developed. Collectively, these findings suggested that modification to our conceptualization of the CBM model might be warranted such that the principle difference between journeymen and experts is represented in terms of increasing accuracy, or from the perspective of item response distributions, decreased variance around the item means. The transition from novice to journeyman would still be associated with shifts in response distributions and means because novices have little, or no, basis for their responses and their responses would be nearly or completely random. This revised model is represented in Panel D in Figure

8.2. To evaluate this model, it is necessary to inspect the response distributions of sizeable samples of individuals from groups varying in level of expertise.

Most databases are not adequate for this purpose because in most non-stratified samples there are very few novice or expert performing individuals, and identifying these individuals would be difficult. However, the TKML database is unique because it contains substantial numbers of novices (355 cadets), experts (50 Lieutenant Colonels) and examinees at the journeyman levels (125 Lieutenants, 117 Captains and 98 Majors). These groups differ on a number of salient dimensions that affect expertise: age, experience, and education. In fact, Cadets have really very little experience of the Army, but they do have some experience with interpersonal events and problems, and issues of authority, caring, and obedience that underlie the scenarios in the TKML; so although they are novices, they do have pertinent knowledge.

It should not be too surprising, then, that when the means of 355 Cadet item response distributions were correlated with the means of 50 Lieutenant Colonels (experts), the overall correlation was quite high ($r = .96$) *and* the slope was close to one (0.99). The slope indicates a similar level of variance across the two sets of item means. Thus, despite the difference in expertise between Cadets (with 0 years of experience) and Lieutenant Colonels (with an average of 18 years of military experience), the use of the group's average as the standard is indistinguishable from an expert-based score. And yet, the same standard still cleanly discriminates between these two groups. Although the overall item mean for each of the scenarios' alternatives was practically the same for Cadets and Colonels, even the top 25% of Cadets scored significantly lower than the Colonels on the overall TKML scale. Overall, the mean of the top 25% of the Cadets was 0.73, whereas the colonels' mean score was 0.82 ($t = 4.27, \mathrm{df} = 132, p < .01$), which is equivalent to a difference of 0.36 standard deviation units, demonstrating that consensus based standards are effective in assessing what the scale was intended to assess: military leadership.

Differences between scoring standards can be demonstrated using the TKML dataset, but only by isolating a group associated with a very low level of expertise and comparing their means with values based on the other groups. Figure 8.3 shows exactly this sort of difference between the top and bottom 25% of the Cadets at USMA.

For the top 25%, the correlation with the experts is $r = .95$ and the slope is 1.00. But for the bottom 25%, the correlation with the experts is $r = .85$ and the slope is 0.31. The low slope indicates less variance in item means computed using the lowest 25% of the cadets. Only by artificially restricting the examinee sample to the lowest quartile of the cadet sample can substantial changes in the standards be effected, and even then, the correlation is still $r = .85$.

If our notions of how expert knowledge is tapped in these consensual scales are accurate, not only should novices have a lower correlation with experts, than journeymen with intermediate levels of expertise, but the slope of the regression line should also be lower. To understand this prediction, think of how the many different, and less correct, opinions of novices should combine. In the absence of systematic biases, components of the novices' thinking should

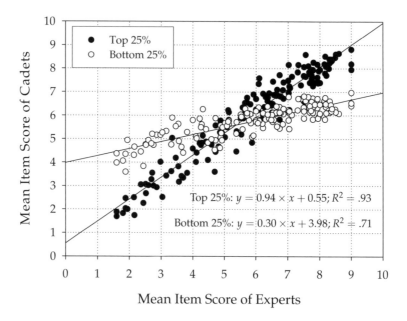

Figure 8.3   The relationship between the top 25% of Cadets, the bottom 25%, and the Expert Senior Officers used to standardize the TKML, showing that the top 25% are practically indistinguishable as a group for setting the standards of the test.

be in error in different ways, but the components that are on the road to expertise should be similar. As there is more and more error, the overall regression to the mean should be stronger and stronger, giving rise to lower slopes. Thus, the TKML data are most consistent with a model in which experts and journeymen differ primarily in variance, with changes in central tendency being more closely related to differences between novices and journeymen; this model is illustrated in Panel D in Figure 8.2.

8.6   CONCEPTUALIZING CBM: TOWARDS A WORKING MODEL

To describe CBM and summarize data describing its effectiveness and utility were two goals of this chapter. But the initial model was more descriptive than theoretical, and the concept that expert knowledge can be approximated by surveying large numbers of non-experts must have some limitations. So a more theoretical explanation of CBM is warranted. To understand consensus based scoring, it is useful to consider that for most knowledge domains, and especially for procedural knowledge domains, knowledge accumulates as the result of experience (see Anderson & Lebiere, 1998). As a greater range of events is experienced, greater levels of knowledge and associated skills will be acquired, and reactions to a new event or situation may reflect increasing levels of sophistication.

When presented with a situation to analyze, novices will have little basis for their opinions, and they will frequently disagree among themselves as well as with experts. Disagreement among novices is expected because the knowledge and cognitive structures associated with an individual novice will reflect either the action of a few unique experiences or the actions of experiences that have marginal relevance to the depicted situation. Thus, novices will reference different experiences and expectations, and their opinions will tend to be inconsistent, both among themselves as well as with experts.

In contrast, experts will generally have well-developed, mature knowledge structures reflecting broad, extensive sets of experiences. While each expert will have a slightly different set of experiences, these sets will largely overlap across individual experts. Moreover, with increasing levels of expertise, knowledge structures and related opinions will become progressively more consistent. Journeymen with partially developed and varying levels of expertise will agree at a moderate level both among themselves and with experts, and this moderate level of agreement is based on developing cognitive structures that reflects a modest but not extensive array of experience. From a mathematical perspective, the correlation of knowledge between individual A and individual B can be conceptualized as the product of the correlation of individual A with the "truth" and of individual B with the "truth". As individuals A and B become more knowledgeable and their opinions more "truthful", their opinions and responses will become more highly correlated (see Romney & Weller, 1984).

In theory this progression is reasonable, but in some domains experts frequently disagree with each other, and expert performance may not be very impressive in comparison to non-expert performance: Clinical psychology, graduate admissions, and economic forecasting are all examples of domains in which it has been suggested that experts do not perform much better than novices (Chi, Glaser, & Farr, 1988). Thus, expectations concerning levels of expert agreement may easily be overstated and a more realistic perspective is to expect experts to differ quantitatively and not qualitatively from journeymen. In fairness to experts in these domains, these individuals may perform better than novices.

Because procedural knowledge is experientially based and because these experiences are dependent on the occurrence of real-world events, various journeymen may have different types of experiences and knowledge, although much of this knowledge will be most relevant to those situations that frequently occur. It follows that the breadth of experience associated with a single expert, while more extensive than that of an individual journeyman, will often be exceeded by the variety of experiences associated with a substantial number of journeymen. The implication of this view for CBM, as well as for other knowledge engineering applications, is that more information might be present in the knowledge structures of a large number of journeymen than a small number of experts.

The concept that expertise represents the sum total of many small components relates well to theories of intelligence to the extent that intelligence can be viewed as reflecting general life expertise. Thomson (1928, 1939) conceptualized psychometric g as arising from the separate action of many connections that sum to represent one's level of intelligence, and this view is based on the application of sampling theory to the measurement of intelligence. Under this model of intelligence, no single individual would perform perfectly across all connections, but across individuals, all connections would occasionally be closed. IQ tests were viewed as sampling these connections to estimate one's overall level of connectivity or general intelligence. A high IQ would evidence a high proportion of connections, and a low IQ would evidence a low proportion. However, low and moderate IQ scores could easily result from separate and sometimes non-overlapping sets of connections, for example when different individuals are knowledgeable regarding facts in different domains but unable to respond to many other queries. In modern parlance, g might be viewed as the sum of a very large number of separate factors or cognitive structures.

Because learning theories associate knowledge and experience, Thomson's view of intelligence as representing the sum of many small parts or connections has relevance. Expertise can be conceptualized as reflecting one's overall number and strength of cognitive structures; just as intelligence might reflect the presence of connections. Across individuals, lower levels of expertise can reflect cognitive structures reflecting largely non-overlapping sets of events, with higher levels of expertise reflecting more complete sets of cognitive structures and experiences. As in Thomson's analysis, no single individual can be expected to have experienced the universe of events associated with a domain of expertise. However, a large number of individuals, each with a moderate level of experience, could be expected to experience most, if not all, classes of events and to have cognitive structures correspondent with those events.

These learning theories are most relevant to understanding CBM when cognitive structures and related knowledge reflect the experience of largely unpredictable events, as does much procedural and tacit knowledge. In contrast, academic knowledge reflects more formal instruction, which is often structured to provide a systematic, highly ordered set of experiences based on objective information, and the surveying of students on topics not yet covered is unlikely to identify much information. However, all of the domains described in the current chapter correspond to incidental, tacit, or procedural knowledge. With respect to the SJT methodology (see e.g., McDaniel et al., 2001), a similar set of conditions prevail, as appears the case, we suspect, in many soft, poorly defined domains of psychological inquiry.

Thus, cognitive theories related to the acquisition of procedural knowledge support the contention that the opinions of a large number of journeymen can be used to approximate those opinions of a smaller number of experts for these types of domains, and this notion is the heart of CBM. In this chapter, we addressed the utility of CBM for scenario-based scales, on which examinees might respond on Likert scales. It is important that our results are consistent with simulations using dichotomous items when examinees are available but the objective answers are not specified (Batchelder & Romney, 1988). These analyses show highly accurate answer keys can be constructed using relatively small sets of respondents with the number of respondents in balance with the expertise of the group. These data also show that a majority rule may be used to infer correct responses given a large number of respondents. Of course it is rare for this procedure to be required for a dichotomous scale developed for a conventional knowledge domain, but these results are entirely consistent with our findings and the conclusion that CBM is ideal for poorly specified, emergent knowledge domains. It seems likely that this approach will remain relevant to developing scales for emerging domains, especially those based on experience, such as EI, until these emerging domains become much better specified.

8.7   CONSENSUS BASED MEASUREMENT: LIMITATIONS AND IMPLICATIONS

Consensual scoring has several important implications for studying individual differences. First, the approach allows the construction and scoring of scales for knowledge domains for which experts do not exist, or cannot be easily identified. This allows an expansion of the domains for which knowledge tests may be developed, an expansion beyond traditional formal domains into everyday knowledge areas that are meaningful and important in our daily lives. Thus, consensus based scoring allows the assessment of knowledge domains that have not been traditionally addressed in psychological or educational research, and broadens the domain of psychological assessment and intelligence research into horizontal aspects of intelligence, one of which may be emotional or social intelligence. This perspective is consistent with theories of implicit and tacit knowledge acquisition and relates well to conceptualizations of social knowledge.

A second important implication is that CBM provides economy to test development. The approach allows questions to be posed, answered, and scored without the correct responses known a priori. Thus, the scale development cycle is shortened because expert responses are not required to construct scoring standards. In addition, costs associated with the production of scoring standards and rubrics are minimized because expert judgments can be expensive to collect while the examinee data are incidental to scale administration. A related implication results from the use of the Likert format to support CBM. Likert scales allow distances to be computed at the item level, thus allowing a more complete analysis of available information. As might be expected based on the use of additional information, comparisons of scores based on the distance information versus those based on a dichotomous format associates higher levels of reliability with the distance-based measures (Legree, 1995), and therefore the Likert format supports improved testing efficiency.

In addition, distance items can be correlated, and factors extracted from these correlations have been sensible (see Legree et al., 2003).

Third, consensus based scoring has the potential to allow the same protocol to be scored against multiple standards. This approach could be useful in studying controversial domains associated with groups that may adopt different perspectives. This approach might relate well to understanding controversial views differing over gender, political affiliation, race, age, or sexual orientation or in identifying the basis for competing theories to explain some phenomenon. Who knows, it might even be applied to the development of formal theories of scaling and item measurement, such as consensual scaling, in an interesting recursive cycle!

Fourth, consensual scoring explicitly invokes the notion of disagreement and inconsistency in the coherence of knowledge structures. Ill-defined domains are characterized by disagreement even among experts. Factorial analysis and multidimensional scaling of their responses (Psotka et al., 2004) using such powerful technologies as Latent Semantic Analysis not only brings order to these disagreements, but provides the prospect of being able to define the source of differences and create new conjunctions in the informal frameworks. To paraphrase an oft-cited opinion:[2] "An intuitive inconsistency is the muse of great minds".

Fifth, consensus-based scoring emphasizes that *under at least some conditions*, standards based on a body of relatively informed individuals approximate the standards of experts. SJTs are sometimes called "low fidelity simulations" because they provide the minimum stimulus cues needed to evoke responses representing the phenomenon targeted for measurement. As such, SJTs present somewhat ambiguous situations. Our principal interpretation suggests that judgments to these ambiguous situations are direct reflections of existing knowledge. A complementary explanation inspired by Gestalt psychology, is that abstract stimulus situations do not create all cues needed for a response, instead forcing interpretation or induction of meaning. Thus, rather than directly reflecting the qualities of existing knowledge structures, responses reflect the existing structures mediated by the understanding reached about the abstract situations. Superior performance would then reflect greater access to commonality in forcing interpretation and induction of meaning.

Under conditions when paradigm shifts develop or when information is distributed that differentially influences either expert or journeyman opinions, or when these conditions result in group divisions that retard rather than further group goals, then it seems less likely that CBM will produce a useful metric of group agreement needed to evaluate expertise. Whether a multimodal approach could be used to develop multiple metrics is an open question, but this approach might have relevance to understanding interactions between groups that sometimes conflict.

---

[2]"A foolish consistency is the hobgoblin of small minds"—Ralph Waldo Emerson.

Much social knowledge represents the convergence between many perspectives and truth is commonly believed to exist at the intersection of these perspectives. Thus, the American legal system, with one side designated as prosecutor and the opposing side as defendant is a manifestation of this view, as are all democratic institutions. The perspective that knowledge is rooted in widely diverse opinion is reflected in Tolstoy's observation that "Happy families are all alike; every unhappy family is unhappy in its own way", and from a cross-cultural perspective, the African proverb, "It takes a village to raise a child". The success of these institutions and the relevance of these statements reflect the notion that much useful knowledge can be distributed over individuals. To take full advantage of this knowledge, CBM techniques are needed to analyze this type of knowledge and its evidentiary sources for emerging fields such as social and emotional intelligence.

8.8   EPILOGUE

We would like feedback from our readers. Using a 9-point Likert scale, please email your ratings of the extent (1 = not at all . . . 9 = completely) to which you believe:

1. You are very knowledgeable concerning test development.
2. Traditional test development methods are appropriate for well-specified knowledge domains.
3. Traditional test development methods are appropriate for emerging, ill-specified knowledge domains.
4. CBM methods are appropriate for well-specified knowledge domains.
5. CBM methods are appropriate for emerging, ill-specified knowledge domains.
6. Academic knowledge can be accurately measured using multiple-choice measures.
7. Academic knowledge can be accurately measured using Likert based items.
8. Procedural knowledge can be accurately measured using multiple-choice measures.
9. Procedural knowledge can be accurately measured using Likert based items.
10. It is reasonable to expect that happy families are more similar than unhappy families.

If we collect sufficient information, we will compare the response distributions of readers of this chapter for these items to those collected from test-developers who have not reviewed this information. If our theory is correct, then a greater level of agreement for CBM related items should be apparent for the chapter readers than for the non-readers as evidenced by decreased variance yet similar means over those items. Please respond to the first author by email: legree@ari.army.mil.

Author Note

The views, opinions, and/or findings contained in this article are solely those of the authors and should not be construed as an official Department of the Army or DOD position, policy, or decision, unless so designated by other documentation.

REFERENCES

Anastasi, A., & Urbina, S. (1997). *Psychological testing* (7th ed.). Upper Saddle River, NJ: Prentice Hall.

Anderson, J. R., & Lebiere, C. (1998). *The atomic components of thought.* Mahwah, NJ: Lawrence Erlbaum.

Arthur, J., W., Barrett, G. V., & Alexander, R. A. (1991). Prediction of vehicular accident analysis: A meta–analysis. *Human Performance, 4,* 89–105.

Batchelder, W. H., & Romney, A. K. (1988). Test theory without an answer key. *Psychometrica, 53,* 71–92.

Cantor, N., & Kihlstrom, J. F. (1987). *Personality and social intelligence.* Englewood Cliffs, NJ: Prentice-Hall.

Carroll, J. B. (1993). *Human cognitive abilities: A survey of factor–analytic studies.* New York: Cambridge University Press.

Chi, M. T. H., Glaser, R., & Farr, M. J. (1988). *The nature of expertise.* Hillsdale, NJ: Lawrence Erlbaum.

Detterman, D. K., Caruso, D. R., Mayer, J. D., Legree, P. J., & Conners, F. (1992). Assessment of basic cognitive abilities in relation to cognitive deficits; mopping up: Relation between cognitive processes and intelligence. *American Journal on Mental Retardation, 97,* 251–286.

Hedlund, J., Forsythe, G. B., Horvath, J. A., Williams, W. M., Snook, S., & Sternberg, R. J. (2003). Identifying and assessing tacit knowledge: Understanding the practical intelligence of military leaders. *Leadership Quarterly, 14,* 117–140.

Heffner, T. S., & Porr, W. B. (2000, August). *Scoring situational judgment tests: A comparison of multiple standards using scenario response alternatives.* Paper presented at the Annual Conference of the American Psychological Association, Washington, DC.

James, L. R. (1998). Measurement of personality via conditional reasoning. *Organizational Research Methods, 1,* 131–163.

Jensen, A. R. (1998). *The g factor.* Westport, CT: Praeger.

Legree, P. J. (1995). Evidence for an oblique social intelligence factor. *Intelligence, 21,* 247–266.

Legree, P. J., & Grafton, F. C. (1995). *Evidence for an interpersonal knowledge factor: The reliability and factor structure of tests of interpersonal knowledge and general cognitive ability* (ARI Technical Report No. 1030). Alexandria, VA: U.S. Army Research Institute for the Behavioral and Social Sciences.

Legree, P. J., Heffner, T. S., Psotka, J., Martin, D. E., & Medsker, G. J. (2003). Traffic crash involvement: Experiential driving knowledge and stressful contextual antecedents. *Journal of Applied Psychology, 88,* 15–26.

Legree, P. J., Martin, D. E., & Psotka, J. (2000). Measuring cognitive aptitude using unobtrusive knowledge tests: A new survey technology. *Intelligence, 28,* 291–308.

Mayer, J. D., Caruso, D. R., & Salovey, P. (1999). Emotional intelligence meets traditional standards for an intelligence. *Intelligence, 27,* 267–298.

Mayer, J. D., Salovey, P., Caruso, D. R., & Sitarenios, G. (2003). Modeling and measuring emotional intelligence with the MSCEIT V2.0. *Emotion, 3,* 97–105.

McDaniel, M. A., Morgeson, F. P., Finnegan, E. B., Campion, M. A., & Braverman, E. P. (2001). Use of situational judgement tests to predict job performance: A clarification of the literature. *Journal of Applied Psychology, 86,* 730–740.

Psotka, J. (1977). Syntely: Paradigm for an inductive psychology of memory, perception, and thinking. *Memory and Cognition, 3,* 553–600.

Psotka, J., Streeter, L. A., Landauer, T. K., Lochbaum, K. E., & Robinson, K. (2004). *Augmenting electronic environments for leadership.* In Advanced Technologies for Military Training: Proceedings No. RTO-MP-HFM-101-21 of the Human Factors and Medicine Panel, Genoa, Italy, October 13, 2003 (pp. 287–301). Neuilly-sur-Seine, France: Research and Technology Organization.

Roberts, R. D., Zeidner, M., & Matthews, G. (2001). Does emotional intelligence meet traditional standards for an intelligence? Some new data and conclusions. *Emotion, 1,* 196–231.

Romney, A. K., & Weller, S. C. (1984). Predicting informant accuracy from patterns of recall among informants. *Social Networks, 6,* 59–77.

Schaie, K. W. (2001). Emotional intelligence: Psychometric status and developmental characteristics—Comment on Roberts, Zeidner, and Matthews. *Emotion, 1,* 243–248.

Sternberg, R. J., Forsythe, G. B., Hedlund, J., Horvath, J. A., Wagner, R. K., Williams, W. M., et al. (2000). *Practical intelligence in everyday life.* New York: Cambridge University Press.

Thomson, G. H. (1928). A worked out example of the possible linkages of four correlated variables on the sampling theory. *The British Journal of Psychology, 18,* 68–76.

Thomson, G. H. (1939). *The factorial analysis of human ability.* New York: Houghton-Mifflin Company.

Veling, I. H. (1982). Measuring driving knowledge. *Accident, Analysis, & Prevention, 14,* 81–85.

Zeidner, M., Matthews, G., & Roberts, R. D. (2001). Slow down you move too fast: Emotional intelligence remains an elusive intelligence. *Emotion, 1,* 265–275.

9

Measuring Trait Emotional Intelligence

Juan Carlos Pérez
Faculty of Education, Universidad Nacional de Educación a Distancia (UNED), Spain

K. V. Petrides
Institute of Education, University of London, UK

Adrian Furnham
Department of Psychology, University College London, UK

Summary

This chapter provides a brief introduction to the construct of emotional intelligence (EI), focusing on the conceptual distinction between trait EI (or emotional self-efficacy) and ability EI (or cognitive-emotional ability). The former encompasses emotion-related behavioral dispositions and self-perceived abilities measured via self-report, whereas the latter concerns actual emotion-related cognitive abilities and must be measured via maximum-performance tests. Salient measures of both types of EI are succinctly reviewed. It is argued that in terms of measurement most success has been achieved in relation to trait EI rather than ability EI. The overarching message of the chapter is that progress in the field is contingent on recognizing the fundamental differences between the two EI constructs.

9.1　INTRODUCTION

In *Sense and Nonsense in Psychology*, Hans J. Eysenck posed the question whether personality could ever be measured. He noted: "the answer depends on what we mean by personality, what we mean by measurement, and, indeed, one might even maintain that it depends on the meaning of the term 'can' " (Eysenck, 1958, p. 175). Although emotional intelligence (EI) has been the subject of much attention, both at the popular as well as at the academic level, only now are we beginning to provide answers to some of the fundamental questions posed about the construct. This chapter reviews the status of the EI field, with special reference to the distinction between trait EI and ability EI, and focuses specifically on the measurement of the former construct.

9.2　BRIEF HISTORY OF EI

The distal roots of EI can be traced back to Thorndike's (1920) social intelligence, which concerned the ability to understand and manage people and to act wisely in human relations. Its proximal roots lie in Gardner's (1983) work on multiple intelligences and, more specifically, his concepts of intrapersonal and interpersonal intelligence. According to Gardner (1999), "*interpersonal intelligence* denotes a person's capacity to understand the intentions, motivations, and desires of other people and, consequently, to work effectively with others" (p. 43). By contrast, "*intrapersonal intelligence* involves the capacity to understand oneself, to have an effective working model of oneself—including one's own desires, fears, and capacities —and to use such information effectively in regulating one's own life" (p. 43).

As a term, *emotional intelligence* appeared several times in the literature (Greenspan, 1989; Leuner, 1966; Payne, 1986), before the first formal model and definition were introduced by Salovey and Mayer (1990). These researchers also carried out the first relevant empirical studies (Mayer, DiPaolo, & Salovey, 1990). Goleman's (1995) influential book popularized the construct and strongly influenced most subsequent scientific conceptualizations of EI. Thus, following the model proposed by Salovey and Mayer, and especially after Goleman's best-selling book, many models of EI emerged. However, the correspondence between models and data has been weak in the majority of cases, with most models being dissociated from empirical evidence and most studies carried out in a theoretical vacuum.

9.3　TRAIT EI VERSUS ABILITY EI

In the rush to create measures of this emerging construct, researchers and theorists overlooked the fundamental difference between *typical* versus *maximal* performance (e.g., Ackerman & Heggestad, 1997; Cronbach, 1949; Hofstee, 2001. Thus, while some researchers developed and used self-report questionnaires, others embarked on the development of maximum-performance tests of EI. All, however, assumed they were operationalizing the same construct. Unsurprisingly, this led to conceptual confusion and numerous, seemingly conflicting, findings.

The manner in which individual differences variables are measured (self-report versus maximum-performance) has a direct impact on their operationalization. In recognition of this basic fact, Petrides and Furnham (2000a, 2000b, 2001) distinguished between *trait EI* (or emotional self-efficacy) and *ability EI* (or cognitive-emotional ability). It is important to understand that trait EI and ability EI are two *different* constructs. The former is measured through self-report questionnaires, whereas the latter ought to be measured through tests of maximal performance. This measurement distinction has far-reaching theoretical and practical implications. For example, trait EI would not be expected to correlate strongly with measures of general cognitive ability (g) or proxies thereof, whereas ability EI should be unequivocally related to such measures.

9.4   MIXED VERSUS ABILITY MODELS OF EI

The distinction between trait EI and ability EI is predicated on the method used to measure the construct and *not* on the elements (facets) that the various models are hypothesized to encompass. As such, it is unrelated to the distinction between mixed and ability models of EI (Mayer, Salovey, & Caruso, 2000), which is based on whether or not a theoretical model mixes cognitive abilities and personality traits.

Unlike the distinction between trait EI and ability EI, that between mixed and ability models pays no heed to the most crucial aspect of construct operationalization (i.e., the method of measurement) and is perfectly compatible with the idea of assessing cognitive ability variables via self-report (see Mayer et al. 2000; Tapia, 2001). However, it should be clear that cognitive abilities cannot be successfully assessed through self-report procedures. Indeed, correlations between actual and self-estimated scores tend to hover around $r = .30$ (Furnham, 2001; Paulhus, Lysy, & Yik, 1998).

Mayer et al.'s (2000) distinction between mixed versus ability models is at variance both with established psychometric theory, because it neglects the issue of the measurement method, as well as with all available empirical evidence, which clearly shows that self-report measures of EI tend to intercorrelate strongly, irrespective of whether or not they are based on mixed or ability models. All incoming data continue to highlight the need to distinguish between two EI constructs, namely, trait EI and ability EI (O'Connor & Little, 2003; Warwick & Nettelbeck, 2004).

9.5 MEASUREMENT OF ABILITY EI

The most prominent measures of ability EI are the Multifactor Emotional Intelligence Scale (MEIS Mayer, Caruso, & Salovey, 1999) and its successor, the Mayer-Salovey-Caruso Emotional Intelligence Test (MSCEIT; Mayer, Salovey, and Caruso, 2002). However, other measures of this construct are slowly starting to emerge. Table 9.1 presents a summary of ability EI measures, along with basic information about their reliability, validity, and factor structure.

The problem that ability EI tests have to tackle is the inherent subjectivity of emotional experience (e.g., Spain, Eaton, & Funder, 2000; Watson, 2000). Unlike standard cognitive ability tests, tests of ability EI cannot be objectively scored because, in most cases, there are no clear-cut criteria for what constitutes a correct response. Ability EI tests have attempted to bypass this problem by relying on alternative scoring procedures, which had also been used in the past for addressing similar difficulties in the operationalization of social intelligence, but without marked success (see Matthews, Zeidner, & Roberts, 2002). It is perhaps still too early to pass final judgment on the effectiveness of these procedures and it should be noted that some progress has been achieved over the many iterations that the best of these tests have undergone (e.g., Mayer et al., 2002). Indeed, some researchers argue that ability EI tests have improved considerably over the years (Matthews, Zeidner, & Roberts, in press). In our view, the fact that ability EI tests, after over a decade of research and development, continue to grapple with questions about internal consistency and factor structure does not augur well for their future.

9.6 MEASUREMENT OF TRAIT EI

The explosion in the number of trait EI measures may have given the impression that the construction of psychometrically sound questionnaires is an easy business. Anyone cognizant of the basic elements of psychometrics, particularly those relating to the validation process, knows that this is not the case. The fact is that few trait EI measures have been developed within a clear theoretical framework and even fewer have sturdy empirical foundations. Indicative of the confusion in the field is that most self-report questionnaires purport to measure EI as a cognitive ability. Table 9.2 presents a summary of trait EI measures, along with basic information about their reliability, validity, and factor structure. The entries have been organized by year of publication and principal author surnames. Some additional information for each measure is presented in the text.

Table 9.1 Summary of Ability EI Measures

Measure	Authors	α	r_{tt}	Pred. Val.	Incr. Val.	Conv./Discr. Val.	Structure
EARS. Emotional Accuracy Research Scale	Mayer & Geher (1996)	Low (.24 for target scoring and .53 for consensus scoring	?	?	?	Small and unstable correlations with self-report empathy	Unclear (4 factors?)
EISC. Emotional Intelligence Scale for Children	Sullivan (1999)	Low to moderate	?	?	?	?	?
MEIS. Multifactor Emotional Intelligence Scale	Mayer et al. (1999)	Good for global ability EI (.70–.80), but low (.35–.66) for branches 3 & 4 (better for consensus than for expert scoring)	?	Unclear	?	Small to moderate correlations with crystallized intelligence (Gc) Low correlations with the Big Five	Unclear (3 factors?)

table continues

Table 9.1 Summary of Ability EI Measures

Measure	Authors	α	r_{tt}	Pred. Val.	Incr. Val.	Conv./Discr. Val.	Structure
MSCEIT. Mayer-Salovey-Caruso Emotional Intelligence Test	Mayer et al. (2002)	Better for Version 2 than Version 1 (.68–.71)	?	Well-being, verbal SAT scores	Social deviance (over personality and verbal intelligence)	Convergence between general consensus and expert consensus scoring. Very low correlations (< .30) with trait EI measures	Unclear (4 factors?)
FNEIPT. Freudenthaler & Neubauer Emotional Intelligence Performance Test	Freudenthaler & Neubauer (2003)	Moderate: .69 for "managing own emotions" and .64 for "managing others' emotions"	?	?	?	"Managing own emotions" correlated with self-reported intrapersonal EI (.51), and "managing others' emotions" correlated with self-report interpersonal EI (.25). Both subscales correlated with the Big Five (.18 to −.51)	Unclear (2 factors?)

Note. Information in this table is necessarily succinct and readers are encouraged to consult the original sources for specific details. Entries designated "unclear" do not necessarily indicate conflicting evidence, as they may also refer to lack of adequate data. Question marks indicate that we have been unable to obtain data for the relevant entry.

α = Reliability estimate Cronbach's α, r_{tt} = Test-retest reliability estimate, Pred. Val. = Predictive validity, Incr. Val. = Incremental validity, Conv./Discr. Val. = Convergent/discriminant validity, Structure = Factor structure.

Trait Meta-Mood Scale (TMMS; Salovey et al., 1995)

The first measure of EI, in general, and of trait EI, in particular, the TMMS is loosely based on the original model by Salovey and Mayer (1990). It comprises 30 items, which are responded to on a 5-point Likert scale. The TMMS produces scores on three factors, namely, "attention to emotion", "emotional clarity", and "emotion repair". Contrary to the assumption of many users, the TMMS was not designed to yield a global score, which should be taken into account when analyzing data and interpreting results. Another point to keep in mind is that the TMMS was not designed to cover the entire trait EI sampling domain and, thus, overlooks many core facets of the construct.

BarOn Emotional Quotient Inventory (EQ-i; Bar-On, 1997)

The EQ-i is one of the most widely used measures of trait EI in the literature. Its theoretical background is somewhat vague, having been converted from a well-being inventory to an EI questionnaire. The a-priori structure of the EQ-*i* is 133 items, 15 subscales, and 5 higher-order factors: "intrapersonal", "interpersonal", "adaptation", "stress management", and "general mood". Empirically, however, there is no evidence for a higher-order structure, as the questionnaire seems to be unifactorial (Petrides & Furnham, 2001). Furthermore, in an item-level factor analysis, Palmer, Manocha, Gignac, and Stough (2003) identified a solution comprising six subscales, instead of the 15 reported in the technical manual of the inventory. Another limitation of the EQ-*i* is that it includes several irrelevant facets (e.g., "problem solving", "reality testing", "independence") and neglects many relevant ones (e.g., "emotion perception", "emotion expression", "emotion regulation"). The EQ-*i* covers the sampling domain of trait EI better than many other inventories, as can be seen by a comparison of Tables 1 and 2 in Petrides and Furnham (2001).

Schutte Emotional Intelligence Scale (SEIS Schutte et al., 1998)

The SEIS consists of 33 items responded to on a 5-point Likert scale. Its psychometric properties have been scrutinized in several papers (e.g., Austin, Saklofske, Huang, & McKenney, 2004; Petrides & Furnham, 2000b; Saklofske, Austin, & Minski, 2003) and it has been found to have between three and four factors. The main shortcoming of the SEIS is that it provides incomplete coverage of the trait EI domain, being exclusively based on the three dimensions postulated in the early Salovey and Mayer (1990) model. Nevertheless, it has been used extensively in the literature and can be employed as a short measure of global trait EI (Schutte et al., 2001).

Emotional Competence Inventory (ECI; Boyatzis et al., 1999)

The ECI measures "emotional competencies" broadly related to EI. It has two forms (self-report and 360 degree). Currently, there exist two versions: Version 1 (110 items, 7-point Likert scale) and Version 2 (73 items, 6-point Likert

Table 9.2 Summary of Trait EI Measures

Measure	Authors	α	r_{tt}	Pred. Val.	Incr. Val.	Conv./Discr. Val.	Structure
TMMS. Trait Meta Mood Scale	Salovey, Mayer, Goldman, Turvey, & Palfai (1995)	.70–.85	?	Depression, mood recovery, goal orientation	?	Moderate correlations with the Big Five	3 factors, but no global score
EQ-i. Emotional Quotient Inventory	Bar-On (1997)	Generally good (about .85)	Good	Mental health, coping, work and marital satisfaction	?	Moderate to high correlations with the Big Five	Unclear
SEIS. Schutte Emotional Intelligence Scales	Schutte et al. (1998)	.70–.85	?	Social support, life and marital satisfaction, depression, performance on cognitive tasks	Some evidence vis-à-vis the Big Five	Medium-to-high correlations with the Big Five	Unclear (3 or 4 factors?) global score
ECI. Emotional Competence Inventory	Boyatzis, Goleman, & Hay/McBer (1999)	.70–.85 for global score, > .85 for social skills	Adequate, but based on small samples	Moderate correlations with managerial styles and organizational climate. Low correlations with career success	?	Unclear (small samples); uncorrelated with critical thinking and with analytical reasoning	Unclear (4 factors?)
EI-IPIP. Emotional Intelligence-based IPIP-Scales	Barchard (2001)	.70–.85	?	?	?	?	?

table continues

Table 9.2   Summary of Trait EI Measures

Measure	Authors	α	r_{tt}	Pred. Val.	Incr. Val.	Conv./Discr. Val.	Structure
EISRS. Emotional Intelligence Self-Regulation Scale	Martinez-Pons (2000)	.75–.94	?	Depression, life satisfaction, positive affect	?	Unclear	Unclear (1 factor?)
DHEIQ. Dulewicz & Higgs Emotional Intelligence Questionnaire	Dulewicz & Higgs (2001)	Low to moderate (.54–.71)	?	Organizational level advancement	?	Unclear	Unclear
TEIQue. Trait Emotional Intelligence Questionnaire	For example, Petrides (2001), Petrides, Pérez, & Furnham (2003)	Generally good (about .85)	Good (.50–.82; global score .78; 12-month period)	Mental health (depression, personality disorders, dysfunctional attitudes), adaptive coping styles, job stress, job performance, organizational commitment, deviant behavior at school, sensitivity to mood induction	Good vis-à-vis Giant Three, Big Five, and positive and negative affect	The TEIQue can be isolated in Giant Three and Five-Factor space (Petrides, 2001)	4 factors, global score

table continues

Table 9.2 Summary of Trait EI Measures

Measure	Authors	α	r_{tt}	Pred. Val.	Incr. Val.	Conv./Discr. Val.	Structure
SPTB. Sjöberg Personality Test Battery (EI Scale)	Sjöberg (2001)	.70–.85	?	Anti-authoritarian attitudes, emotion identification skills, social orientation	?	Moderate correlations with Extraversion (.37) and Neuroticism (−.50)	?
TEII. Tapia Emotional Intelligence Inventory	Tapia (2001)	.70–.85	Good (.60–.70)	?	?	?	4 factors, global score
SUEIT. Swinburne University Emotional Intelligence Test	Palmer & Stough (2002)	Generally good (about .85)	Good (.82–.94, 1-month period)	Well-being, occupational stress	?	Moderate correlations with Neuroticism (−.41), Extraversion (.44), Openness (.27)	?
WEIP-3. Workgroup Emotional Intelligence Profile (Version 3)	Jordan, Ashkanasy, Härtel, & Hooper (2002)	.70–.85	?	Self-Monitoring, empathy	?	Small to moderate correlations with TMMS	Unclear (7 factors?)

table continues

MEASUREMENT OF TRAIT EI   191

Table 9.2 Summary of trait EI Measures

Measure	Authors	α	r_{tt}	Pred. Val.	Incr. Val.	Conv./Discr. Val.	Structure
EIS. Emotional Intelligence Scales	Van der Zee, Schakel, & Thijs (2002)	Adequate for "other ratings" (.70–.85) Low for self-ratings (< .60)	?	Academic performance, social success	Some evidence vis-à-vis the Big Five	Low correlations with IQ. Moderate to high correlations with the Big Five	Unclear (3 factors?)
WLEIS. Wong & Law Emotional Intelligence Scales	Wong & Law (2002)	.70–85	?	Job performance and satisfaction. Organizational commitment, turnover intention	?	Small negative correlations with IQ	4 factors, global score
LEIQ. Lioussine Emotional Intelligence Questionnaire	Lioussine (2003)	.70–85	?	?	?	Moderate correlations with the Big Five	Unclear (7 factors?)

Note. Information in this table is necessarily succinct and readers are encouraged to consult the original sources for specific details. Entries designated "unclear" do not necessarily indicate conflicting evidence, as they may also refer to lack of adequate data. Question marks indicate that we have been unable to obtain data for the relevant entry.

α = Reliability estimate Cronbach's α, r_{tt} = Test-retest reliability estimate, Pred. Val. = Predictive validity, Incr. Val. = Incremental validity, Conv./Discr. Val. = Convergent/discriminant validity, Structure = Factor structure.

scale; Sala, 2002). The ECI consists of 20 dimensions (called competencies) that are organized into four clusters: "self-awareness", "self-management", "social awareness", and "social skills". Although it has proved popular in the field of human resources management, there seems to be little information about its psychometric properties in scientific journals.

Emotional Intelligence IPIP Scales (EI-IPIP; Barchard, 2001)

The EI-IPIP appears in the International Personality Item Pool web site (http://www.ipip.org). It comprises 68 items organized into seven components: "positive expressivity", "negative expressivity", "attending to emotions", "emotion-based decision making", "responsive joy", "responsive distress", and "empathic concern". Barchard (2001) presents gender-specific internal consistency values for each of the seven components, ranging from .59 to .83. To our knowledge, the EI-IPIP has not yet been used in the scientific literature.

Emotional Intelligence Self-Regulation Scale (EISRS; Martinez-Pons, 2000)

This instrument is based on Martinez-Pons's self-regulation model of EI, which attempts to integrate Bandura's social-cognitive theory with the original EI model by Salovey and Mayer (1990). The EISRS consists of 52 items, responded to on a 7-point Likert scale, 10 subscales and four higher-order dimensions: "motivation", "goal setting", "strategy usage", and "self-evaluation of strategy effectiveness and adjustment". Martinez-Pons (2000) presents data based on a sample of 100 adults showing adequate internal consistency reliabilities for the EISRS. To our knowledge, this scale has not yet been used in other studies in the literature.

Dulewicz & Higgs Emotional Intelligence Questionnaire (DHEIQ; Dulewicz & Higgs, 2001; Higgs & Dulewicz, 1999)

The DHEIQ is based on Goleman's (1995, 1998) books and was designed for use in organizational settings. It consists of 69 items organized into seven dimensions: "self-awareness", "influence", "decisiveness", "interpersonal sensitivity", "motivation", "conscientiousness and integrity", and "resilience". The DHEIQ has not been used much in the scientific literature and there is little information about its reliability and validity.

Trait Emotional Intelligence Questionnaire (TEIQue; Petrides, 2001; Petrides & Furnham, 2003; Petrides et al., 2003)

Over the past six years, the various forms and translations of the TEIQue are being developed, adapted, and validated within the context of an academic research program,[1] focusing primarily on trait EI (e.g., Furnham & Petrides, 2003; Pérez, 2003; Petrides, Frederickson, & Furnham, 2004). The TEIQue is predicated on the trait EI theory and model, which conceptualizes emotional intelligence as a personality trait, located at the lower levels of personality hierarchies (e.g., Petrides & Furnham, 2000b, 2001, 2003). The latest version of the long form of the TEIQue comprises 153 items, providing scores on 15 subscales, four factors, and global trait EI. The dimensionality of the TEIQue is currently under investigation. Early analyses appear to support a four-factor structure comprising "well-being", "self-control skills", "emotional skills", and "social skills". Empirical studies using various TEIQue forms and versions have been reported in Furnham and Petrides (2003); Petrides and Furnham (2003); Petrides et al. (2004).

Sjöberg Personality Test Battery (SPTB; Sjöberg, 2001)

The SPTB is a large battery measuring many different personality constructs and facets, including trait EI. The complete battery comprises 789 items, responded to on a 4-point Likert scale. In an exploratory factor analysis of the 21 SPTB scales, one of the four factors obtained encompassed seven traits which the author interpreted as dimensions of EI: "introversion", "empathy", "emotional inhibition", "machiavellianism", "alexithymia", "self-actualization", and "external attribution".

Tapia Emotional Intelligence Inventory (TEII; Tapia, 2001)

The TEII epitomizes the theoretical confusion permeating the field, purporting to operationalize the cognitive ability model of Mayer and Salovey (1997) via self-report items. It should be clear that the TEII is a measure of trait EI because its items attempt to operationalize self-perceptions and dispositions, rather than emotion-related cognitive abilities. The TEII consists of 41 items that factor into four dimensions: "empathy", "utilization of feelings", "handling relationships", and "self-control".

Work-Place Swinburne University Emotional Intelligence Test (Work-place SUEIT; Palmer & Stough, 2002)

This is another measure of the construct designed for use in the workplace. The Work-place SUEIT comprises 64 items, responded to on a 5-point Likert scale. It produces a global score as well as scores on five, empirically determined, subscales: "emotional recognition and expression", "understanding emotions", "emotions direct cognition", "emotional management", and "emotional control". The Work-place SUEIT is relatively new and its reliability and validity are currently under investigation.

---

[1]All TEIQue forms and translations are available from the second author of this chapter, free of charge, for research purposes only.

Workgroup Emotional Intelligence Profile (WEIP; Jordan et al., 2002)

This measure was designed to profile the EI of individuals in workgroups. It consists of 27 items, responded to on a 7-point Likert scale and measuring seven facets organized into two broad dimensions ("intrapersonal" and "interpersonal"). Early research with the WEIP has shown that work teams comprising high trait EI employees tend to perform better than work teams comprising low trait EI employees (Jordan et al., 2002).

Emotional Intelligence Scale (EIS; Van der Zee et al., 2002)

The EIS comprises 85 items responded to on a 5-point Likert scale and measuring 17 subscales. It appears to have a three-factor structure comprising "empathy", "autonomy", and "emotional control". The internal consistencies for most EIS subscales are relatively low, with several values below the .50 mark. Consistent with the conceptual distinction between trait and ability EI, Van der Zee et al. (2002) found that the EIS is related to personality traits, but not to cognitive ability.

Wong & Law Emotional Intelligence Scale (WLEIS; Wong & Law, 2002)

The WLEIS was designed as a short measure of EI for use in organizational research. It comprises 16 items, responded to on a 7-point Likert scale and measuring four dimensions: "self-emotion appraisal", "emotion appraisal of others", "use of emotion", and "regulation of emotion". Wong and Law (2002) report good internal consistency reliabilities for their measure. In terms of validity, they present data showing that scores on the WLEIS are related to job performance and job satisfaction.

Lioussine Emotional Intelligence Questionnaire (LEIQ; Lioussine, 2003)

This is a trait EI questionnaire developed in the Russian language. It consists of 38 items based on a 4-point Likert scale. Its structure includes eight subscales and two broad dimensions ("intrapersonal" and "interpersonal"). The LEIQ is also relatively new and its reliability and validity are currently under investigation.

9.7   GENERAL COMMENTS ON THE MEASUREMENT OF EI

In most cases, the existence of alternative measures for the same construct is a sign of research progress. We suspect the main reason why this is not the case with trait EI is that the field remains stuck in a pre-paradigmatic state in which questionnaires are being developed without adequate reference to underlying theory; psychometric or substantive. Indeed, most authors and users of these instruments are still under the impression that EI is a unitary construct that can be measured via self-report questionnaires or via maximum-performance tests or via makeshift tasks, without any implications for its conceptualization, or its nomological network, or the interpretation of the resultant findings.

It should be pointed out that not all trait EI measures are open to the foregoing criticisms. However, instead of concentrating on the relative strengths and weaknesses of the various inventories, it would be more profitable briefly to counter a criticism that continues to be levelled against trait EI as a construct. Thus, it is sometimes construed as a serious shortcoming that trait EI is related to the basic personality dimensions and does not always contribute incrementally to the prediction of criterion variance (e.g., MacCann, Matthews, Zeidner, & Roberts, 2004; Salovey, Woolery, & Mayer, 2001). This criticism must be put into perspective by emphasizing once again that the conceptualization of EI as a lower-order personality trait (Petrides & Furnham, 2001) evidently implies that it will be associated with higher-order personality dimensions. Indeed, it would be rather odd if a lower-order personality construct were unrelated to the higher-order personality dimensions that define the factor space it occupies. It is both true and repeatedly noted by researchers (e.g., Petrides et al., 2004) that neither type of EI has effects that are in line with expectations that have been built up in the popular literature (e.g., Cooper & Sawaf, 1997). However, it is also the case that the discriminant and incremental validity of the construct are beyond empirical doubt (Saklofske et al., 2003). In any event, it is important to realize that the issue of incremental validity, as currently discussed, is of limited theoretical significance for the understanding of the construct (see Petrides & Furnham, 2003).

A related issue concerns the sampling domain on which the various EI measures (trait and ability) are based. The first step in the operationalization of a psychological construct entails defining its sampling domain, that is, the facets (elements) that the construct encompasses (e.g., Cattell, 1973). Virtually all EI models, questionnaires, and tests have bypassed this step, providing arbitrarily defined sampling domains. This is evident in Table 9.3, which presents a concise summary of salient EI models, along with the main facets that they encompass.

In the vast majority of cases, the inclusion or exclusion of facets in a model is the result of unstated or arbitrary processes. Also worth noting here is the fact that many facets may sound different, but are operationally the same ("jangle fallacy"; see Block, 1995).

With respect to the elements they encompass, the various models of EI tend to be complementary rather than contradictory (Ciarrochi, Chan, & Caputi, 2000). Moreover, salient EI models tend to share many core facets, even though they also include ones that are prima facie irrelevant to the construct. The commonalities between models provided the basis for the systematic identification of the first sampling domain of trait EI, which included the shared facets, but excluded the peculiar ones (Petrides & Furnham, 2001). The TEIQue is modeled directly on this sampling domain.

As regards the view that trait EI measures are little more than proxies for the Giant Three or the Big Five (e.g., Brackett & Mayer, 2003; Matthews et al., in press), we believe that it is overly pessimistic. There is compelling evidence

Table 9.3   Summary of EI Models

Salovey & Mayer (1990)	Goleman (1995)	Mayer & Salovey (1997)	Bar-On (1997)	Cooper & Sawaf (1997)
– Appraisal and expression of emotion – Utilization of emotion – Regulation of emotion	– Self-awareness – Self-regulation – Self-motivation – Empathy – Handling relationships	– Perception, appraisal, and expression of emotion – Emotional facilitation of thinking – Understanding and analyzing emotions; employing emotional knowledge – Reflective regulation of emotions to promote emotional and intellectual growth	*Intrapersonal* – Emotional self-awareness – Assertiveness – Self-regard – Self-actualization – Independence *Interpersonal* – Empathy – Interpersonal relationship – Social responsibility *Adaptation* – Problem solving – Reality testing – Flexibility *Stress management* – Stress tolerance – Impulse control *General mood* – Happiness – Optimism	– Emotional literacy – Emotional fitness – Emotional depth – Emotional alchemy

table continues

Table 9.3   Summary of EI Models

Goleman (1998)	Weisinger (1998)	Higgs & Dulewicz (1999)	Petrides & Furnham (2001)
Self-awareness – Emotional self-awareness – Accurate self-assessment – Self-confidence	– Self-awareness – Emotional management	*Drivers* – Motivation – Intuitiveness	– Adaptability – Assertiveness
Self-regulation – Self-control – Trust worthiness – Conscientiousness – Adaptability – Innovation	– Self-motivation – Effective communication skills	*Constrainers* – Conscientiousness – Emotional resilience	– Emotion appraisal (self & others) – Emotion expression
Self-motivation – Achievement orientation – Commitment – Initiative – Optimism	– Interpersonal expertise – Emotional coaching	*Enablers* – Self-awareness – Interpersonal sensitivity – Influence – Trait	– Emotion management (others) – Emotion regulation
Empathy – Empathy – Organizational awareness – Service orientation – Developing others – Leveraging diversity			– Impulsiveness (low) – Relationship skills – Self-esteem
Social Skills – Leadership – Communication – Influence – Change catalyst – Conflict management – Building bonds – Collaboration and co-operation – Team capabilities			- Self-motivation – Social competence – Stress management – Trait empathy – Trait happiness – Trait optimism

Note. This table cannot always include all the elements and relevant information in the various models. Interested readers are encouraged to consult the original sources and other chapters in this book (e.g., Chapter 2 by Neubauer and Freudenthaler).

in support of the discriminant and incremental validity of trait EI, including the isolation of an oblique trait EI factor in Eysenckian as well as Big Five factor space and mounting data showing that several of the measures used to operationalize the construct are able to predict criteria in the presence of the basic personality traits (e.g ., Furnham & Petrides, 2003; Saklofske et al., 2003).

We had three aims in writing this chapter. First, to describe the latest research findings in the EI field, with special reference to the measurement of trait EI. Second, to provide a useful listing of existing EI measures, along with basic information about their structure, reliability, and validity. As regards the first two aims, although some measures are still new, the rationale and theoretical background upon which they are based, in combination with the context within which they have been developed gives a clear indication of their potential for achieving construct validity. Our final aim was to motivate the reader critically to reflect on the extant literature by sifting facts from opinions and speculation. The most basic conclusion to be drawn from such reflection is that the operationalization of EI as a cognitive ability leads to a different construct than its operationalization as a personality trait.

REFERENCES

Ackerman, P. L., & Heggestad, E. D. (1997). Intelligence, personality, and interests: Evidence for overlapping traits. *Psychological Bulletin, 121*, 219–245.

Austin, E. J., Saklofske, D. H., Huang, S. H. S., & McKenney, D. (2004). Measurement of trait emotional intelligence: Testing and cross-validating a modified version of Schutte et al.'s (1998) measure. *Personality and Individual Differences, 36*, 555–562.

Barchard, K. A. (2001). *Seven components potentially related to emotional intelligence.* Retrieved August 11, 2003 from http://ipip.ori.org.

Bar-On, R. (1997). *BarOn Emotional Quotient Inventory (EQ–i): Technical manual.* Toronto, Canada: Multi-Health Systems.

Block, J. (1995). A contrarian view of the five-factor approach to personality description. *Psychological Bulletin, 117*, 187–215.

Boyatzis, R. E., Goleman, D., & Hay/McBer. (1999). *Emotional competence inventory.* Boston: HayGroup.

Brackett, M. A., & Mayer, J. D. (2003). Convergent, discriminant, and incremental validity of competing measures of emotional intelligence. *Personality and Social Psychology Bulletin, 29*, 1147–1158.

Cattell, R. B. (1973). *Personality and mood by questionnaire.* San Francisco: Jossey-Bass.

Ciarrochi, J., Chan, A. Y. C., & Caputi, P. (2000). A critical evaluation of the emotional intelligence construct. *Personality and Individual Differences, 28*, 539–561.

Cooper, R. K., & Sawaf, A. (1997). *Executive EQ: Emotional intelligence in leadership and organizations.* New York: Grosset/Putnam.

Cronbach, L. J. (1949). *Essentials of psychological testing.* New York: Harper & Row.

Dulewicz, S. V., & Higgs, M. J. (2001). *EI general and general 360 user guide.* Windsor, UK: NFER-Nelson.

Eysenck, H.-J. (1958). *Sense and nonsense in psychology.* Middlesex, UK: Penguin.

Freudenthaler, H. H., & Neubauer, A. C. (2003, July). *The localization of emotional intelligence within human abilities and personality.* Poster presented at the 11th Biennial Meeting of the International Society for the Study of the Individual Differences (ISSID), Graz, Austria.

Furnham, A. (2001). Self-estimates of intelligence: Culture and gender differences in self and other estimates of both general (*g*) and multiple intelligences. *Personality and Individual Differences, 31,* 1381–1405.

Furnham, A., & Petrides, K. V. (2003). Trait emotional intelligence and happiness. *Social Behavior and Personality, 31,* 815–823.

Gardner, H. (1983). *Frames of mind: The theory of multiple intelligences.* New York: Basic Books.

Gardner, H. (1999). *Intelligence reframed: Multiple intelligence for the 21st century.* New York: Basic Books.

Goleman, D. (1995). *Emotional intelligence: Why it can matter more than IQ.* New York: Bantam Books.

Goleman, D. (1998). *Working with emotional intelligence.* New York: Bantam.

Greenspan, S. I. (1989). Emotional intelligence. In K. Field, B. J. Cohler, & G. Wool (Eds.), *Learning and education: Psychoanalytic perspectives* (pp. 209–243). Madison, CT: International Universities Press.

Higgs, M. J., & Dulewicz, S. V. (1999). *Making sense of emotional intelligence.* Windsor, UK: NFER-Nelson.

Hofstee, W. K. B. (2001). Intelligence and personality: Do they mix? In J. Collis & S. Messick (Eds.), *Intelligence and personality: Bridging the gap in theory and measurement* (pp. 43–60). Mahwah, NJ: Lawrence Erlbaum.

Jordan, P. J., Ashkanasy, N. M., Härtel, C. E. J., & Hooper, G. S. (2002). Workgroup emotional intelligence scale development and relationship to team process effectiveness and goal focus. *Human Resource Management Review, 12,* 195–214.

Leuner, B. (1966). Emotionale Intelligenz und Emanzipation [Emotional intelligence and emancipation]. *Praxis der Kinderpsychologie und Kinderpsychiatry, 15,* 196–203.

Lioussine, D. V. (2003, July). *Gender differences in emotional intelligence.* Poster presented at the 11th Biennial Meeting of the International Society for the Study of the Individual Differences (ISSID), Graz, Austria.

MacCann, C., Matthews, G., Zeidner, M., & Roberts, R. D. (2004). The assessment of emotional intelligence: On frameworks, fissures, and the future. In G. Geher (Ed.), *Measuring emotional intelligence: Common ground and controversy* (pp. 21–52). Hauppauge, NY: Nova Science.

Martinez-Pons, M. (2000). Emotional intelligence as a self-regulatory process: A social cognitive view. *Imagination, Cognition and Personality, 19,* 331–350.

Matthews, G., Zeidner, M., & Roberts, R. D. (2002). *Emotional intelligence: Science and myth.* Cambridge, MA: MIT Press.

Matthews, G., Zeidner, M., & Roberts, R. D. (in press). Measuring emotional intelligence: Promises, pitfalls, solutions? In A. D. Ong & M. vanDulmen (Eds.), *Handbook of methods in positive psychology.* Oxford, UK: Oxford University Press.

Mayer, J. D., Caruso, D. R., & Salovey, P. (1999). Emotional intelligence meets traditional standards for an intelligence. *Intelligence, 27,* 267–298.

Mayer, J. D., DiPaolo, M., & Salovey, P. (1990). Perceiving affective content in ambiguous visual stimuli: A component of emotional intelligence. *Journal of Personality Assessment, 54*, 772–781.

Mayer, J. D., & Geher, G. (1996). Emotional intelligence and the identification of emotion. *Intelligence, 22*, 89–113.

Mayer, J. D., & Salovey, P. (1997). What is emotional intelligence? In P. Salovey & D. J. Sluyter (Eds.), *Emotional development and emotional intelligence: Educational implications* (pp. 3–31). New York: Basic Books.

Mayer, J. D., Salovey, P., & Caruso, D. R. (2000). Models of emotional intelligence. In R. J. Sternberg (Ed.), *The handbook of intelligence* (pp. 396–420). New York: Cambridge University Press.

Mayer, J. D., Salovey, P., & Caruso, D. R. (2002). *The Mayer-Salovey-Caruso Emotional Intelligence Test (MSCEIT): User's manual.* Toronto, Canada: Multi-Health Systems.

O'Connor, R. M., & Little, I. S. (2003). Revisiting the predictive validity of emotional intelligence: Self-report versus ability-based measures. *Personality and Individual Differences, 35*, 1893–1902.

Palmer, B. R., Manocha, R., Gignac, G., & Stough, C. (2003). Examining the factor structure of the Bar-On Emotional Quotient Inventory with an Australian general population sample. *Personality and Individual Differences, 35*, 1191–1210.

Palmer, B. R., & Stough, C. (2002). *Swinburne University Emotional Intelligence Test (Workplace SUEIT). Interim technical manual (Version 2).* Victoria, Australia: Swinburne University of Technology.

Paulhus, D. L., Lysy, D. C., & Yik, M. S. N. (1998). Self-report measures of intelligence: Are they useful as proxy IQ tests? *Journal of Personality, 66*, 525–554.

Payne, W. L. (1986). A study of emotion: Developing emotional intelligence, self-integration, relating to fear, pain, and desire. *Dissertation Abstracts International, 47*, 203.

Petrides, K. V. (2001). *A psychometric investigation into the construct of emotional intelligence.* University College London: Doctoral dissertation.

Petrides, K. V., Frederickson, N., & Furnham, A. (2004). The role of trait emotional intelligence in academic performance and deviant behavior at school. *Personality and Individual Differences, 36*, 277–293.

Petrides, K. V., & Furnham, A. (2000a). Gender differences in measured and self-estimated trait emotional intelligence. *Sex roles, 42*, 449–461.

Petrides, K. V., & Furnham, A. (2000b). On the dimensional structure of emotional intelligence. *Personality and Individual Differences, 29*, 313–320.

Petrides, K. V., & Furnham, A. (2001). Trait emotional intelligence: Psychometric investigation with reference to established trait taxonomies. *European Journal of Personality, 15*, 425–448.

Petrides, K. V., & Furnham, A. (2003). Trait emotional intelligence: Behavioural validation in two studies of emotion recognition and reactivity to mood induction. *European Journal of Personality, 17*, 39–57.

Petrides, K. V., Pérez, J. C., & Furnham, A. (2003, July). *The Trait Emotional Intelligence Questionnaire (TEIQue): A measure of emotional self-efficacy.* Paper presented at the

11th Biennial Meeting of the International Society for the Study of the Individual Differences (ISSID). Graz, Austria.

Pérez, J. C. (2003). Adaptación y validación espa nola del Trait Emotional Intelligence Questionnaire (TEIQue) en población universitaria [Spanish adaptation and validation of the Trait Emotional Intelligence Questionnaire (TEIQue) in a university population]. *Encuentros en psicología social, 1,* 278–283.

Saklofske, D. H., Austin, E. J., & Minski, P. S. (2003). Factor structure and validity of a trait emotional intelligence measure. *Personality and Individual Differences, 34,* 707–721.

Sala, F. (2002). *Emotional Competence Inventory: Technical manual.* Boston: Hay/McBer Group.

Salovey, P., & Mayer, J. D. (1990). Emotional intelligence. *Imagination, Cognition and Personality, 9,* 185–211.

Salovey, P., Mayer, J. D., Goldman, S., Turvey, C., & Palfai, T. (1995). Emotional attention, clarity, and repair: Exploring emotional intelligence using the Trait Meta–Mood Scale. In J. W. Pennebaker (Ed.), *Emotion, disclosure, and health* (pp. 125–154). Washington, DC: American Psychological Association.

Salovey, P., Woolery, A., & Mayer, J. D. (2001). Emotional intelligence: Conceptualization and measurement. In G. Fletcher & M. Clark (Eds.), *The blackwell handbook of social psychology* (pp. 279–307). London: Blackwell.

Schutte, N. S., Malouff, J. M., Bobik, C., Coston, T. D., Greeson, C., Jedlicka, C., et al. (2001). Emotional intelligence and interpersonal relations. *Journal of Social Psychology, 141,* 523–536.

Schutte, N. S., Malouff, J. M., Hall, L. E., Haggerty, D. J., Cooper, J. T., Golden, C. J., et al. (1998). Development and validation of a measure of emotional intelligence. *Personality and Individual Differences, 25,* 167–177.

Sjöberg, L. (2001). Emotional intelligence: A psychometric analysis. *European Psychologist, 6,* 79–95.

Spain, J. S., Eaton, L. G., & Funder, D. C. (2000). Perspectives on personality: The relative accuracy of self versus others for the prediction of emotion and behavior. *Journal of Personality, 68,* 837–867.

Sullivan, A. K. (1999). The emotional intelligence scale for children. *Dissertation Abstracts International, 60,* 68.

Tapia, M. (2001). Measuring emotional intelligence. *Psychological Reports, 88,* 353–364.

Thorndike, E. L. (1920). Intelligence and its use. *Harper's Magazine, 140,* 227–235.

Van der Zee, K., Schakel, L., & Thijs, M. (2002). The relationship of emotional intelligence with academic intelligence and the big five. *European Journal of Personality, 16,* 103–125.

Warwick, J., & Nettelbeck, T. (2004). Emotional intelligence is…? *Personality and Individual Differences, 37,* 1091–1100.

Watson, D. (2000). *Mood and temperament.* New York: Guilford.

Weisinger, H. (1998). *Emotional intelligence at work: The untapped edge for success.* San Francisco: Jossey-Bass.

Wong, C.-S., & Law, K. S. (2002). The effects of leader and follower emotional intelligence on performance and attitude: An exploratory study. *The Leadership Quarterly, 13,* 243–274.

10

Social Intelligence—A Review and Critical Discussion of Measurement Concepts

Susanne Weis
Heinz-Martin Süß
Otto-von-Guericke University Magdeburg, Germany

Summary

This chapter provides a description of theoretical and empirical approaches to sketch the nature and scope of the social intelligence construct. Detailed attention is given to the empirical investigations of the structure and validity of this construct. Research designs and outcomes of these studies are described along a classification of the applied measurement procedures that affect the validity of the studies. Our considerations support the assumption that method-related variance can explain a substantial part of the results. Therefore, we suggest applying multitrait-multimethod designs to control for this bias. In addition, past theoretical and empirical accounts are integrated into a performance model of social intelligence with the main focus on the cognitive facets of the construct: social understanding, social memory, social perception, and social creativity. Some empirical data is provided that supports this model. The chapter concludes by discussing important conceptual and measurement issues for future research: the importance of thoroughly specifying the intended measurement construct and the corresponding task requirements, the construction of tests that reflect the real-life significance of the construct, and a well-considered validation strategy (construct and predictive validity) that also takes related constructs like emotional intelligence into account.

10.1   INTRODUCTION

Psychological research has been concerned with the study of human intelligence for over a century. From its inception on up through the present time, academic (i.e., abstract or general) intelligence represents the most examined and clearly defined construct investigated as part of this scientific enterprise. Recently, however, the concept of human intelligence has been expanded with the introduction of so-called new intelligences, that is, social, emotional, and practical. The chapters contained in this book give detailed attention to theoretical and measurement issues of emotional intelligence. Nevertheless, a comprehensive scientific treatment of emotional intelligence cannot ignore the apparently related concept of social intelligence. Apart from common acceptance that both concepts receive in all parts of contemporary society (see e.g., Gardner, 1983; Goleman, 1995; Matthews, Zeidner, & Roberts, 2002), substantial overlap can also be perceived in theoretical definitions and measurement approaches. Relying on the long research tradition of social intelligence, future research in both fields may benefit from past lessons learned. In return, it seems essential for research on social intelligence to profit from the scientific interest and concerted endeavors that are currently concentrated, to a large measure, on emotional intelligence. Despite the long tradition of research on social intelligence, both theory and measurement issues remain unresolved at a (fairly) low level of sophistication. Further examination is also indispensable to eventually identifying a viable and discriminable domain of social intelligence.

The purpose of this chapter is to provide an overview of scientific investigations in the domain of social intelligence. Comparable approaches date back many years (see Orlik, 1978; Walker & Foley, 1973, for reviews). Since then, the research landscape has changed with respect to some aspects. For example, empirical studies have begun to make use of multitrait-multimethod designs, used structural equation modeling for data analysis, and various situational judgment testing paradigms to assess the so-called "construct space". In this chapter, we review the literature on social intelligence, including findings that have been obtained recently with these newer approaches.

10.2   THEORIES AND DEFINITIONS OF SOCIAL INTELLIGENCE

Thorndike (1920) postulated a framework of human intelligence differentiating between ideas, objects, and people as the contents that human intellect has to deal with. In other words, he discriminated between academic, mechanical, and social intelligence. In this framework, Thorndike (1920) defined the latter as "the ability to understand and manage men and women, boys and girls, and to act wisely in human relations" (p. 228). Thorndike's idea of social intelligence is still fundamental to, and even more extensive than, any other given definition. Indeed, most contemporary research efforts appear to cite

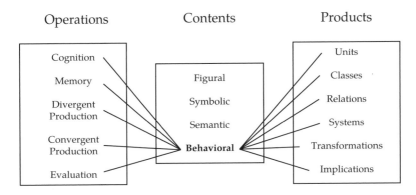

Figure 10.1   Structural Model of Human Intellect (Guilford, 1967); the domain of social intelligence (behavior) is highlighted in bold letters and the lines.

(and subsequently rely) on this definition when examining the concept of social intelligence. Notably, his distinction between cognitive (i.e., understand other people) and behavioral (i.e., to act wisely in human relations) components has been specified in only one other definition of social intelligence. Thus, Vernon (1933) defined social intelligence as "knowledge of social matters and insight into the moods or personality traits of strangers" (cognition) and as the ability to "get along with others and ease in society" (behavior) (p. 44). Other definitions focus either on cognitive or behavioral aspects. Some of these definitions, along with their chief protagonists, are listed as follows: "the ability to get along with others" (Moss & Hunt, 1927, p. 108); "judge correctly the feelings, moods, and motivation of individuals" (Wedeck, 1947, p. 133); "ability to judge people with respect to feelings, motives, thoughts, intentions, attitudes, etc." (O'Sullivan, Guilford, & deMille, 1965, p. 6); "individuals fund of knowledge about the social world" (Cantor & Kihlstrom, 1987).

Indeed, the establishment and subsequent empirical application of broad theoretical frameworks of social intelligence appear scant in the literature. The most prominent and broadest conceptualization was introduced by Guilford (1967). In his Structural Model of Human Intellect, the three dimensions of *operations, contents,* and *products* are pivotal. The dimension of *operations* describes the cognitive requirements participants need to accomplish a task and contains five elements. The *content* dimension, with four elements, refers to the properties of task material. Finally, the *product* dimension comprises six elements, each describing a type of outcome associated with a certain task. The model, which relies on a complex interaction between these three dimensions, is depicted in Figure 10.1.

Guilford's conceptualization resulted in 120 factors that described distinct human intellectual abilities. For Guilford, the behavioral content facet, along with its cross-classification in terms of both operations and products, represented the domain of social intelligence, thus comprising 30 (= 5 × 6) distinct abilities as demarcated in Figure 10.1. Guilford and his colleagues (Hendricks,

Guilford, & Hoepfner, 1969; O'Sullivan et al., 1965) focused on the operational domains of *cognition* and *divergent production* to construct possible measures of social intelligence. O'Sullivan and Guilford's efforts in the domain of behavioral *cognition* resulted in two test publications: the Six Factor Test (O'Sullivan & Guilford, 1966) and the Four Factor Test (O'Sullivan & Guilford, 1976) of Social Intelligence. The task material consisted, above all, of pictures. Only a few purely verbal measures were constructed. These test batteries of the *cognitive* behavioral domain received wide interest in the research community. At about the same time, Hendricks et al. (1969) specified the domain of *divergent* or "creative" production of behavioral contents according to the six possible *products*. Thus, they postulated the following constructs: the ability to engage in behavioral acts that communicate internal mental states (units), the ability to create recognizable categories of behavioral acts (classes), the ability to perform an act that has a bearing on what another person is doing (relations), the ability to maintain a sequence of interactions with another person (systems), the ability to alter an expression or a sequence of expressions (transformations), and the ability to predict many possible outcomes of a setting (implications). Although this domain of "creative" social intelligence appeared to be a meaningful facet of social intelligence performance, further reaching investigations relying on these types of operationalizations have not been forthcoming in the literature.

Both Thorndike (1920) and Guilford (1967), in their theoretical frameworks, located the domain of social intelligence as equal and discriminable on one level with the traditional domain of academic intelligence. However, empirical results suggesting the autonomy of social intelligence from academic intellectual abilities are equivocal, seemingly dependent on the measurement procedures adopted. Indeed, empirical evidence for the relation of social to emotional (or practical) intelligence barely exist. Instead, the relation of social to emotional intelligence has largely been examined using rather specific measures of social and emotional skills. For example, Davies, Stankov, and Roberts (1998) operationalized social intelligence with the Interpersonal Perception Task–15 (IPT-15 Costanzo & Archer, 1993), a performance measure of social perception presented on videotape. Additionally, they employed a performance measure of emotional intelligence, that is, the Emotion Perception in Faces Test (Mayer, DiPaolo, & Salovey, 1990). However, the two measures correlated $r = -.09$. A subsequent factor analysis showed that these measures had bipolar loadings on one factor. Given this constitutes one of the few published studies of its kind, we contend that empirical approaches investigating the relation of the two constructs, particularly those that rely on performance data, are not readily apparent in the literature.

10.3   THE ASSESSMENT OF SOCIAL INTELLIGENCE

10.3.1   Multiple Test Batteries of Social Intelligence

Two broad attempts to assess social intelligence using comprehensive test batteries are discussed in the passages that follow. These represent approaches that seem to address problematic features put forward by various critiques of social intelligence (Orlik, 1978; Walker & Foley, 1973). These attempts aside, we note from the outset that the idea of developing tests of social intelligence from an a priori theoretical framework remains an outstanding problem in the long research tradition on social intelligence.

One of the first broad measures of social intelligence constructed is the George Washington Social Intelligence Test (GWSIT; Moss, Hunt, Omwake, & Woodward, 1955). This test is based on the authors' definition of social intelligence as "the ability to get along with others" (p. 108). A revised (short) form of the test, containing five subscales, comprises the following abilities:

Judgment in Social Situations: Find possible solutions for a social problem.

Memory for Names and Faces: Recognize target photographs previously studied and presented later among a larger group of photographs.

Observation of Human Behavior: Answer questions about human functioning on a true-false basis.

Recognition of the Mental States Behind Words: Choose the correct mental state or emotion, among four, reflected in a given statement.

Sense of Humor: Select the best ending to a joke.

Despite the authors' claim, performance in these subscales appears to be less dependent on socially intelligent behavior and more on understanding the importance of certain social milieu. Moreover, as Orlik (1978) points out, several validation studies show that variance in performance data may be explained, to a large extent, by verbal measures of academic intelligence. Whereas performance in the GWSIT has been shown to correlate up to .70 with academic (verbal) intelligence, correlations with other social intelligence indicators show no evidence for convergent validity.

A second major approach to the assessment of social intelligence was introduced by Guilford and colleagues, under the framework provided by the previously elucidated Structural Model of Human Intellect (Guilford, 1967). The following list briefly describes some examples of tasks out of the Six and the Four Factor Test of Social Intelligence (O'Sullivan & Guilford, 1966, 1976) and their classification in that model:

Expression Grouping (Classes): Participants find one facial expression, out of four alternatives, which best fit a group of three other facial expressions.

Missing Pictures (Systems): Participants are presented with a sequence of events, pictured in photographs, and have to complete the sequence by choosing the correct last photograph.

Missing Cartoons (Systems): Participants are required to fill-in a blank, in a sequence of cartoons, by selecting the correct cartoon out of four choice alternatives.

Picture Exchange (Transformations): A sequence of photographs is presented that tells a story. Participants are required to replace one marked photograph of this sequence, with one of four alternatives, in order to give the story a different meaning.

Social Translations (Transformations): This test is the only verbal measure of social intelligence in this battery. Participants are given a verbal statement made between a pair of people, in a defined social relation. They have to choose one pair of people out of three alternatives, for whom the given statement has a different meaning.

Cartoon Prediction (Implications): Participants are required to select one cartoon, out of three alternatives, that most appropriately completes a cartoon series.

As O'Sullivan et al. (1965) recognized, these tests were measures of cognitive rather than behavioral skills. The authors themselves reported no substantial correlations with general intellectual abilities (O'Sullivan & Guilford, 1966). More recent studies have focused on the construct validity of these test batteries. For example, Probst (1982) applied the Six Factor Test in an extensive study of social intelligence, finding empirical support for an independent ability construct. However, factor analysis did not yield a common social intelligence factor comprising different types of assessment methods. In another study, Riggio, Messamer, and Throckmorton (1991) neither found evidence for convergent nor for discriminant construct validity. They applied the Four Factor Test of Social Intelligence, along with a measure of academic intelligence, that is, the Wechsler Adult Intelligence Scale—Revised Edition (WAIS-R), Vocabulary Subscale (Wechsler, 1981). Furthermore, the Social Skills Inventory (SSI; Riggio, 1989) was administered as a measure of self-reported social skills. In an exploratory factor analysis, the subscales of the Four Factor Test loaded on one factor with the WAIS-R, showing near to zero correlations with the SSI. Thus, neither convergent nor discriminant construct validity were evidenced in this investigation.

10.3.2   Individual Tests of Social Intelligence

Empirical approaches that occurred after Walker and Foley's (1973) and Orlik's (1978) summarizing works, somewhat surprisingly, appear less theory-guided than those discussed in the aforementioned passages. More specific, but seemingly related concepts like social skills, nonverbal decoding skills, or nonverbal communication skills have subsequently been operationalized as indicators of social intelligence (Barnes & Sternberg, 1989; Feldman, Tomasian, & Coats, 1999; Riggio, 1986; Sternberg & Smith, 1985). With every consideration of the contributive value of these investigations, it seems somehow less difficult to find appropriate indicators of these concepts, as task requirements are more explicit and less complex. It appears necessary to classify these more narrow approaches in order to facilitate the interpretation of research results. For this purpose, operationalizations can be cross-classified along two dimensions. One is defined by the content under examination (i.e., cognitive vs. behavioral social skills), while the other dimension describes the method of assessment (i.e., performance vs. self-report data). In the following subsections, we provide a critical analysis of tests represented by this classification scheme. Note that the treatment of self-report measures will include attempts to assess both the cognitive and behavioral dimensions of social intelligence.

Cognitive performance measures.   Keating (1978) employed three verbal indicators of social intelligence performance designed previously (e.g., Chapin Social Insight Test, Chapin, 1967; Gough, 1968), as well as three measures of academic intelligence (both verbal and nonverbal material). Neither correlational nor factor analytic results supported construct validity. Within-domain correlations did not exceed across-domain correlations, and no coherent factor structure was observed. Furthermore, the social intelligence performance measures did not predict effective social functioning (assessed by peer-reports) to a larger extent than academic intelligence. Sternberg and colleagues (Barnes & Sternberg, 1989; Sternberg & Smith, 1985) operationalized the concept of nonverbal decoding skills as an indicator of social intelligence. They developed two tasks relying on similar principles. One was the so-called "Couples" Test, which contained photographs of heterosexual couples that were either in a close relationship or were strangers. Participants had to judge each photograph for the kind of relation depicted (i.e., close relationship or strangers). The second task consisted of photographs of a supervisor and his or her supervisee. In this instance, participants had to judge who the supervisor was. Barnes and Sternberg (1989) used self-report inventories of social competence, as well as performance measures of academic intelligence, to ascertain construct validity. Correlational analyses showed an unequivocal pattern with only significant convergent and non-significant discriminant validity coefficients.

Along with studies by Riggio et al. (1991) as well as O'Sullivan and Guilford (1966), these results alone only allow ambiguous conclusions about the validity of social intelligence based on performance measurement. At first blush, it seems that applying verbal performance measures results in substantial overlap between social intelligence and academic (especially verbal) abilities (Keating, 1978). Thus, investigations using nonverbal measures as indicators of socially intelligent performance succeed somewhat better in identifying a conceptually coherent domain of social intelligence (O'Sullivan & Guilford, 1966; Barnes & Sternberg, 1989). However, this result is not always demonstrated (Sternberg & Smith, 1985; Riggio et al., 1991).

The difficulties of both verbal and nonverbal cognitive performance measures in defining an unequivocal social intelligence construct could be attributed to a methodological problem. According to Schneider, Ackerman, and Kanfer (1996), certain characteristics of social cognitive tasks increase the overlap with academic intellectual abilities by matching their typical measurement features. These characteristics include: when participants encounter social stimuli that are inconsistent with their expectancies, when participants are faced with novel stimuli, and when participants are faced with highly structured tasks (Schneider et al., 1996, p. 469). Among cognitive performance measures of social intelligence, above all, those relying on verbal material seem to meet all three criteria. The sequential type of presentation inherent to written language does not seem to be an adequate operationalization of more or less complex social stimuli. Instead, written language appears to be distinct from socially relevant stimuli found in real-life settings. Plausibly, this type of presentation confronts the participants with novel (or thus far unexperienced) stimuli that implicate cognitive functions that parallel those necessary for the accomplishment of academic intelligence tests.

Behavioral performance measures.   Ford and Tisak (1983) applied a performance measure of socially intelligent behavior as an indicator of social intelligence. Participants' behavior in an interview situation was rated along certain criteria (e.g., the ability to speak effectively, to be appropriately responsive to the interviewer's questions, to display appropriate nonverbal behaviors). Additionally, the authors assessed self- and other-reported social behavioral skills and academic intelligence. Correlational, as well as factor analytic, results suggested a distinct social intelligence construct. Within-domain correlations exceeded across-domain correlations, and social intelligence measures loaded on a separate, interpretable factor.

A comparable study was conducted by Frederiksen, Carlson, and Ward (1984). Again, performance in an interview setting served as an indicator of social intelligence. Participants had to take the role of a doctor who was interviewing his/her patient. Additionally, Frederiksen et al. (1984) applied various measures of academic intelligence and problem-solving abilities. Results showed only a few substantial correlations between interview performance and academic intelligence measures. These correlations were partly negative in sign, suggesting that high academic intelligence was accompanied by low social behavioral skills.

Finally, Stricker and Rock (1990) applied a technique similar to the interview settings described thus far. Stricker developed his own measure of socially intelligent behavior, the Interpersonal Competence Inventory (ICI). The ICI was based on video scenes containing an interview situation between a subordinate and his superior. In the Replies section, participants had to respond orally to the subordinate in place of a superior. Answers were judged in terms of effectiveness and originality. In the Judgment section, participants had to write down their description of the situation and its important features. The performance criterion was accuracy. Conceptually, the Replies section operationalized socially intelligent behavior, whereas the Judgment section assessed, for the most part, cognitive skills. Along with the ICI, Stricker and Rock (1990) assessed non-verbal social skills, academic intelligence, and self-reported social intelligence. Results from correlational and multidimensional scaling analyses showed no coherent structure either within the domain of social intelligence or concerning the relation of social intelligence measures to academic intelligence. Social intelligence performance measures correlated inconsistently with each other (between $r = -.08$ and .37) and the Judgment section of the ICI correlated substantially with the verbal measure of academic intelligence ($r = .30$).

The interpretation of results in the aforementioned studies allows us to draw some tentative conclusions concerning the validity of social intelligence. Both Ford and Tisak (1983) as well as Frederiksen et al. (1984) succeeded in separating social from academic intelligence thus proving discriminant construct validity. However, Frederiksen et al.'s (1984) findings—partly negative correlations with academic performance—raise doubts about the nature of the performance construct of social intelligence. It should be expected that a so-called "intelligence" construct would at least be slightly positively correlated with traditional measures of academic intelligence. Furthermore, a strict account would note that the generalization of the findings is restricted to a rather specific (albeit practically meaningful) instantiation of the social context in which humans interact: interview settings. Finally, it must be stated that the convergent construct validity was not convincingly proven in these studies, neither for the restricted interview settings as indicators of social intelligence nor for a possibly more general social intelligence construct.

Self-reported social intelligence.   Numerous studies have applied self-report inventories as measures of social intelligence. In several of these investigations self-reported social skills serve as psychologically meaningful validation criteria (Barnes & Sternberg, 1989; Ford & Tisak, 1983; Frederiksen et al., 1984; Riggio et al., 1991). However, there are a large number of studies that rely *only* on self-reported social skills as indicators of social intelligence (Brown & Anthony, 1990; Marlowe, 1986; Riggio, 1986).

We have already described Riggio et al.'s (1991) study in the context of the O'Sullivan and Guilford (1976) test battery. In this investigation, the subscales of the Four Factor Test of Social Intelligence loaded on one factor together with academic intellectual abilities, whereas the subscales of the Social Skills Inventory (SSI; Riggio, 1989) loaded on a separate factor. Self-reported social skills and performance measures of social intelligence did not correlate substantially and only one correlation (viz., the Social Translation Subtest with the SSI) reached significance. However, other studies employing both self-reported social skills and social intelligence performance tests report evidence of convergent validity (Barnes & Sternberg, 1989; Ford & Tisak, 1983).

Riggio (1986) validated the SSI using the traditional personality scales of the 16 Personality Factor Questionnaire (16PF). The SSI contained six subfacets that resulted from a cross-classification of contents (viz., social vs. emotional contents) and postulated skills (viz., sensitivity, expressivity, and control). Summarizing these results, the SSI subfacets correlated substantially with various personality traits (e.g., social expressivity: outgoing, happy-go-lucky, venturesome, group dependent; social sensitivity: affected by feelings, shy, astute, apprehensive, conservative, tense, undisciplined). Moreover, participants scoring high on the different SSI subfacets could be described by a differing personality structure. According to Riggio (1986), these results proved the convergent validity of SSI as a measure of nonverbal social skills. His conclusion was also supported by further validity evidence: high scorers on the SSI tended to report more socially effective behavior and richer social contacts

(Riggio, 1986). The aforementioned findings of Riggio et al. (1991) put some ambiguity into this interpretation. In terms of Schneider et al.'s (1996) criticisms, the subscales of the Four Factor Test of Social Intelligence embodied operationalizations that were conceptually too close to academic intelligence performance measures. Thus, they represent no valid operationalization of the social intelligence ability construct. From another viewpoint, it is also possible that these results could be attributed to common method-related variance in self-report and performance data.

To examine these propositions more closely, two other studies are worth noting. Marlowe (1986) operationalized social intelligence via a self-report instrument. He intended to demonstrate that social intelligence would show independence from academic intelligence. Secondly, Marlowe postulated the multidimensionality of social intelligence. He extracted four dimensions from the empirical literature. Along these dimensions, social intelligence includes social interest, social self-efficacy, empathy skills, and social performance skills. Factor analytic results of the social intelligence measures yielded five separate factors labeled pro-social attitudes, social skills, empathy skills, emotionality, and social anxiety. The postulated dimensions could thus not be instantiated, though there was clear evidence for the multidimensionality of social intelligence. Correlational analyses suggested construct independence, showing near to zero correlations with academic intellectual abilities assessed by performance data. Anyway, evidence for the convergent construct validity was again missing.

Subsequently, Brown & Anthony (1990) found similar results. They assessed self- and peer ratings of both social behavior and personality traits, along with general intellectual performance. A factor analysis resulted in a clearly defined factor structure. The three factors were identified as: (a) academic intelligence, (b) peer ratings of both social behavior and personality, and (c) self-reported social behavior and personality. However, it seems plausible that these findings point to meaningful method-related variance, which is inherent to different measurement approaches.

10.3.3   Recent MTMM Studies

Most of the aforementioned approaches did not clarify the role of the intended measurement constructs in a putative higher-order framework of social intelligence. During the past decade, however, attempts have been made to apply multitrait-multimethod (MTMM) designs for a better understanding of the structure and construct validity of social intelligence (Jones & Day, 1997; Lee, Day, Meara, & Maxwell, 2002; Lee, Wong, Day, Maxwell, & Thorpe, 2000; Wong, Day, Maxwell, & Meara, 1995). All these investigations have assessed verbal and nonverbal performance measures, as well as self- and sometimes other-report data, of the respective trait-facets. Furthermore, the use of confirmatory factor analysis in these studies allowed the separation of trait- and method-related variance to derive an empirically defensible structural model of social intelligence.

In the first of these studies, Wong et al. (1995, Study 1) set out to measure academic intelligence, social perception as a cognitive facet of social intelligence, and socially intelligent behavior (operationalized as effective heterosexual interaction). The latter included ratings of both verbal and nonverbal behavior in a first encounter between a male and a female (recorded on videotape). Verbal social perception was operationalized by a subtest of the George Washington Social Intelligence Test (i.e., recognition of the mental state behind words, see above). The Expression Grouping subtest of the Four Factor Test of Social Intelligence (O'Sullivan & Guilford, 1976) was also used as a measure of nonverbal social perception. Results yielded a model with four uncorrelated method-factors (viz., verbal, nonverbal, self-report, and other-report) and three correlated trait-factors (viz., academic intelligence, social perception, and effective heterosexual interaction). However, both zero-order correlations as well as trait-factor intercorrelations pointed to substantial overlap between social perception and academic intellectual abilities ($r = .67$), a value that exceeded the intercorrelation between social perception and effective heterosexual interaction ($r = .54$).

In the second of these studies, Wong et al. (1995, Study 2) postulated three facets of social perception, social insight, and social knowledge. In the verbal measures of social knowledge, participants had to identify the best solution for a social problem. The nonverbal measure demanded the identification of etiquette mistakes, pictured in drawings. Verbal social perception was operationalized by the Social Translation Test of the Four Factor Test of Social Intelligence (O'Sullivan & Guilford, 1976), while the nonverbal measure of this facet was again the Expression Grouping subtest of the same test battery. The verbal measure of social insight was the Judgment in Social Situations subtest of the GWSIT (Moss et al., 1955). The nonverbal measure was the Cartoon Prediction subtest of O'Sullivan and Guilford (1976). The authors successfully identified the cognitive facets of social insight and social knowledge as trait-factors separable from, but positively related to, academic intelligence. Social perception could not be separated from social insight.

In yet another study, Jones and Day (1997) applied Cattell's distinction of fluid versus crystallized intelligence on the social intelligence construct and thus operationalized verbal and nonverbal social cognitive flexibility (fluid intelligence) and verbal and nonverbal social knowledge (crystallized intelligence). The nonverbal measure of social cognitive flexibility contained short video clips of ambiguous social situations. Participants had to list all possible interpretations of each scene. The verbal task of this facet included written descriptions of ambiguous social situations. Participants had again to list all possible interpretations. The Expression Grouping subtest of O'Sullivan and Guilford (1976) represented the nonverbal measure of social knowledge. The Social Translation subtest (O'Sullivan & Guilford, 1976) was used as the verbal measure of social knowledge. Jones and Day (1997) could show a trait-factor of social cognitive flexibility again separable from, but positively related to, academic problem solving, whereas social knowledge could not be separated from academic problem solving.

Extending on these findings, Lee et al. (2000) operationalized both fluid and crystallized social and academic intelligence. The authors specified fluid and crystallized social intelligence as social inference and social knowledge, respectively. Results showed that all four postulated trait-factors were discriminable from each other. Lee et al. (2002) diverged from the just described approaches by using tasks with open-ended questions to operationalize social knowledge and the flexible application of it. Thus, they rather represented the ideas of Cantor and Kihlstrom (1987), who claimed that open-ended questions would be more indicative of real-life social problems than tasks with just one correct answer. The verbal measure of social knowledge was the Role Category Questionnaire (see Lee et al., 2002). Participants had to write detailed descriptions of persons fitting into a certain kind of social role (e.g., liked same sex friend). In the nonverbal measure of social knowledge, participants had to describe as fully as they could well-known target persons (e.g., Oprah Winfrey), whose photos were presented on screens. Answers were scored in terms of the number of different personality and behavioral characteristics identified. The verbal and nonverbal measure of social cognitive flexibility represented the same as applied in the study of Jones and Day (1997). Results of this study showed separable social intelligence trait-factors distinct from, but positively correlated with, (general) creativity.

In summary, these MTMM-studies provide clear evidence for the multi-dimensionality of social intelligence. However, although the method-related variance of self- and other-report data was controlled by the introduction of method-factors or correlations among the respective measures, trait-factor loadings vary strikingly between performance measures and self- and other-report data. Moreover, the different measurement procedures exhibit no coherent loading pattern on one trait-factor. Consequently, it remains uncertain what influence the inclusion of self- and other-report data has on the identified trait-structure. Particularly, no further (convergent) validity evidence was available since self-report data were already included in the social intelligence models.

10.3.4   Summary

In spite of the early, extensive work of Guilford and his colleagues on social intelligence and their attempts to establish a theoretical framework, not many comparable systematic approaches may be found in the literature. Most empirical studies focus on a single, very specific *cognitive* aspect of social intelligence. These operational definitions seldom clarify the role of measurement constructs within the context of a higher-order framework. In addition, MTMM approaches do not conceptually integrate lower-order facets of social intelligence (and their concomitant cognitive determinants) into a comprehensive model of social intelligence. Since there is clear evidence for the multi-dimensionality of social intelligence (Lee et al., 2000, 2002; Wong et al. 1995), it seems important for future studies to locate constructs within a coherent, taxonomic model of social intelligence. The same kind of critique might be addressed to approaches focusing on the measurement of social *behavioral effectiveness*. Neither the role of effective social behavior in a framework of social intelligence nor an internal classification of relevant social settings appears to underlie extant approaches.

Empirical evidence for the construct validity of social intelligence varies strikingly across the measurement procedures that have been adopted. For example, self-report inventories and behavioral effectiveness criteria suggest a distinct domain of social intelligence. Approaches relying on verbal (and sometimes also nonverbal) tasks fail to provide incontrovertible evidence of a discriminable performance construct. However, the problems associated with the various types of measurement procedures remains an empirical issue. It is relatively self-evident that self-report data better serve as measures of typical social intellectual performance in comparison to measures of a performance construct that is based on the idea of maximal performance. Approaches relying on pure performance measurement should carefully consider the nature of the task material, both with respect to the selection of convergent validity criteria and to real-life congruence (Schneider et al., 1996).

10.4   FACETS OF SOCIAL INTELLIGENCE

In this section, we will attempt to integrate past theoretical and empirical work into a performance model of social intelligence. This model is based on the idea of a faceted intelligence model as a framework for the description and classification of variables or tests (Süß & Beauducel, 2005), the main focus of which will be various *cognitive* facets. It does not lay claim on completeness or conclusiveness and will need to be supported by empirical data. In any event, considering the diversity of past empirical approaches, it seems necessary to classify the theoretical and operational definitions of social intelligence in a unified framework. The model is based on five cognitive facets: social understanding, social memory, social perception, social creativity (or flexibility), and social knowledge. After a description of this model, we will provide some preliminary results of a study based on this performance model.

10.4.1   A Taxonomy of Cognitive Facets of Social Intelligence

The facet of *social understanding* (or insight) was included in a large number of theoretical and operational definitions, given different labels but comprising similar requirements. It can be perceived as the pivotal facet of social intelligence in past investigations. Thus, several definitions of social intelligence referred to in Section 10.2, namely, the ability to understand people (Thorndike, 1920), the ability to define a given situation in terms of the behavior imputed to others present (Chapin, 1942), and to judge correctly the feelings, moods, and motivations of individuals (Wedeck, 1947) could all be subsumed under the facet of social understanding or social insight. Additionally, both broad and specific operationalizations of socially intelligent cognition may be classified under this facet: the GWSIT (Moss et al., 1955), the Chapin Social Insight Test (Chapin, 1967; Gough, 1968), the broad test batteries of O'Sullivan and Guilford (1966, 1976), nonverbal decoding skills (Barnes & Sternberg, 1989), and so forth. Social understanding abilities thus require individuals to interpret or understand given social stimuli, which may vary according to their complexity, in terms of the implications for the situation and their underlying features. The point is well illustrated by a sample test requirement: understand correctly what a person wants to express via verbal or nonverbal means of communication.

The facet of *social memory* (i.e., behavioral memory) was included in the Structural Model of Human Intellect (Guilford, 1967). Kosmitzki and John (1993) also discovered a social memory factor in laypersons' implicit theories about social intelligence, that is, memory for names and faces. One documented operationalization is that provided by Moss et al. (1955) in the GWSIT (see also Probst, 1982). They operationalized social memory as memory for names and faces. The facet of social memory requires the intentional storing and recall of both episodic and semantic memory contents. Correspondingly, social memory performance is determined by the conscious recall of objectively and explicitly given social information that can vary along a continuum of complexity.

So far, the facet of *social perception* has not been reflected in theoretical accounts of social intelligence. Nevertheless, according to our view, the ability to perceive socially relevant information should play a role in a performance model of social intelligence. The ability to (quickly) perceive social information in a given situation could determine further information processing that is relevant for the exhibition of socially intelligent behavior. Only Wong et al. (1995) attempted to operationalize social perception. However, they did not succeed in separating social perception from social understanding abilities. These results could be attributed to the requirements of the selected tasks. The tasks also included interpretational demands that, in our view, cannot be subsumed under the facet of pure perceptual abilities. To meet these conceptual requirements, social perception can be specified as social perceptual speed, analogous to the idea of perceptual speed in models of academic intelligence (Carroll, 1993; Thurstone, 1938).

Social creativity (or flexibility) was conceptualized in Guilford's Structural Model of Human Intellect (Guilford, 1967) as divergent production of behavioral contents. Recent empirical work (Jones & Day, 1997; Lee et al., 2002) operationalizes social cognitive flexibility as the fluent production of possible interpretations of, or solutions for, a given social situation. Importantly, participants' performance is not based on one correct answer but on the number and diversity of ideas. The measures used by both Jones and Day (1997) and Lee et al. (2002) to define this construct were partly in line with Guilford's early propositions. Note that these authors were capable of successfully distinguishing the domain of social cognitive flexibility from academic intellectual abilities.

Social knowledge has been given credence in the definitions of Vernon (1933, viz., knowledge of social matters) and Cantor and Kihlstrom (1987, viz., individual's fund of knowledge about the social world). The concept of social knowledge also plays a substantial role in recent conceptualizations of practical intelligence and the related concept of wisdom (Baltes, Staudinger, Maercker, & Smith, 1995; Staudinger, Lopez, & Baltes, 1997; Sternberg, 1998; Sternberg et al., 2000). So far, social knowledge has mostly been operationalized by measures relying on knowledge of good etiquette (Lee et al., 2000; Wong et al. 1995). Contrary to these operationalizations, Kihlstrom and Cantor (2000) differentiated between procedural (or so-called tacit knowledge) and declarative social knowledge. They postulated that procedural knowledge could not be taught or recalled explicitly, in contrast to declarative knowledge and the corresponding memory components of episodic and semantic memory. With respect to these considerations, social knowledge can be specified as contents stored in the procedural memory component that cannot be taught or recalled explicitly.

Given these constraints, social knowledge becomes conceptually distinct from social memory. However, social knowledge, as specified in these considerations, is dependent on the influence of the cultural environment in general or the specialty of the situation (Weber & Westmeyer, 2001). The assessment of social knowledge, thus, would require a comprehensive classification of possible social situations. Still, any assessment would be subject to respective cultural values and standards.

From this description, it is not possible to conclude how these facets interact to enable people to exhibit socially intelligent behavior, in general. These cognitive determinants need not necessarily stand on one and the same level and, thus, contribute to higher-order performance to the same extent. Figure 10.2 portrays the proposed model of social intelligence including the cognitive facets, their possible interactions with each other, and with social behavior as the outcome of social cognitive intelligence.

In this illustration, the just described facets constitute the social (cognitive) intelligence construct. However, the facet of social knowledge, as depicted in Figure 10.2, does not play the same role as the other four facets. It seems reasonable to assume that social knowledge (as a kind of meta-concept) might also influence the performance, for example, in social understanding or social perception abilities. Furthermore, it is questionable whether social knowledge only contains cognitive requirements, following the aforementioned considerations of Weber and Westmeyer (2001). Altogether, the social cognitive facets surely determine social behavior performance to an important degree. However, the extent of this determination and, hence, the final exhibition of socially intelligent behavior is also influenced by some other, at this point indeterminate, array of person and environmental variables (i.e., situational demands, moods, personality, aims, etc.), as indicated in the figure.

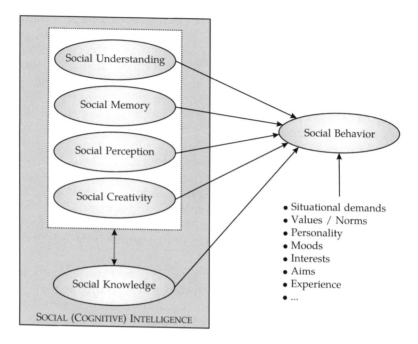

Figure 10.2   A possible performance model of social intelligence, including five cognitive facets.

10.4.2   A Preliminary Test of the Model

The focus of the present investigation (Weis & Süß, 2004) was to assess three cognitive facets of social intelligence: social understanding, social memory, and social knowledge, based on performance measures. To control possible effects of task material, we used verbal tasks, pictures, and videos. The verbal measures of social understanding were the Chapin Social Insight Test (SIT; Chapin, 1967; Gough, 1968) and the Social Translation subtest (O'Sullivan & Guilford, 1976). The pictorial measure of social understanding was the Faces Test (Mayer, Salovey, Caruso, and Sitarenios, 2002), while the video-based measure was the Interpersonal Perception Task–15 (Costanzo & Archer, 1993). The tasks for the social memory facet were all newly constructed. The Tacit Knowledge Inventory for Managers (TKIM; Wagner & Sternberg, 1991) served as the verbal measure of social knowledge. A confirmatory factor analysis supported the postulated trait structure within the social intelligence performance measures, when variance due to verbal content was controlled. The fit indices for model with best data fit were as follows: CFI = .964; $\chi^2(26)$ = 30.277, p = .256; RMSEA = .037 with a 90% confidence interval of [.000, .085]; SRMR = .056. The model is depicted in Figure 10.3. It postulated three correlated trait-factors corresponding to the design of the study (viz., social understanding, memory, and knowledge) and a verbal factor with loadings from all measures based on verbal material.

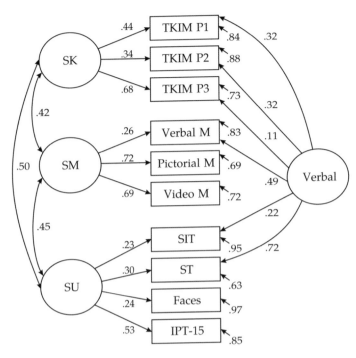

Figure 10.3   Structural model of social intelligence (standardized solution; ML). SK = Social Knowledge; SM = Social Memory; SU = Social Understanding; TKIM P1–3 = Tacit Knowledge Inventory for Managers Parcel 1–3; SIT = Chapin Social Insight Test; ST = Social Translation Test; Faces = Faces Test; IPT–15 = Interpersonal Perception Test–15.

The social knowledge factor correlated significantly with the social memory and the social understanding factor (.42 and .50, respectively). The social memory and social understanding factors also correlated significantly (i.e., .45). The factor loadings of the manifest variables on the respective trait-factors showed a coherent pattern. The loadings on the verbal method factor were heterogeneous, but all verbal indicators loaded positively on this factor.

We further investigated whether social intelligence was separable from academic intelligence, as specified by the Berlin Intelligence Structure Test (BIS-Test; Jäger, Süß, & Beauducel, 1997). Correlational and multiple regression analysis showed domain-specific overlap of the social intelligence trait-factors with specific domains of the BIS (Weis & Süß, 2004). Results from confirmatory factor analysis suggested still separable trait-factors of social and academic intelligence. Additionally, several social intelligence self-report inventories and scales of Extraversion, Openness, and Agreeableness were assessed. However, just as in past studies, results did not show any evidence for the convergent construct validity of performance based social intelligence with self-reported social skills. Furthermore, self-report data on social intelligence could be explained, to large measure, by the personality traits that we assessed.

10.5   SOCIAL INTELLIGENCE: CURRENT AND FUTURE PERSPECTIVES

Despite arguably uncritical acceptance of social or emotional intelligence as relevant individual differences constructs, the introduction of new statistical methods (e.g., structural equation modeling) provides opportunities for clarifying formerly unresolved problems. Furthermore, recent advances in technology, including digital means of stimulus recording, preparation, and presentation, allow the application of task material that is closer to real-life scenarios than paper-and-pencil drawings or black and white copies of photographs. However, future research on social intelligence is still faced with overcoming the failures and difficulties of past research and, thus, the challenge of proving the nature, structure, convergent and discriminant validity, and predictive value of the social intelligence construct.

10.5.1   Importance of Resolving Conceptual Issues

Ford (1994) claimed that social intelligence could not be specified as a pure ability construct. According to Ford, individual differences in socially intelligent performance should not be specified without considering situational demands, social values, and personal aims. Weinstein (1969) also related socially intelligent behavior to its underlying intentions. For Weinstein, one aspect of social intelligence is the ability to manipulate the responses of others. As a matter of course, the eventual exhibition of social behavior cannot be specified without considering, and perhaps specifying in advance, the relevant delimiting conditions in which social intelligence operates. Nevertheless, it is necessary to differentiate between the fundamental cognitive ability structure and the conditions that allow or influence the final performance of social behavior. If not, this criticism might justifiably be applied to the construct of academic intelligence. Of course, intelligent performance in real-life situations certainly depends on present moods or motivation, and/or on peer group values (Steele, 1997). So do socially relevant personality traits (e.g., Agreeableness, Extraversion), while social interests clearly influence socially intelligent behavior in everyday-life. Even so, certain cognitive determinants of socially intelligent behavior are necessary requirements for the accomplishment of social tasks and need to be identified by empirical research. Consequently, concepts like social engagement, social interests, or Machiavellian world views should not be confounded with a pure social (cognitive) intelligence construct.

No matter whether future studies rely on broad measurement approaches or rather focus investigation on specific domains of social intelligence, the conceptualization of the design demands a thorough specification of the intended measurement constructs and the corresponding task requirements. This approach has proven useful in the academic intelligence domain and we argue that it is equally important when considering social intelligence. Thus, even when the focus is on a narrow constructs, which claim to measure social intelligence in terms of specific social skills, there will be a need to place these constructs within a higher-order framework. Analogous to Carroll's idea to systematically integrate the various specific and more general constructs of academic intelligence in his hierarchical Three-Stratum-Theory (1993), it might be possible to establish a framework of social intelligence with comparable characteristics. In his late work, Guilford (1981, 1985) already recognized the possibility of several higher-order factors within his Structure of Intellect Model. Anyway, empirical studies and theoretical accounts are far away from solving these questions that are thus still subject to speculations.

10.5.2   Resolving Measurement Issues

Design issues.   Besides these fundamental conceptual concerns, past research has clearly demonstrated that the application of MTMM designs is inevitable for avoiding any effects of task material on the research results. Additionally, the construction of new tests appears necessary for all different facets of social intelligence. The latest technical developments, (i.e., DVD, digital cameras, web-based test delivery, and so forth) allow the development of task materials that are closer to real-life scenarios than only verbal performance measures. Relying on spoken language (auditory stimuli) seems just one way to realize the assessment of socially relevant attributes. Furthermore, new tests should take into account the topicality of the social milieu (just as intelligence tests need to be modified to take into account emerging historical events, technologies, and the like).

Validation.   According to the postulated performance model of social intelligence, social behavior appears to be an adequate criterion to validate social cognitive intelligence. However, considering the aforementioned criticisms, the conceptualization of appropriate indicators of social behavior seems to be a difficult obstacle to traverse. The exhibition of intelligent social behavior is certainly influenced by the social environment, present moods, prevailing social norms, values, and so forth. In this respect, it appears difficult, if at all possible, to assess performance in real-life contexts under the control of all relevant boundary conditions constituting the social world. This point notwithstanding, it appears important not to lose sight of the need to specify limiting conditions in advance. Consequently, future studies need to establish a more comprehensive classification of social settings and both universally and specifically valid criteria for the judgment of socially intelligent behavior.

Investigating the construct validity of social intelligence also needs to match the latest state-of-the-art in scientific research in terms of the selection and specification of validation criteria. Certainly, the replication of past findings by applying similar or the same measures of academic intellectual skills is valuable. However, in order to gain further information about construct validity, validating social intelligence performance with what are now thought of as relatively obsolete indicators of academic intelligence (e.g., simple grade point average) or apparently deficient operationalizations of g appears inadequate. In any case, it should be stated clearly, in correspondence with underlying theory, what type of academic intelligence is purportedly assessed (i.e., g, crystallized intelligence, reasoning abilities, or some other constellation of measurement constructs) and the strata upon which the construct resides (see Carroll, 1993).

Building the bridge to the main topic of this book, certainly, empirical investigations are required that allow conclusions about the overlap of social intelligence to the purportedly related concept of emotional intelligence (Matthews et al., 2002). As mentioned at the beginning of this chapter, at an empirical level, few data is available that provides evidence for the relation of the two constructs (Davies et al., 1998). At a theoretical level, some commentators see the constructs as positively interrelated (Salovey & Mayer, 1990; Sternberg et al., 2000). More specifically, Salovey and Mayer (1990) defined "emotional intelligence as a subset of social intelligence" (p. 189). At the same time, emotional intelligence was conceptualized as a kind of metacognitive ability (Goleman, 1995) with effects on all kinds of cognitive tasks, including tasks from the domain of social intelligence. Anyway, the absence of a common model of social intelligence and the elusiveness of emotional intelligence (Zeidner, Matthews, & Roberts, 2001) inhibits a more detailed theoretical description of construct overlap.

Consequently, any statement about the relation of these two constructs can, at present, only be derived from a comparison of operationalizations. For example, the Mayer-Salovey-Caruso Emotional Intelligence Test (MSCEIT; Mayer et al., 2002) is based on a performance model of emotional intelligence (Mayer & Salovey, 1997) containing four branches of different classes of abilities: perception of emotion (Branch 1), emotional facilitation of thought (Branch 2), understanding emotions (Branch 3), and managing emotions (Branch 4). A detailed description of the model and the four branches can be found in Chapter 2 by Neubauer and Freudenthaler in this volume. Table 10.1 contrasts the operationalizations of the MSCEIT with some traditional operationalizations of social intelligence.

Table 10.1 Operationalizations of the MSCEIT (Mayer et al., 2002) and Corresponding Tests of Social Intelligence

Tasks	Operationalizations of the MSCEIT	Operationalizations of social intelligence	
	Description	Exemplary description	Test
Branch 1: Faces	Test-takers are asked to identify how a person feels based upon their facial expression.	**Faces**: Choose the one of four photographed men's faces that expresses the same feeling as that of a woman's face. **Picture Exclusion**: Choose the one of four photographed expressions that does not belong to the other three. **IPT-15**: Judge a social situation presented on videotape in terms of the depicted meaning (e.g., the relation of two persons, possible deception, etc.). **Couples Test**: Recognize whether a photograph of a man and a woman represents a couple or two strangers.	Faces; Expression Grouping*; Picture Exclusion; Expression Exchange (O'Sullivan et al., 1965) IPT-15 (Constanzo & Archer, 1993) Couples Test (Barnes & Sternberg, 1989)
Branch 1: Pictures	Test-takers have to indicate the extent to which certain images or landscapes express various emotions.	≠	
Branch 2: Synesthesia	Test-taker are asked to compare different emotions to different sensations, such as light, color, and temperature.	≠	

table continues

Table 10.1   Operationalizations of the MSCEIT (Mayer et al., 2002) and Corresponding Tests of Social Intelligence

Tasks	Operationalizations of the MSCEIT		Operationalizations of social intelligence	
	Description		Exemplary description	Test
Branch 2: Facilitation	...measures the test-taker's knowledge of how moods interact and support our thinking and reasoning.	⊆	**Cartoon Implications:** Choose the one of four verbal statements that describes what precedes, or will follow a cartoon situation.	Missing Cartoons* Picture Exchange* Social Translation* Cartoon Prediction*
Branch 3: Changes	...measures the test-taker's knowledge of experiencing possibly conflicting emotions in certain situations and understanding "emotional chains", or how emotions transition from one to another.	⊆	**Questions II:** Choose the one of four alternative questions that might have provoked a given photographed facial expression. **Chapin SIT:** Asks the test-taker to select the most logical or intelligent solution or explanation for a given social problem.	Cartoon Implications; Questions II (O'Sullivan et al., 1965); Chapin SIT (Chapin, 1967; Gough, 1968); IPT-15
Branch 3: Blends	...refers to being able to connect situations with certain emotions.	⊆		
Branch 4 EM	...asks the test-taker to rate the effectiveness of alternative actions in achieving a certain result, in situations where a person had to regulate their own emotions.	≈	**Chapin SIT:** Asks the test-taker to select the most logical or intelligent solution or explanation for a given social problem. **TKIM:** Situations in the context of business settings, each is followed by possible actions. Participants have to rate the effectiveness of each action for the solution of the presented problem. According to the manual, the TKIM assessed knowledge about managing oneself, others, and tasks.	Chapin Social Insight Test (SIT; Chapin, 1967; Gough, 1968) TKIM (Wagner & Sternberg, 1991)
Branch 4: EiR	...asks test-takers to evaluate how effective different actions are in achieving an outcome involving other people.	≈		

Notes. EM = Emotion management; EiR = Emotions in relationships.

* The task has already been described in the section about test batteries of social intelligence.

≠ No comparable operationalization in the domain of social intelligence.

⊆ The ability purportedly assessed by this task contributes to the accomplishment of the social intelligence test.

≈ The task requirements rather equal those necessary for the social intelligence test.

Without going too much into detail of the single operationalizations, most of those belonging to the social intelligence domain were included in the test batteries of O'Sullivan and Guilford (1966, 1976) and have already been described in the first part of this chapter. Some aspects of the overview shown in Table 10.1 need to be commented on. Two tests of the MSCEIT (Pictures and Sensations) do not find any equivalent operationalizations in the domain of social intelligence. From our viewpoint, it is not conceivable to construct equivalent measures for the assessment of social intelligence, as can be done for other tests of the MSCEIT. For two tests (Emotion Management [EM] and Emotions in Relationships [EiR]), the TKIM (Wagner & Sternberg, 1991) represents a test with rather equivalent cognitive requirements, only differing with respect to the range of contents of the predetermined aim of actions (EM: regulate one's own emotions; EiR: achieving an outcome involving other people; TKIM: the combination of both for the solution of a given problem). Comparably, the Chapin SIT (Chapin, 1967; Gough, 1968) asks the test-taker to identify the most logical or intelligent solution or explanation for a given social problem and just omits the effectiveness ratings for the alternatives. Furthermore, for most of the MSCEIT tasks the purported task requirements contribute to the accomplishment of several social intelligence tests. For example, the ability to identify how a person feels based upon their facial expression (Faces, MSCEIT) contributes to the performance in the Faces Test of O'Sullivan et al. (1965) (choose one of four photographs of men's faces that expresses the same feeling as that of a woman's face). Moreover, the ability to perceive emotions as specified in the Faces Test of the MSCEIT surely contributes to the accomplishment of the Couples Test (Barnes & Sternberg, 1989) where test-takers have to decide whether a pictured couple represents a real or a faked couple. Furthermore, the knowledge of how moods interact (Facilitation Task) surely contributes to the ability to choose the one of four verbal statements that describes what precedes, or will follow a cartoon situation (Cartoon Implications; O'Sullivan et al., 1965). The knowledge of experiencing possibly conflicting emotions in certain situations and understanding emotional chains (Changes Task) might also help test-takers to accomplish the Chapin SIT where solutions or explanations for given problems have to be identified. At a scale level, the SIT intends to measure the ability to evaluate others, to foretell what may occur in interpersonal and social situations, and the ability to rectify disturbing tensions or conflicts. Conceptually, this definition certainly contains the requirements of the scale definition of Branch 3 (Understanding Emotions), that is, the ability to understand emotional information, how emotions combine and progress through relationship transitions, and to reason about such emotional meanings.

Obviously, several abilities belonging to the emotional intelligence construct form a subset of those abilities belonging to the domain of social intelligence. This supports the early conceptualization of Salovey and Mayer (1990). As a matter of course, the last considerations only represent statements about the face validity of the compared tests and only with respect to the constructs as assessed by the given operationalizations. Any further going conclusions must be subject to empirical investigations. Hence, at present, many questions concerning the overlap of social and emotional intelligence remain unanswered. For example, do the tasks with no corresponding social intelligence test assess a facet of emotional intelligence independent from social intelligence? That is, is emotional intelligence not only a subset of social intelligence, but contains distinct abilities? Or is it possible to regard social and emotional intelligence as constructs comprising the same cognitive requirements based on two different kinds of contents (social vs. emotional contents)?

10.6 CONCLUDING REMARKS

To conclude the chapter, we would like to provide some summarizing statements on the assessment of social intelligence, the associated problems and expected future challenges. Without repeating in detail future requirements as already outlined in this chapter, elements that appear most important for successful studies are (a) a theory-guided approach to the conceptualization of the construct with respect to higher- and lower-order facets and necessary task requirements, (b) the control of method-related variance (e.g., by MTMM-designs), and (c) the application of nonverbal and auditory task material to enhance real-life equivalence. When the construct can be conceptually delineated and adequately operationalized, examining the construct and finally predictive validity must be the focus of research. It appears inevitable for the conduct of useful studies to provide evidence for the convergent validity as an essential step for the establishment of a new ability construct (Süß, 2001). Moreover, it should be noted that the subfacets of a new hierarchical concept are in need of support by evidence of convergent validity. Last but not least, a discussion about the position of social and emotional intelligence within the field of individual differences research appears indispensable. In our view, it does not appear convincing to generate practical relevance only by the lexical introduction of new ability constructs. The apparent gold rush associated with the introduction and exploration of emotional intelligence might easily seduce researchers to adopt its importance from laypersons' theories without supporting the relevance by meaningful empirical evidence, especially for the convergent and incremental validity (Süß, 2001). In this respect, Schaie (2001) elaborates necessary steps towards the establishment of the emotional intelligence construct like a comprehensive convergent and discriminant validation, a well-founded selection of the validation sample, and the application of multivariate statistics for data analysis. Besides the already mentioned further duties as elaborated in this chapter, these methodological challenges might inspire researchers to come up with—as a seemingly overdue step—a book on social intelligence in the near future.

REFERENCES

Baltes, P. B., Staudinger, U. M., Maercker, A., & Smith, J. (1995). People nominated as wise: A comparative study of wisdom-related knowledge. *Psychology and Aging, 10,* 155–166.

Barnes, M. L., & Sternberg, R. J. (1989). Social intelligence and decoding of nonverbal cues. *Intelligence, 13,* 263–287.

Brown, L. T., & Anthony, R. G. (1990). Continuing the search for social intelligence. *Personality and Individual Differences, 11,* 463–470.

Cantor, N., & Kihlstrom, J. F. (1987). *Personality and social intelligence.* Englewood Cliffs, NJ: Prentice Hall.

Carroll, J. B. (1993). *Human cognitive abilities: A survey of factor-analytic studies.* New York: Cambridge University Press.

Chapin, F. S. (1942). Preliminary standardization of a social insight scale. *American Sociological Review, 7,* 214–225.

Chapin, F. S. (1967). *The Social Insight Test.* Palo Alto, CA: Consulting Psychologists Press.

Costanzo, M., & Archer, D. (1993). *The Interpersonal Perception Task-15 (IPT–15)* [Videotape]. Berkeley, CA: University of California Extension Media Center.

Davies, M., Stankov, L., & Roberts, R. D. (1998). Emotional intelligence: In search of an elusive construct. *Journal of Personality and Social Psychology, 75,* 989–1015.

Feldman, R. S., Tomasian, J. C., & Coats, E. J. (1999). Nonverbal deception abilities and adolescents social competence: Adolescents with higher social skills are better liars. *Journal of Nonverbal Behavior, 23,* 237–249.

Ford, M. E. (1994). A new conceptualization of social intelligence. In R. J. Sternberg (Ed.), *Encyclopedia of human intelligence* (pp. 974–978). New York: Macmillan Publishing Company.

Ford, M. E., & Tisak, M. S. (1983). A further search for social intelligence. *Journal of Educational Psychology, 75,* 196–206.

Frederiksen, N., Carlson, S., & Ward, W. C. (1984). The place of social intelligence in a taxonomy of cognitive abilities. *Intelligence, 8,* 315–337.

Gardner, H. (1983). *Frames of mind: The theory of multiple intelligences.* New York: Basic Books.

Goleman, D. (1995). *Emotional intelligence: Why it can matter more than IQ.* New York: Bantam Books.

Gough, H. G. (1968). *Manual for the Chapin Social Insight Test.* Palo Alto, CA: Consulting Psychologists Press.

Guilford, J. P. (1967). *The nature of human intelligence.* New York: McGraw-Hill.

Guilford, J. P. (1981). Higher-order structure-of-intellect abilities. *Multivariate Behavioral Research, 16,* 411–435.

Guilford, J. P. (1985). The structure-of-intellect model. In B. B. Wolmn (Ed.), *Handbook of intelligence. Theories, measurements, and applications* (pp. 225–266). New York: John Wiley & Sons.

Hendricks, M., Guilford, J. P., & Hoepfner, R. (1969). *Measuring creative social intelligence* (Psychological Laboratory Reports No. 42). Los Angeles: University of Southern California.

Jäger, A. O., Süß, H.-M., & Beauducel, A. (1997). *Berliner Intelligenzstruktur-Test* [Berlin Intelligence Structure Test]. Göttingen, Germany: Hogrefe.

Jones, K., & Day, J. D. (1997). Discriminations of two aspects of cognitive-social intelligence from academic intelligence. *Journal of Educational Psychology, 89*, 486–497.

Keating, D. P. (1978). A search for social intelligence. *Journal of Educational Psychology, 70*, 218–223.

Kihlstrom, J. F., & Cantor, N. (2000). Social intelligence. In R. J. Sternberg (Ed.), *Handbook of intelligence* (pp. 359–379). New York: Cambridge University Press.

Kosmitzki, C., & John, O. P. (1993). The implicit use of explicit conceptions of social intelligence. *Personality and Individual Differences, 15*, 11–23.

Lee, J.-E., Day, J. D., Meara, N. M., & Maxwell, S. E. (2002). Discrimination of social knowledge and its flexible application from creativity: A multitrait-multimethod approach. *Personality and Individual Differences, 32*, 913–928.

Lee, J.-E., Wong, C.-M. T., Day, J. D., Maxwell, S. E., & Thorpe, P. (2000). Social and academic intelligences: A multitrait-multimethod study of their crystallized and fluid characteristics. *Personality and Individual Differences, 29*, 539–553.

Marlowe, H. A. (1986). Social intelligence: Evidence for multidimensionality and construct independence. *Journal of Educational Psychology, 78*, 52–58.

Matthews, G., Zeidner, M., & Roberts, R. D. (2002). *Emotional intelligence: Science and myth.* Cambridge, MA: MIT Press.

Mayer, J. D., DiPaolo, M., & Salovey, P. (1990). Perceiving affective content in ambiguous visual stimuli: A component of emotional intelligence. *Journal of Personality Assessment, 54*, 772–781.

Mayer, J. D., & Salovey, P. (1997). What is emotional intelligence? In P. Salovey & D. J. Sluyter (Eds.), *Emotional development and emotional intelligence: Educational implications* (pp. 3–31). New York: Basic Books.

Mayer, J. D., Salovey, P., Caruso, D. R., & Sitarenios, G. (2002). *The Mayer, Salovey, and Caruso Emotional Intelligence Test: Technical manual.* Toronto, Canada: Multi-Health Systems.

Moss, F. A., & Hunt, T. (1927). Are you socially intelligent? *Scientific American, 137*, 108–110.

Moss, F. A., Hunt, T., Omwake, K. T., & Woodward, L. G. (1955). *Manual for the George Washington University Series Social Intelligence Test.* Washington, DC: The Center for Psychological Service.

Orlik, P. (1978). Soziale Intelligenz [Social intelligence]. In K. J. Klauer (Ed.), *Handbuch der Pädagogischen Diagnostik* (pp. 341–354). Düsseldorf, Germany: Schwann.

O'Sullivan, M., & Guilford, J. P. (1966). *Six Factor Test of Social Intelligence: Manual of instructions and interpretations.* Beverly Hills, CA: Sheridan Psychological Services.

O'Sullivan, M., & Guilford, J. P. (1976). *Four Factor Tests of Social Intelligence: Manual of instructions and interpretations.* Orange, CA: Sheridan Psychological Services.

O'Sullivan, M., Guilford, J. P., & deMille, R. (1965). *The measurement of social intelligence* (Psychological Laboratory Reports No. 34). Los Angeles: University of Southern California.

Probst, P. (1982). Empirische Untersuchung zum Konstrukt der "sozialen Intelligenz" [Empirical investigation on the 'social intelligence' construct]. In K. Pawlik (Ed.), *Multivariate Persönlichkeitsforschung* (pp. 201–226). Bern, Switzerland: Hans Huber.

Riggio, R. E. (1986). Assessment of basic social skills. *Journal of Personality and Social Psychology, 51*, 649–660.

Riggio, R. E. (1989). *Manual for the Social Skills Inventory.* Palo Alto, CA: Consulting Psychologists Press.

Riggio, R. E., Messamer, J., & Throckmorton, B. (1991). Social and academic intelligence: Conceptually distinct but overlapping constructs. *Personality and Individual Differences, 12*, 695–702.

Salovey, P., & Mayer, J. D. (1990). Emotional intelligence. *Imagination, Cognition and Personality, 9*, 185–211.

Schaie, K. W. (2001). Emotional intelligence: Psychometric status and developmental characteristics—Comment on Roberts, Zeidner, & Matthews (2001). *Emotion, 1*, 243–248.

Schneider, R. J., Ackerman, P. L., & Kanfer, R. (1996). To "act wisely in human relations": Exploring the dimensions of social competence. *Personality and Individual Differences, 4*, 469–481.

Süß, H.-M. (2001). Prädiktive Validität der Intelligenz im schulischen und außerschulischen Bereich [The predictive validity of intelligence in the scholastic and non-scholastic domain]. In E. Stern & J. Guthke (Eds.), *Perspektiven der Intelligenzforschung* (pp. 109–136). Lengerich, Germany: Pabst Science Publisher.

Süß, H.-M., & Beauducel, A. (2005). Faceted models of intelligence. In O. Wilhelm & R. Engle (Eds.), *Handbook of understanding and measuring intelligence* (pp. 313–332). Thousand Oaks, CA: Sage.

Staudinger, U. M., Lopez, D. F., & Baltes, P. B. (1997). The psychometric location of wisdom-related performance: Intelligence, personality or more? *Personality and Social Psychology Bulletin, 23*, 1200–1214.

Steele, C. M. (1997). A threat in the air: How stereotypes shape the intellectual identities and performance of women and African-Americans. *American Psychologist, 52*, 613–629.

Sternberg, R. J. (1998). A balance theory of wisdom. *Review of General Psychology, 2*, 347–365.

Sternberg, R. J., Forsythe, G. B., Hedlund, J., Horvath, J. A., Wagner, R. K., Williams, W. M., et al. (2000). *Practical intelligence in everyday life.* New York: Cambridge University Press.

Sternberg, R. J., & Smith, C. (1985). Social intelligence and decoding skills in nonverbal communication. *Social Cognition, 3*, 168–192.

Stricker, L. J., & Rock, D. A. (1990). Interpersonal competence, social intelligence, and general ability. *Personality and Individual Differences, 11*, 833–839.

Thorndike, E. L. (1920). Intelligence and its use. *Harper's Magazine, 140*, 227–235.

Thurstone, L. L. (1938). *Primary mental abilities.* Chicago: University of Chicago Press.

Vernon, P. E. (1933). Some characteristics of the good judge of personality. *Journal of Social Psychology, 4*, 42–57.

Wagner, R. K., & Sternberg, R. J. (1991). *Tacit knowledge inventory for managers*. San Antonio, TX: The Psychological Corporation Harcourt Brace & Company.

Walker, R. E., & Foley, J. M. (1973). Social intelligence: Its history and measurement. *Psychological Reports, 33*, 839–864.

Weber, H., & Westmeyer, H. (2001). Die Inflation der Intelligenzen [The inflation of intelligences]. In E. Stern & J. Guthke (Eds.), *Perspektiven der Intelligenzforschung* (pp. 251–266). Lengerich, Germany: Pabst Science Publisher.

Wechsler, D. (1981). *Wechsler Adult Intelligence Scale—Revised*. New York: Psychological Corporation.

Wedeck, J. (1947). The relationship between personality and 'psychological ability'. *British Journal of Psychology, 37*, 133–151.

Weinstein, E. A. (1969). The development of interpersonal competence. In D. A. Goslin (Ed.), *Handbook of socialization theory and research* (pp. 753–775). Chicago: Rand McNally.

Weis, S., & Süß, H.-M. (2004). *Social intelligence—Investigating its structure and construct validity in a multitrait-multimethod design*. Manuscript submitted for publication.

Wong, C.-M. T., Day, J. D., Maxwell, S. E., & Meara, N. M. (1995). A multitrait-multimethod study of academic and social intelligence in college students. *Journal of Educational Psychology, 87*, 117–133.

Zeidner, M., Matthews, G., & Roberts, R. D. (2001). Slow down, you move too fast: Emotional intelligence remains an "elusive" intelligence. *Emotion, 1*, 265–275.

Part III
Applications of Emotional Intelligence

11

Emotional Intelligence in the Context of Learning and Achievement

Thomas Goetz
Anne C. Frenzel
Reinhard Pekrun
Institute of Educational Psychology
University of Munich, Germany

Nathan Hall
Department of Psychology
University of Manitoba, Canada

Summary

This chapter is concerned primarily with emotional intelligence (EI) as it relates to learning and achievement in an academic setting. It aims to assist researchers, educators, and politicians alike to decide what aspects of EI are worthwhile to promote and are possible to teach in school. We first discuss the conceptualization of EI on which the present contribution is based, and provide an overview of existing programs for fostering EI in schools. Based on some major flaws we have identified in these programs, we present a framework of antecedents, "intelligent" processing, and effects of academic emotions. Subsequently, a model for fostering EI in academic learning and achievement situations is presented, and tangible instructional suggestions are provided. The chapter closes with implications for research and scholastic applications.

11.1 INTRODUCTION

"I am not that good at emotions." This real-life response is what a male student wrote on the top of a questionnaire on academic emotions (emotions directly linked to academic learning, classroom instruction, and achievement; see Goetz, Zirngibl, Hall, & Pekrun, 2003; Pekrun, Goetz, Titz, & Perry, 2002); most likely as an excuse for not completing the survey (Molfenter, 1999). What does it mean to "not be good at emotions"? How could we have prevented this student from developing such poor judgment of his emotional self? With respect to the first question, the student perhaps thought his knowledge about emotions was too limited, that he was not aware of his own emotions, or that he could not adequately deal with them. The latter question is also a difficult one to answer. Perhaps, apart from socialization authorities such as parents, it is the task of educational institutions to teach students knowledge and skills concerning one of the most important areas of human functioning: emotions.[1]

11.2 CONCEPTUALIZATION OF EMOTIONAL INTELLIGENCE

In light of the host of diverse conceptualizations of emotional intelligence (EI; see Matthews, Zeidner, & Roberts, 2002), one must first decide on a definition of this construct that is adequate to apply to learning and achievement. Studies investigating EI in the classroom usually lack a theoretical framework (Zeidner, Roberts, & Matthews, 2002), or do not explicate the bases for the choice of their employed construct (cf. Cohen, 2001; Elias, Hunter, & Kress, 2001). In choosing an adequate theory of EI for academic learning and achievement situations, we considered the following criteria. The theory should:

1. be consistent with the cognitively referenced conceptualization of intelligence (see Mackintosh, 2001; Sternberg, 1997),

2. need a minimal number of context-specific modifications and supplements,

3. be suitable for operationalization and evaluation, and

4. be conducive to the development of intervention programs.

We consider Mayer and Salovey's (1997; Salovey & Mayer, 1990) revised ability model of EI to be particularly suitable for meeting Criteria 1 through 4. Consistent with standard conceptualizations of intelligence, Mayer and Salovey (1997) explicitly define EI as a mental ability concept (see also Chapter 2 by Neubauer & Freudenthaler). Specifically, the authors integrate four branches (i.e., facets) of emotional abilities in their model:

---

[1]For the pros and cons of emotion education in school, see Elias et al. (1997); Zeidner, Roberts, and Matthews (2002). Concerning the promotion of emotional intelligence by parents, see Martinez-Pons (1998).

- Branch I: Perception, appraisal, and expression of emotion.
- Branch II: Emotional facilitation of thinking.
- Branch III: Understanding and analyzing emotions; employing emotional knowledge.
- Branch IV: Reflective regulation of emotions to promote emotional and intellectual growth.

For our conceptualization of EI, we focus on those aspects of this model that appear to be most important within our framework that is explicitly intervention oriented. These include (1) perceiving emotions (Mayer and Salovey's Branch I), (2) reflecting on emotions (knowledge about emotions; e.g., knowledge about the causes of emotions, their manifestations and effects, as well as knowledge about methods of emotion regulation, Mayer and Salovey's Branch III), and (3) managing one's own emotions in the sense of being able to regulate them (Mayer and Salovey's Branch IV). We omit Mayer and Salovey's Branch II (emotional facilitation of thinking) because we think this aspect is less applicable for intervention. Overall, we thus define EI, within our framework, as a person's cognitive ability for the perception, reflection, and regulation of emotions.

11.3   PROGRAMS FOR FOSTERING EMOTIONAL INTELLIGENCE IN STUDENTS

At the time of writing, a literature search constrained to the German language revealed only occasional, primarily practice-oriented publications concerning the topic of EI at school (e.g., Hofer, 2000). However, Klauer's research does suggest some valuable techniques for the promotion of students' "classical" intelligence (see Klauer, 1988; Klauer & Phye, 1994). In the U.S.A., there have been numerous practice-oriented publications on this topic since the 1990s (for a description of intervention programs and their evaluation, see Zeidner, Roberts, & Matthews, 2002), with most of these studies published in the context of Social and Emotional Learning (SEL; Cohen, 1999, 2001).

SEL programs were developed in response to an increasing body of research showing that children's and adolescents' socio-emotional competencies are important to foster (cf. the terms *social and emotional literacy*, Cohen, 2001; (Elias et al., 1997)). It has been further acknowledged that these competencies need to be taught in educational institutions, above all, in our schools (Mayer & Salovey, 1997). SEL is a comprehensive approach that attempts to encompass numerous, rather heterogeneous, approaches. Typical SEL programs involve social skills training, cognitive-behavioral modification programs, self-management and conflict-solving programs, general promotion of problem-solving skills, and also prevention programs against suicide, drug abuse, and violence (see Elias et al., 2001; Topping, Holmes, & Bremner, 2000).

Due to the popularity of EI in the past 10 years, many of the SEL programs in wide-spread use in the U.S.A. have post-hoc been declared as EI programs, despite not having been explicitly developed for the promotion of EI. Nevertheless, many of these programs do address some of the pivotal components of EI. Zeidner, Roberts, and Matthews (2002) list six central aspects of programs for the promotion of EI:

1. Problem solving—a term used extensively in the context of SEL and EI programs that is partially related to aspects comprising Points 2 to 6 below (i.e., it encompasses multiple ways of solving problems or the ability to take someone else's perspective; e.g., ICPS [I can problem solve] program, Shure & Glaser, 2001);

2. Perception and understanding of emotions in oneself and in others;

3. Controlling of impulses;

4. Emotion regulation;

5. Coping with stress and negative emotions; and

6. Being able to take someone else's perspective (i.e., empathy).

The degree to which these programs actually foster EI is dependent on the underlying definition of the construct. Very few programs, however, have explicitly been designed to foster EI (e.g., the PATHS program [Promoting Alternative Thinking Strategies]; Greenberg, Kusche, Cook, & Quamma, 1995).

EI programs can also be distinguished as being either intra- or extracurricular in nature. Intra-curricular programs integrate socio-emotional learning into classroom activities by promoting the idea of dealing with the emotion-oriented aspects of specific subject areas (Cohen, 1999). Works of literature, art, or musical pieces are particularly suitable as starting points for discussions. By contrast, extracurricular programs explicitly and exclusively deal with the topic of socio-emotional learning outside the regular classroom setting.

From our perspective, existing programs for the promotion of EI in schools have the following central problems:

1. The programs usually lack a clear definition of the construct of EI.

2. Evaluations are problematic because there are no adequate instruments for the measurement of EI in a classroom setting (cf. the evaluation of SEL programs; Elias et al., 1997).

3. In these programs, negative emotions, and how to deal with them, is almost exclusively the topic of discussion, with positive emotions seen as irrelevant to coping. However, more recent findings show that positive emotions—in spite of their predominantly positive effects—can in specific circumstances also have detrimental effects. When making a decision, for example, people in a positive mood may not take negative, albeit important, aspects of a situation into account in order to maintain their positive feelings (*mood maintenance*; for a critical discussion, see Aspinwall, 1998). Although selecting exclusively positive aspects can maintain "pleasing" emotions in the short term, it may also lead to wrong decisions, resulting in prolonged negative emotions in the long run.

4. The question of whether EI may be emotion-specific, meaning that some-one could be good at perceiving, reflecting on, or regulating certain emo-tions (e.g., anger) and not others (e.g., anxiety), remains to be addressed.

5. This is also true for the question of EI being situation-specific (e.g., that someone would be differentially skilled at regulating their emotions in social vs. academic situations).

6. The confounding of maturation with external influences is also rarely taken into consideration.

7. Theories and empirical findings of research on emotions are often over-looked (e.g., findings on the phenomenology of emotions and on the ef-fects of emotions on learning and achievement).

8. These programs predominantly address the importance of emotions in social contexts, with the consequences of emotions on learning and achievement remaining largely unexplored.

Overall, even though it is intuitively plausible that EI needs to be fostered during school hours, existing programs lack persuading and operationalizable theoretical frameworks. Consequently, as for their evaluation, many of these programs lack clear, testable hypotheses. To make matters worse, we also lack instruments for the assessment of students' EI that are reliable, valid, and sen-sitive to change. As such, in the drive to foster EI in students, practice appears to have surpassed supporting research, making the results of these programs theoretically questionable.

11.4 FRAMEWORK OF ANTECEDENTS, "INTELLIGENT" PROCESSING, AND EFFECTS OF ACADEMIC EMOTIONS

Our framework of antecedents, "intelligent" processing, and effects of acad-emic emotions in a school setting is based on three central components that are presented below.

11.4.1 Focus on Academic Emotions

The model is focused on a person's academic emotions and is thus different from other models of EI that are predominantly concerned with social emo-tions (cf. models in the context of SEL; e.g., Elias et al., 1997). As mentioned earlier, the literature on EI in schools almost exclusively deals with social as-pects.[2] In this chapter, we focus on the perception, reflection, and regulation of academic emotions such as enjoyment of learning, hope for success in an exam, and boredom during instruction.

---

[2]For example, classroom climate or social competence (Cohen, 2001) and the assessment of intra- and interpersonal aspects of emotional intelligence with the BarOn Emotional Quotient Inventory (BarOn EQ-i; Bar-On, 1997).

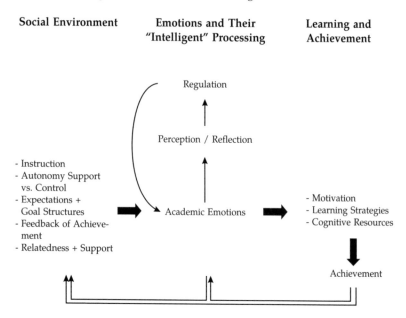

Figure 11.1   Antecedents, "intelligent" processing, and effects of academic emotions.

11.4.2   Integration of Emotional Intelligence Into the Emotion Research Tradition

It is interesting to note that models and theories of EI rarely refer to previous findings from the emotion research tradition (cf. Mayer, Salovey, & Caruso, 2002). Standard works in emotion psychology, which are central in terms of both content and research heuristics (e.g., Frijda, 1998; Scherer, 1984), are rarely cited in the literature on EI. However, knowledge concerning taxonomies and the phenomenology of emotions is highly applicable to the study of perception and regulation of emotions. Moreover, without a fundamental knowledge of the achievement-related effects of specific emotions, their regulation toward achievement goals is impossible. Within our framework, we deliberately integrate EI into an existing model from the emotion research tradition.

11.4.3   Emotion-Focused Regulation

Following the classical coping literature (e.g., Lazarus & Folkman, 1984), one can differentiate between two basic types of regulatory processes: emotion-focused and problem-focused regulation. The first refers to the direct regulation of one's own emotions, the latter to the goal-directed modification of emotion-inducing circumstances (e.g., leaving or restructuring the situation). Basically, both emotion- and problem-focused regulation are applicable in a classroom setting and may be used alternatively, or in parallel, depending on the situation. In our model (depicted in Figure 11.1), we concentrate on emotion-focused regulation processes.

The model presented in Figure 11.1 is based on Pekrun and colleagues' framework that incorporates the antecedents and effects of academic emotions (Pekrun, 2000; Pekrun et al., 2002) and integrates our described conceptualization of EI with that outlined by Mayer and Salovey (1997). In this model, variables concerning the social environment are primarily conceptualized as emotional *antecedents*. At the same time, emotions are also assumed to influence a person's social environment. Previous exploratory and confirmatory analyses (structural equation models) confirm relationships between the social environment and students' emotional experiences as postulated in our model (Goetz, 2004; Titz, 2001). A cognitive-motivational model (Pekrun et al., 2002) provides the theoretical basis for understanding the *effects* of emotions on learning and achievement. Specifically, this model suggests that emotions affect students' motivation, quality of learning strategies, and the mobilization of cognitive resources which, in turn, affect scholastic achievement (itself recursively affecting emotions and aspects of the social environment).

The middle section of the model, emotions and their "intelligent" processing, is considered to be a self-regulatory process closely intertwined with social antecedents and the effects of emotions (on the topic of self-regulation in the context of learning and achievement see Boekaerts, Pintrich, & Zeidner, 2000; concerning EI as a self-regulatory process see Martinez-Pons, 2000, 2001). According to this model, emotionally intelligent behavior means applying one's cognitive abilities for perceiving and reflecting on emotion-related information in learning and achievement situations, and regulating these emotions in a goal-directed way. Perception represents the identification of one's own emotions related to learning and achievement situations (e.g., anger about overly difficult tasks); reflection refers to knowledge about these emotions (e.g., knowledge about their positive or negative consequences for learning and achievement); and regulation stands for knowledge concerning the goal-directed modification of one's current emotion.

11.5   A MODEL FOR THE PROMOTION OF EI IN LEARNING AND ACHIEVEMENT SITUATIONS

In this section, we present possibilities for the promotion of EI in the context of learning and achievement situations at school (for increasing positive emotions and decreasing negative emotions in students during instruction, see Astleitner's Fear, Envy, Anger, Sympathy, and Pleasure [FEASP] approach, 2000). We refer to the conceptualization of EI as described above and outline a model that focuses attention on the three components of EI (perceiving emotions, reflecting on emotions, and regulating emotions) comprising our theoretical framework (see Section 11.4). This model allows for numerous implications and should be seen as a heuristic for the development of EI-based intervention and promotion programs. Figure 11.2 shows a model incorporating facets of expectancy-value theory that originates from the motivational-psychological research tradition (Atkinson, 1957, 1964).

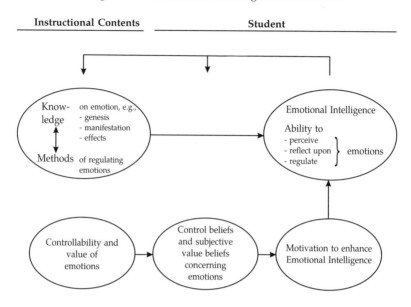

Figure 11.2   A model for the promotion of EI in learning and achievement situations.

In this tradition, it is typically argued that motivation is based on subjective appraisals of the probability of action outcomes and the values of these outcomes. These two aspects are assumed to be multiplicatively combined, implying that both components have to be above some minimum level for motivation to arise. Following this approach, our model considers subjective perceptions of control and value of emotions as antecedents of the motivation to enhance EI. According to this model, students' EI can be fostered by teaching them both knowledge and methods of regulation concerning emotional experiences, while making clear to them at the same time that emotional experiences are valuable and controllable. The students' levels of EI, in turn, recursively affect their subjective perceptions of control and value. Further, the content of instruction is dependent on the level of EI among the students in a given class.

The instructional content of EI training programs can generally be taught by all socialization authorities, including teachers, parents, and peers, but also the media (on the promotion of EI by teachers, see Mayer & Salovey, 1997; Zins, Travis, & Freppan, 1997; on the promotion by parents, see Martinez-Pons, 1998). As such, we suggest possibilities for the promotion of students' EI at school, focusing exclusively on individuals' academic emotions in the scholastic environment, and specifically the promotion of students' EI as pertaining to emotion-focused regulation (see above). Corresponding to our model (Figure 11.2), our discussion also concerns the following: (a) knowledge about academic emotions, (b) knowledge of affective self-regulation, (c) perceived controllability of emotions, as well as (d) perceived value of emotions related to learning and achievement situations. Because previous programs for the promotion of EI have been poorly integrated into the emotion research tradition, we will also attempt to highlight potentially related points and cross-linkages with research on emotions and clinical psychology.

11.5.1   Teaching Knowledge About Academic Emotions

Having knowledge about emotions related to learning and achievement is helpful for their regulation. In the following sections, we list core components of this knowledge that can be imparted during instruction and scholastic interactions directed toward the promotion of EI.

Definition of emotions related to learning and achievement.   First, it can be discussed with students what the phenomenon of *emotion* actually represents. Within the numerous definitions of emotions (see Van Brakel, 1994), component theories or definitions are highly applicable, with knowledge concerning the differential components of emotions contributing to a multi-dimensional, and thus differentiated, perception of emotions. Scherer (1993), for example, suggests the following five components of emotions: cognition, physiology, motivation, motor expression, and affect. Selected emotions can be discussed in terms of these components. To this end, individually experienced emotions described in interviews from emotion research (e.g., Titz, 2001) can be used. Conducting sample interviews with students based on existing interview manuals may also be considered (e.g., Kusche Affective Interview Revised, KAI-R; Kusche, Greenberg, & Beilke, 1988). After a general definition of emotions on the basis of their components, subsequent discussions may involve a greater focus on academic emotions specifically.

Extension of the emotion vocabulary.   Included in the descriptive knowledge of emotions, one's understanding of emotion-related terminology appears to be an important subcomponent of EI. To be able to adequately talk about and discuss emotions, it is necessary that students have a broad emotion vocabulary. Thus, it is important to teach students a diverse vocabulary of emotion words (e.g., adjectives like blithe, cheery, glad, or bright for the differentiated description of the experience of joy). Extending students' emotion vocabulary is an important goal that can be incorporated into the study of nearly all academic subjects. Particularly suitable are language-related courses and subjects in the arts (music, art education) where the expression of emotions in pieces of art or fictitious persons found in works of literature can be discussed. An example for extracurricular teaching of emotional words is Greenberg's PATHS program (see also Kusche & Greenberg, 2001). In a subsection of that program, students are taught approximately 35 affective states by means of so-called "Feeling Units" where students learn emotion words in a hierarchical way, beginning with common emotions (e.g., happiness, sadness, anger) and proceeding to more complex emotional experiences (e.g., jealousy, guilt, pride).

Mimicked and gesticulated representations of emotions and discussion of their messages may also build a basis for extracurricular activities aimed at extending students' emotion vocabulary. For example, a group of students might be encouraged to express specific emotions through pantomime, while their classmates try to figure what they mean. In another exercise, two students might act as politicians discussing a certain topic, with the audience taking notes on their impressions of the emotional experiences of the actors. Further, students could be given very specific emotion words (like hope, tenderness, loneliness, rage) which they should assign to pictures. Extensive material from emotion research is applicable to this end (e.g., Facial Action Coding System [FACS], Ekman & Friesen, 1978; Emotional Facial Action Coding System [EFACS], Friesen & Ekmann, 1984; Self-Evaluative Emotions Coding System [SEECS], Geppert, Schmidt, & Galinowski, 1997; International Affective Picture System [IAPS], Lang, Bradley, & Cuthbert, 1995; see also pictures and stories from the MSCEIT, Mayer et al., 2002).

Teaching emotion taxonomies.   To be able to categorize emotions, it is important to teach students taxonomies of emotional experiences that reduce complexity. Classic criteria for building emotion taxonomies are qualitative aspects such as mood versus emotion (e.g., differentiating between "being in a bad temper" vs. "being angry at something or someone"; see Abele, 1996), as well as quantitative aspects like intensity (e.g., differentiating being enraged vs. being annoyed; see Ricci-Bitti & Scherer, 1986). For teaching emotion taxonomies, educators can rely on classification schemes derived from emotional research such as Plutchik's (1980) circumplex model of basic emotions, or other categorizations considering valence, expression, and physiological activity (Ekman & Davidson, 1994) or their cognitive appraisal (Smith & Ellsworth, 1985). Watson and Tellegen (1985) suggest a categorization of emotions based on the dimensions of activation and valence. Using these dimensions, emotions relevant for the context of learning and achievement can be classified as follows: positive activating emotions (e.g., enjoyment, hope), positive deactivating emotions (e.g., relaxation, relief), negative activating emotions, (e.g., anxiety, anger), and negative deactivating emotions (e.g., hopelessness, boredom). A further categorization of emotions suggested by Pekrun et al. (2002) categorizes emotions according to the dimensions of valence (positive vs. negative emotions), point of reference (task-related vs. self-related emotions), as well as a temporal factor (process-oriented, prospective, and retrospective emotions). Basically, such schemas can be starting points for teaching the ability to categorize emotions. Emotion taxonomies can, for example, be taught by asking students to work together to categorize various emotions and to explain the criteria for their arrangement. Subsequently, their taxonomies can be compared and contrasted with existing taxonomies from the literature on emotions.

Knowledge about the effects of academic emotions on learning and achievement.   For the goal-oriented regulation of emotions, it is helpful for students to have personal goal statements about their emotional experiences. As pointed out by Boekaerts (1999), the choice of goals is a prerequisite of self-regulation. To this end, students can be advised to make up their minds about their emotional goals (i.e., desirable emotional experiences) before they start regulating their emotions. In academic settings, this means that it is beneficial for students to know about the consequences of specific emotional experiences for learning and achievement; for example, how positive and negative emotions influence the way they think and solve problems at school (on the effects of moods and emotions on thinking and problem solving, see Ellis & Ashbrook, 1988; Fiedler, 1988). Bases for discussing the effects of emotions on learning and achievement can be Pekrun et al.'s (2002) emotion taxonomy, which classifies the effects of emotions based on a 2×2 factorial cross of the activation and valence of emotions. Similarly, Pekrun et al.'s (2002) cognitive-motivational mediation model, which outlines the effects of emotions on motivation/volition, learning strategies, and cognitive resources, may be helpful.

11.5.2   Knowledge of Methods for the Self-Regulation of Academic Emotions

Definition of emotional self-regulation.   Before discussing the teaching of knowledge and methods of emotional self-regulation, the term self-regulation should be clarified and illustrated. Self-regulation can be seen as a form of problem-solving in the sense of reducing the difference between the actual value and the target value of a given internal state (Anderson, 2000; see also Self-Regulation Scale of Emotional Intelligence [SRSEI], Martinez-Pons, 2001). In this case, emotion-related self-regulation activities are directed towards changing actual emotional states into target emotional states.

Teaching knowledge about methods of emotion regulation and their application.   Of the numerous potential methods for the regulation of emotions, we review four in the present context. Emotion regulation in the context of learning and achievement can be understood as involving areas of research from both the educational and clinical psychological domains. Emotion regulation can take place, first, by means of a change of meta-levels (for meta-emotions in the context of EI, see Gohm, 2003). In this respect, students can observe and analyze their emotional experiences in a concrete situation. For example, if a student feels ashamed during instruction, he or she can consider the potential reasons for this emotion or analyze it in terms of its structural components. Inspecting an emotion at a meta-level may be helpful in order to distance oneself from the emotion. On the other hand, clinical research suggests that meta-levels of emotion may also be the starting point of a self-intensifying circle of emotional experiences (e.g., phobophobia).

Second, students could also be taught a repertoire of relaxation techniques (e.g., breathing techniques, autogenic training, and/or progressive muscle relaxation). This can be particularly helpful for the regulation of negative emotions such as anxiety or anger.

Third, positive self-instruction (self-communication) concerning the valence and controllability of academic emotions should also be encouraged; factors that can significantly influence one's emotional experiences. Becoming aware of the controllability of emotions, and meta-emotions, may be crucial for students' motivation to alter their emotional experience. When lacking control beliefs, a student can, for example, get excessively anxious over an increase in test anxiety, especially if perceived as uncontrollable in nature. Moreover, meta-anxiety due to a perceived lack of control can be more intense and thus even more performance-inhibiting than the initial anxiety surrounding an exam.

Finally, students should try to reduce their subjectively experienced work-play dichotomy (Covington & Wiedenhaupt, 1995). For example, if a student gets angry during her mathematics homework because a problem is hard to solve, she can try to deliberately see the problem as a game.

11.5.3   Teaching That Academic Emotions Are Controllable

The development of subjective perceptions of control related to emotions is very important for the promotion of students' EI (for a developmental-psychological examination of subjective perceptions of control related to emotions, see Stegge & Terwogt, 1998). Emotional control beliefs significantly determine the interpretation of previous emotional experiences. For example, intense anger surrounding a previous exam can simply be interpreted as uncontrollable, or as a result of poor self-regulation of this potentially controllable emotion. Such interpretations influence subsequent emotional goals, expectations, the application of emotion-regulation strategies, and in turn, future emotional experiences (Covington, 1997). Subjective interpretations of preceding events are far-reaching both within and outside an achievement context, as has been shown in the literature on attribution theory (Möller & Köller, 1996; Weiner, 1985, 1995), and in the literature on learned helplessness and learned optimism, respectively (Peterson, 2000; Seligman, 1991, 1993).

In terms of teaching the controllability of emotional experiences, methods of attributional retraining (Perry, 1991; Schunk, 1984; Struthers, Perry, & Menec, 2000; Van Overwalle & De Metsenaere, 1990) can be adapted or used as a basis for instructional activities (on attributional emotion theories, see Weiner & Graham, 1985). Specifically, emotion focused attributional retraining may help students to interpret their previous emotional experiences as unstable and potentially controllable in nature. As a starting point, students could be asked to report about a recent exam and explore in detail the phenomenology of their anxiety with respect to this exam, and also elaborate on possible reasons for why they were anxious. Students' attention can also be directed toward the fact that they have not been equally anxious on other exams. Becoming aware that one's emotions need not be perceived as due to immutable, stable traits will help students see that both negative and positive academic emotions may be, in part, controllable (for an empirical examination of emotion-focused attributional retraining in college students, see Hall, Perry, Chipperfield, Clifton, & Haynes, in press).

11.5.4   Teaching That Academic Emotions Are Valuable

According to the model depicted in Figure 11.2, students' EI can be fostered by developing or enhancing their subjective value beliefs concerning emotions through corresponding instructional activities. To do so, in the class room, the importance of emotions to subjective well-being (Ekman & Davidson, 1994; Goleman, 1995) and to one's quality of life should be stressed (for discussion of subjective well-being in the context of positive psychology, see Seligman & Csikszentmihalyi, 2000). Experiencing positive emotions is an essential component within most modern definitions of subjective well-being (Diener, 2000). What matters is not the intensity of positive emotions (overwhelming emotions), but their frequencies of occurrence. Thus, subjective well-being is experienced when positive emotions are predominant over time. In the classroom context, asking students about what is really important in life could lead to topics such as well-being and positive emotional experiences, and serve to highlight the value of emotional experiences both within and outside school. Starting points for a discussion could also be a proverb or a statement such as "That we call Good which is apt to cause or increase pleasure, or diminish pain" (Locke, 1690/1975, p. 2).

It is also important to point out to students the significance of emotions for communication processes at school (see Andersen & Guerrero, 1998; on the significance of emotions in nonverbal communication with numerous examples, see also Molcho, 2001). To this end, students can be instructed to engage in role playing, in which they ask each other simple questions like "What are you doing?" with different emotional undertones. Students will experience that the same sentence can be interpreted as expression of interest, as curiosity, as reproach or as derision. According to the emotional undertone of the questioner, the answers may be quite different in content (e.g., normal answer, lie, justification) and emotional reaction (e.g., neutral, pride, anger, anxiety).

Finally, the importance of emotions for the quality of learning and achievement might be demonstrated to students (Pekrun et al., 2002). Teachers could ask them to imagine the learning process of a happy, proud, bored, anxious, or hopeless person and to estimate the quality of learning and achievement outcomes for each of these persons. Differences in motivation, learning styles, and activation of internal and external resources (e.g., effort as internal resource and seeking help as external resource) can be the focus of discussion. In addition to the value of emotions in the scholastic environment, the value of emotions outside school can be discussed with the students. Popular scientific publications on EI provide numerous issues for discussion (on emotions and occupational success, see Caruso & Wolfe, 2001; Goleman, Boyatzis, & McKee, 2003). An achievement-related situation outside school is, for example, a job interview. A possible starting point for a discussion could be the following situation: There are two job candidates of equal gender, comparable age, and the same high school grades. In the process of generating additional arguments for employing the one person over the other, students will likely suggest qualities like sympathy, openness, and the expression of optimism and positive emotions.

11.6   IMPLICATIONS FOR RESEARCH AND PRACTICE

Based on the preceding models and concepts, we discuss the central implications of EI for researchers and practitioners in the passages that follow.

11.6.1   Becoming More Aware of the Relevance of EI for Achievement

Promoting EI is by no means considered important in all societies (Zins, Elias, Greenberg, & Weissberg, 2000). For researchers and practitioners alike, it is important to discuss the relevance of EI for learning and instruction in school. From an achievement-oriented perspective, it is only important to identify and regulate emotions related to academic achievement. Thus, when arguing in favor of the significance of EI in the classroom, the importance of emotional experiences for learning and achievement should play a major role.

11.6.2   Linking EI with the Psychology of Emotions

It is striking that the literature on EI rarely refers to theories and findings from the psychology of emotions (Mayer et al., 2002). We would like to encourage researchers to integrate knowledge from the field of research on emotions into ongoing research on EI. Conversely, the psychology of emotion should consider incorporating some aspects that are relevant for EI in an academic setting. For example, we still lack knowledge about the differential effects of specific emotions on scholastic learning and achievement, even though this is a central issue for the goal-directed regulation of students' emotions.

11.6.3   Linking EI with Clinical (Child) Psychology

In the context of EI, emotion regulation may be seen to form a central interface with clinical psychology. While many branches of psychology have developed theories on emotions (primarily the discipline of general psychology), it was almost exclusively in clinical research in which diverse techniques for their regulation were explicated and encouraged. Those techniques are, for example, anger management methods (Howells & Day, 2003), aspects of rational emotive behavior therapy (Ellis, 2002), and focusing oriented therapy (Gendlin, 1991, 1997). These methods, most of which have been developed for pathological samples, could be rather easily adapted for use in an academic context for the promotion of EI in students. In an academic setting, findings from research on clinical child psychology could also be incorporated, for example, the Anti-Stress-Training for Children (Hampel & Petermann, 1998; Meichenbaum, Turk, & Burstein, 1975).

11.6.4 Developing Age-Specific Materials

The psychology of emotion provides an extensive array of materials suitable for fostering EI in schools (see above). However, these materials would have to be adapted for specific age groups. For example, emotion pictures used in the context of research on emotions (e.g., the Facial Expression Analysis Tool [FEAT], Kaiser & Wehrle, 1994) could be used in developing age-specific materials for the extension of emotion-related vocabulary. Complexity of the emotions depicted in the pictures might depend on the age-group that the materials are developed for. The affectmeter, often used in research on work satisfaction, could also be tailored to illustrate emotions to younger students in particular (on the utilization of the affectmeter in the context of emotion research in schools, see Helmke, 1993).

11.6.5 Teaching Components of EI Step-by-Step

Because perception and reflection of emotions are key aspects of emotion regulation, these two aspects should be taught to students first, before concrete regulation techniques are dealt with. Similar to other self-regulation models, extensive knowledge is a necessary condition for the successful development of emotional regulation processes (see the hierarchical structure of Boekaerts's, 1999, self-regulation model).

11.6.6 Training Teachers

The promotion of EI at school should be integrated into teacher training at universities, and become a module for advanced training for active teachers. Teachers need a comprehensive repertoire of knowledge and methods, as well as expertise in teaching EI in situations of learning and achievement (Zeidner, Roberts, & Matthews, 2002). Multiplier programs could be an effective method for implementing this knowledge. For example, school principals or selected teachers could attend training sessions on encouraging EI in their students and then act as multipliers, passing their knowledge on to their colleagues, or teachers from other schools, while also exchanging experiences in the application of these skills.

11.6.7 Developing Instruments for the Assessment of EI That Are Age- and Subject-Specific

There is a lack of appropriate instrumentation for the evaluation of programs fostering EI. Because of the complexity of the construct of EI, it would make sense to generate instruments that are suitable for the evaluation of sub-goals for its promotion. Such an instrument might exclusively assess an individual's emotion vocabulary, or comprise a knowledge test on the intensity of certain components of specific emotions.

11.7 CONCLUSION

As the necessity of fostering students' EI makes intuitive sense, a number of EI promotion programs have been conceptualized and realized. However, most of these programs lack a theoretical and scientifically sound basis. It appears that in the realm of academic EI, practitioners have surpassed researchers in developing EI programs without the empirical data required to support and guide such initiatives. As most EI promotion techniques appear to have little or no scientific basis, we recommend that such programs be viewed with greater skepticism. In the present chapter, we presented a theoretical model for the promotion of EI in an academic setting, embedded in a larger framework of antecedents, "intelligent" processing, and the effects of academic emotions. While this theoretical foundation can initiate the theory-directed development of EI promotion programs, the evaluation of such initiatives is limited due to the need for corresponding assessment tools. Consequently, the development of instruments for assessing the effectiveness of EI promotion programs, with respect to theoretically derived subcomponents of EI, is critical to the future success of training programs aimed at fostering emotional intelligence in the classroom.

REFERENCES

Abele, A. E. (1996). Einfluss positiver und negativer Stimmungen auf die kognitive Leistung [On the impact of positive and negative moods on cognitive performance]. In J. Möller & O. Köller (Eds.), *Emotionen , Kognitionen und Schulleistung* (pp. 91–111). Weinheim, Germany: Psychologie Verlags Union.

Andersen, P. A., & Guerrero, L. K. (1998). Principles of communication and emotion in social interaction. In P. A. Andersen & L. K. Guerrero (Eds.), *Handbook of communication and emotion* (pp. 49–96). New York: Academic Press.

Anderson, J. R. (2000). *Cognitive psychology and its implications.* New York: Freeman.

Aspinwall, L. G. (1998). Rethinking the role of positive affect in self-regulation. *Motivation and Emotion, 22,* 1–32.

Astleitner, H. (2000). Designing emotionally sound instruction: The FEASP-approach. *Instructional Science, 28,* 169–198.

Atkinson, J. W. (1957). Motivational determinants of risk-taking behavior. *Psychological Review, 64,* 359–372.

Atkinson, J. W. (1964). *An introduction to motivation.* Princeton, NJ: Van Nostrand.

Bar-On, R. (1997). *BarOn Emotional Quotient Inventory (EQ–i): Technical manual.* Toronto, Canada: Multi-Health Systems.

Boekaerts, M. (1999). Self-regulated learning: Where we are today. *International Journal of Educational Research, 31,* 445–475.

Boekaerts, M., Pintrich, P. R., & Zeidner, M. (Eds.). (2000). *Handbook of self-regulation.* San Diego, CA: Academic Press.

Caruso, D. R., & Wolfe, C. J. (2001). Emotional intelligence in the workplace. In J. Ciarrochi, J. P. Forgas, & J. D. Mayer (Eds.), *Emotional intelligence in everyday life* (pp. 150–167). Philadelphia: Psychology Press.

Cohen, J. (1999). *Educating minds and hearts: Social emotional learning and the passage into adolescence.* New York: Teachers College Press.

Cohen, J. (2001). *Caring classrooms/intelligent schools: The social emotional education of young children.* New York: Teachers College Press.

Covington, M. V. (1997). A motivational analysis of academic life in college. In R. P. Perry & J. C. Smart (Eds.), *Effective teaching in higher education* (pp. 61–100). New York: Agathon Press.

Covington, M. V., & Wiedenhaupt, S. (1995). Turning work into play: The nature and nurturing of intrinsic task engagement. In J. C. Perry & R. Smart (Eds.), *Effective teaching in higher education: Research and practice* (pp. 101–114). New York: Agathon Press.

Diener, E. (2000). Subjective well-being: The science of happiness and a proposal for a national index. *American Psychologist, 55,* 34–43.

Ekman, P., & Davidson, R. J. (1994). Affective science: A research agenda. In P. Ekman & R. J. Davidson (Eds.), *The nature of emotion: Fundamental questions* (pp. 411–434). New York: Oxford University Press.

Ekman, P., & Friesen, W. V. (1978). *The facial action coding system.* Palo Alto, CA: Consulting Psychologist Press.

Elias, M. J., Hunter, L., & Kress, J. S. (2001). Emotional intelligence and education. In J. Ciarrochi, J. P. Forgas, & J. D. Mayer (Eds.), *Emotional intelligence in everyday life* (pp. 133–149). Philadelphia: Psychology Press.

Elias, M. J., Zins, J. E., Weissberg, R. P., Frey, K. S., Greenberg, M. T., Haynes, N. M., et al. (1997). *Promoting social and emotional learning: Guidelines for educators.* Alexandria, VA: Association for Supervision and Curriculum Development.

Ellis, A. (2002). *Overcoming resistance: A rational emotive behavior therapy integrated approach* (2nd ed.). New York: Springer.

Ellis, H. C., & Ashbrook, P. W. (1988). Resource allocation model of the effects of depressed mood states on memory. In K. Fiedler & J. Forgas (Eds.), *Affect, cognition, and social behavior* (pp. 25–43). Toronto, Canada: Hogrefe & Huber.

Fiedler, K. (1988). Emotional mood, cognitive style, and behavior regulation. In K. Fiedler & J. Forgas (Eds.), *Affect, cognition and social behavior* (pp. 25–43). Toronto, Canada: Hogrefe & Huber.

Friesen, W. V., & Ekmann, P. (1984). *EMFACS-7: Emotional facial action coding system.* Unpublished Manual, University of California, San Francisco, CA.

Frijda, N. H. (1998). *The emotions.* Cambridge, UK: Cambridge University Press.

Gendlin, E. T. (1991). On emotion in therapy. In J. D. Safran & L. S. Greenberg (Eds.), *Emotion, psychotherapy, and change* (pp. 255–279). New York: Guilford Press.

Gendlin, E. T. (1997). The use of focusing in therapy. In J. K. Zeig (Ed.), *The evolution of psychotherapy: The third conference* (pp. 197–210). Philadelphia: Brunner/Mazel.

Geppert, U., Schmidt, D., & Galinowski, I. (1997). *Self-evaluative emotions coding system (SEECS)* (Technical Manual No. 19/1997). Munich, Germany: Max-Planck-Institute for Psychological Research.

Goetz, T. (2004). *Emotionen und selbstreguliertes Lernen bei Schülern im Fach Mathematik* [Students' emotions and self-regulated learning in mathematics]. Munich, Germany: Utz.

Goetz, T., Zirngibl, A., Hall, N., & Pekrun, R. (2003). Emotions, learning and achievement from an educational-psychological perspective. In P. Mayring & C. Rhoeneck (Eds.), *Learning emotions. The influence of affective factors on classroom learning* (pp. 9–28). Frankfurt am Main, Germany: Peter Lang.

Gohm, C. L. (2003). Mood regulation and emotional intelligence: Individual differences. *Journal of Personality and Social Psychology, 84*, 594–607.

Goleman, D. (1995). *Emotional intelligence: Why it can matter more than IQ.* New York: Bantam Books.

Goleman, D., Boyatzis, R. E., & McKee, A. (2003). *The new leaders: Transforming the art of leadership into the science of results.* London: Little Brown.

Greenberg, M. T., Kusche, C. A., Cook, E. T., & Quamma, J. P. (1995). Promoting emotional competence in school-aged children: The effects of the PATHS curriculum. *Development and Psychopathology, 7*, 117–136.

Hall, N., Perry, R. P., Chipperfield, J. G., Clifton, R. A., & Haynes, T. (in press). Enhancing primary and secondary control in achievement settings through writing-based attributional retraining. *Journal of Social and Clinical Psychology.*

Hampel, P., & Petermann, F. (1998). *Anti-Stress-Training für Kinder* [Anti-stress training for children]. Weinheim, Germany: Beltz Psychologie Verlags Union.

Helmke, A. (1993). Die Entwicklung der Lernfreude vom Kindergarten bis zur 5. Klassenstufe [The development of enjoyment of learning from kindergarten to fifth grade]. *Zeitschrift für Pädagogische Psychologie, 7*, 77–86.

Hofer, T. (2000). *Emotionale Intelligenz im Schulalltag: Erfahrungen und Anregungen für den Regelklassen- und Spezialunterricht* [Emotional intelligence in the classroom: Experiences and recommendations for regular and special education]. Biel, Germany: Schüler AG.

Howells, K., & Day, A. (2003). Readiness for anger management: Clinical and theoretical issues. *Clinical Psychological Review, 23*, 319–337.

Kaiser, S., & Wehrle, T. (1994). Emotion research and AI: Some theoretical and technical issues. *Geneva Studies in Emotion and Communication, 8*, 1–16.

Klauer, K. J. (1988). Paradigmatic teaching of inductive thinking. In H. Mandl, E. De Corte, N. Bennett, & H. F. Friedrich (Eds.), *Learning and instruction* (2nd ed., pp. 23–45). Oxford, UK: Pergamon Press.

Klauer, K. J., & Phye, G. D. (1994). *Cognitive training for children: A developmental program of inductive reasoning and problem solving.* Toronto, Canada: Hogrefe & Huber.

Kusche, C. A., & Greenberg, M. T. (2001). PATHS in your classroom: Promoting emotional literacy and alleviating emotional distress. In J. Cohen (Ed.), *Caring classrooms/intelligent schools: The social emotional education of young children* (pp. 140–161). New York: Teachers College Press.

Kusche, C. A., Greenberg, M. T., & Beilke, B. (1988). *The Kusche affective interview.* Unpublished manuscript, Department of Psychology, University of Washington, Seattle, WA.

Lang, P. J., Bradley, M. M., & Cuthbert, B. N. (1995). *International affective picture system (IAPS): Technical manual and affective ratings.* Gainesville, FL: University of Florida, The Center for Research in Psychophysiology.

Lazarus, R. S., & Folkman, S. (1984). *Stress, appraisal, and coping.* New York: Springer.

Locke, J. (1975). *Essays concerning human understanding.* Oxford, UK: Clarendon Press. (Original work published 1690)

Mackintosh, N. J. (2001). *IQ and human intelligence.* New York: Oxford University Press.

Martinez-Pons, M. (1998). Parental inducement of emotional intelligence. *Imagination, Cognition and Personality, 18,* 3–23.

Martinez-Pons, M. (2000). Emotional intelligence as a self-regulatory process: A social cognitive view. *Imagination, Cognition and Personality, 19,* 331–350.

Martinez-Pons, M. (2001). *The psychology of teaching and learning: A three step approach.* New York: Continuum.

Matthews, G., Zeidner, M., & Roberts, R. D. (2002). *Emotional intelligence: Science and myth.* Cambridge, MA: MIT Press.

Mayer, J. D., & Salovey, P. (1997). What is emotional intelligence? In P. Salovey & D. J. Sluyter (Eds.), *Emotional development and emotional intelligence: Educational implications* (pp. 3–31). New York: Basic Books.

Mayer, J. D., Salovey, P., & Caruso, D. R. (2002). *The Mayer-Salovey-Caruso Emotional Intelligence Test (MSCEIT): User's manual.* Toronto, Canada: Multi-Health Systems.

Meichenbaum, D., Turk, D., & Burstein, S. (1975). The nature of coping with stress. In I. Sarason & C. Spielberger (Eds.), *Stress and anxiety* (Vol. 2, pp. 337–360). Washington, DC: Hemisphere.

Molcho, S. (2001). *Alles über Körpersprache: Sich selbst und andere besser verstehen* [Everything about body language: Understanding oneself and others better]. München, Germany: Mosaik.

Molfenter, S. (1999). *Prüfungsemotionen bei Studierenden: Explorative Analysen und Entwicklung eines diagnostischen Instrumentariums* [University students' test emotions: Exploratory analyses and development of a diagnostic instrument]. Unpublished doctoral dissertation, University of Regensburg.

Möller, J., & Köller, O. (1996). Attributionen und Schulleistung [Attribution and scholastic performance]. In J. Möller & O. Köller (Eds.), *Emotionen, Kognitionen und Schulleistung* (pp. 115–136). Weinheim, Germany: Psychologie Verlags Union.

Pekrun, R. (2000). A social-cognitive, control-value theory of achievement emotions. In J. Heckhausen (Ed.), *Motivational psychology of human development.* Oxford, UK: Elsevier.

Pekrun, R., Goetz, T., Titz, W., & Perry, R. P. (2002). Academic emotions in students' self-regulated learning and achievement: A program of qualitative and quantitative research. *Educational Psychologist, 37,* 91–105.

Perry, R. P. (1991). Perceived control in college students: Implications for instruction in higher education. In J. Smart (Ed.), *Higher education: Handbook for theory and research* (Vol. 7, pp. 1–56). New York: Agathon Press.

Peterson, C. (2000). The future of optimism. *American Psychologist, 55,* 44–55.

Plutchik, R. (1980). *Emotion: A psychoevolutionary synthesis*. New York: Harper and Row.

Ricci-Bitti, P., & Scherer, K. R. (1986). Interrelations between antecedents, reactions, and coping responses. In K. R. Scherer, H. G. Wallbott, & A. B. Summerfield (Eds.), *Experiencing emotion: A cross-cultural study* (pp. 84–97). Cambridge, UK: Cambridge University Press.

Salovey, P., & Mayer, J. D. (1990). Emotional intelligence. *Imagination, Cognition and Personality, 9*, 185–211.

Scherer, K. R. (1984). On the nature and function of emotion: A component process approach. In K. R. Scherer & P. Ekman (Eds.), *Approaches to emotion* (pp. 293–317). Hillsdale, NJ: Lawrence Erlbaum.

Scherer, K. R. (1993). Neuroscience projections to current debates in emotion psychology. *Cognition and Emotion, 7*, 1–41.

Schunk, D. H. (1984). Sequential attributional feedback and children's achievement behaviors. *Journal of Educational Psychology, 76*, 1159–1169.

Seligman, M. E. P. (1991). *Learned optimism*. New York: Knopf.

Seligman, M. E. P. (1993). *Learned helplessness*. New York: Oxford University Press.

Seligman, M. E. P., & Csikszentmihalyi, M. (2000). Positive psychology: An introduction. *American Psychologist, 55*, 5–14.

Shure, M. B., & Glaser, A. L. (2001). I can problem solve (ICPS): A cognitive approach to the prevention of early high-risk behaviors. In J. Cohen (Ed.), *Caring classrooms/intelligent schools: The social emotional education of young children* (pp. 122–139). New York: Teachers College Press.

Smith, C. A., & Ellsworth, P. C. (1985). Patterns of cognitive appraisal in emotion. *Journal of Personality and Social Psychology, 48*, 813–838.

Stegge, H., & Terwogt, M. M. (1998). Perspectives on the strategic control of emotions: A developmental account. In A. H. Fischer (Ed.), *Proceedings of the Xth conference of the international society for research on emotion*. Amsterdam: International Society for Research on Emotion.

Sternberg, R. J. (1997). The concept of intelligence and its role in lifelong learning and success. *American Psychologist, 52*, 1030–1037.

Struthers, C. W., Perry, R. P., & Menec, V. H. (2000). An examination of the relationships among academic stress, coping, motivation, and performance at college. *Research in Higher Education, 41*, 579–590.

Titz, W. (2001). *Emotionen von Studierenden in Lernsituationen: Explorative Analysen und Entwicklung von Selbstberichtskalen* [Students' emotions in learning situations: Exploratory analyses and development of self-report scales]. Münster, Germany: Waxmann.

Topping, K. J., Holmes, E. A., & Bremner, W. G. (2000). The effectiveness of school-based programs: For the promotion of social competence. In R. Bar-On & J. D. A. Parker (Eds.), *The handbook of emotional intelligence: Theory, development, assessment, and application at home, school, and in the workplace* (pp. 411–432). San Francisco, CA: Jossey-Bass.

Van Brakel, J. (1994). Emotions: A cross-cultural perspective on forms of life. In W. M. Wentworth & J. Ryan (Eds.), *Social perspectives on emotion* (Vol. 2, pp. 179–237). Greenwich, CT: JAI Press.

Van Overwalle, F., & De Metsenaere, M. (1990). The effects of attribution-based intervention and study strategy training on academic achievement in college freshmen. *British Journal of Educational Psychology, 60,* 299–311.

Watson, D., & Tellegen, A. (1985). Toward a consensual structure of mood. *Psychological Bulletin, 98,* 219–235.

Weiner, B. (1985). An attributional theory of achievement motivation and emotion. *Psychological Review, 92,* 548–573.

Weiner, B. (1995). *Judgements of responsibility: A foundation for a theory of social conduct.* New York: Guilford Press.

Weiner, B., & Graham, S. (1985). An attributional approach to emotional development. In E. Izard, J. Kagan, & R. B. Zajonc (Eds.), *Emotions, cognition, and behavior* (pp. 167–191). New York: Cambridge University Press.

Zeidner, M., Roberts, R. D., & Matthews, G. (2002). Can emotional intelligence be schooled? A critical review. *Educational Psychologist, 37,* 215–231.

Zins, J. E., Elias, M. J., Greenberg, M. T., & Weissberg, R. P. (2000). Promoting social and emotional competence in children. In K. M. Minke & G. C. Bear (Eds.), *Preventing school problems—promoting school success: Strategies and programs that work* (pp. 71–99). Bethesda, MD: National Association of School Psychologists.

Zins, J. E., Travis, F., & Freppan, P. A. (1997). Linking research and educational programming to promote social and emotional learning. In P. Salovey & D. J. Sluyter (Eds.), *Emotional development and emotional intelligence* (pp. 168–192). New York: Basic Books.

12

Emotional Intelligence in the Workplace: A Review and Synthesis

Rebecca Abraham

Nova Southeastern University, USA

Summary

In this chapter, emotional intelligence (EI) is viewed as a predictor of success in the workplace through its significant association with transformational leadership, ability to foster workgroup cohesiveness, facilitate accurate feedback during performance review, strengthen commitment to the organization, assist in matching employers and employees, permit feelings of control over work, and enhance self-esteem. Conceptual arguments supplemented by empirical validation are offered to link EI and the above attributes for success in the workplace. Research in the area of personnel selection appears promising, with the ability of emotionally based tools to identify employees who are capable of succeeding in a particular organization.

12.1 INTRODUCTION

After almost a century of neglect, the value of emotions is beginning to take its rightful place alongside normative rational models of organizational behavior. Early references to emotions, which link job dissatisfaction to emotional maladjustment (Fisher & Hanna, 1931), emotional lives with work behavior

(Hersey, 1932), and the Hawthorne studies' conclusion that workplace interaction (presumably derived from emotional feeling) determined worker adjustment (Roethlisberger & Dickson, 1939) were not subjected to rigorous empirical investigation. This appears due to the reorienting of affect at work in terms of job satisfaction and the failure to conceptually ground emotions in relation to other predictors of workplace adjustment (Brief & Weiss, 2002).

Emotions are a core element of organizational life with moments of sorrow, joy, passion, and ennui supporting enduring feelings of satisfaction or commitment (Ashforth & Humphrey, 1995). Specifically, Ashforth and Humphrey (1995) conceptualize emotions as driving motivation, leadership, and group commitment. The greater the immersion of the self in work, the greater is the motivation. Involvement with work exists at three levels. At the lowest, involvement is solely physical sans emotional or cognitive involvement, the next rationalist level is purely cognitive, and the highest is emotional, "typified by the individual who forgets to have dinner and works late into the night, lost in the thrill of her work" (Ashforth & Humphrey, 1995, p. 110). This state of flow, entered into by high achievers 40% of the time versus 16% for low achievers (Csikszentmihalyi, 1990), transcends compensation, title, rank, and perceived power and prestige as it catapults the employee to an emotional peak experience. In this vein, pro-social behaviors including volunteering to assist new employees, being a spokesperson for the organization, and suggesting improvements are manifestations of affective commitment in which trust and altruism overshadow purely contractual relationships based on reward, compensation, and promotion. Enactment theories of leadership posit the creation of a system of shared meanings, which provide a framework for behavior (see Daft & Weick, 1984, for a review). Effective leaders use symbols to invoke feelings of passion in subordinates whereby the sight of a corporate logo or figurehead provokes strong emotional arousal to be expanded into frameworks that embody the organization's history, values, and culture. Emotional contagion, whereby the emotions of a few group members are transmitted throughout the work group, is a formalized designation of team spirit that has been documented in a variety of organizational settings (Hatfield, Cacioppo, & Rapson, 1992; Zurcher, 1982).

From the generalized emotional underpinnings of organizational life, this chapter moves to address the skillful processing of affective information by emotionally intelligent individuals. Salovey and Mayer (1990) provide a comprehensive framework for defining emotional intelligence (EI). First, EI is the accurate appraisal and expression of emotion both in the self and in others. Emotional self-appraisal includes the ability to identify and categorize one's own feelings through words or facial expression. In relation to others, empathy forms the cornerstone of emotional appraisal through gauging of feelings in others, reexperiencing those feelings, and choosing socially adaptive responses. Second, EI includes the adaptive regulation of emotion. In the self, regulation is the product of a regulatory system that monitors, evaluates, and, if necessary, changes moods (Mayer & Gaschke, 1988). People engage in mood self-maintenance in which they try to maintain positive moods and suppress negative moods (Tesser, 1986). The most important dimension of emotional regulation involves regulating emotions in others. Leaders who can arouse desired emotions in others have been termed charismatic (Wasielewski, 1985).

Finally, EI is the ability to use emotions to solve problems. Mood swings may assist people in breaking away from routine and perceiving a wider range of alternative solutions to problems. A positive mood may aid memory organization and problem solving. In Duncker's candlestick experiment, Isen, Daubman, and Nowicki (1987) observed that happier participants had more creative solutions. Heightened self-awareness of emotions helps people to redirect their attention to issues of higher priority. Moods may also motivate persistence in the face of challenge. For some individuals, positive moods inspire confidence in one's ability to succeed at challenging tasks. For others, concern over a negative outcome may spur extra effort and motivate performance.

12.2 PERSONNEL SELECTION

One of the few areas in which EI has been investigated empirically is in the area of personnel selection. Probably the earliest empirical study in this area is that of Aylward's (1985) administration of 10 psychological batteries to applicants to a police department. Given that only 7% of the variance in successful hiring decisions could be attributed to IQ, the relative superiority of emotional, behavioral, and attitudinal predictors, in determining an applicant's psychological adaptability to the rigors of police work, was made apparent. As the gateway to personnel selection is the job interview, Fox and Spector (2000) identified the EI component of positive affect or the ability by an emotionally intelligent interviewee to induce positive feelings in the interviewer as increasing the likelihood of being hired (positive affect being a significant predictor of the interview outcome of decision to hire). Positive affect was also found to enhance the interviewer's perception of candidate qualifications. Highly significant beta coefficient in the regression of qualification of candidate on a series of predictors included general intelligence, practical intelligence, negative and positive affectivity, repair of mood, perspective taking, and personal distress. This predictive ability was strengthened by the positive association of positive affect with yet another predictor, practical intelligence, or the use of judgment by interviewees in creating a positive impression during the interview process. An indirect relationship between EI and hiring decisions was found in the link between positive affect and similarity (interviewers are likely to bond more closely with interviewees whom they perceive as having greater similarity with themselves and those for whom they have genuine liking). Likewise, positive affect and another EI dimension, empathy, jointly influenced liking (interviewers appear more favorably disposed towards those whom they like). Perceptions of greater similarity and liking, in turn, positively influenced the perceptions of superiority of candidate qualifications and the decision to hire.

In a job simulation task, in which participants were asked to complete three activities, Graves (1999) validated Fox and Spector's (2000) prediction of job success (based on interview performance) with their finding that EI predicted 6–10% of the variance in three separate performance composites including energy, forcefulness, initiative, organization and planning, decisiveness, judgment, social sensitivity, leadership, oral communication, and teamwork. When combined with cognitive ability, the two predictors accounted for a significant 10–17% of the variance in the performance composites underscoring the enhanced accuracy of selection by the inclusion of EI.

Other studies (see Van Rooy & Viswesvaran, 2004, for a review) have consistently reported correlations between EI and performance. In an effort to promote coherence among multiple empirical investigations, Van Rooy and Viswesvaran (2004) performed meta-analysis on 69 independent studies finding that the correlation of EI and actual job performance ($\rho = .24$) is higher than that of other selection methods such as letters of reference. As their sample employed participants from different countries and occupations, these results are robust across both populations and job classifications. In concurrence with the Graves (1999) results, it was found that EI was strongly correlated with general mental ability ($r = .33$), and each of these predictors incrementally predicted performance over the other; suggesting their combined, rather than separate, importance as predictors of performance.

12.3   LEADERSHIP

George (2000) theorized that EI facilitates dimensions of leadership, including 1) the development of a unified sense of goals and objectives, 2) inculcating the value of work in subordinates, 3) creating a climate of excitement, enthusiasm, cooperation, optimism, and trust, 4) fostering adaptability to change, and 5) creating and sustaining an identity for the organization (Conger & Kanungo, 1998; Locke, 1991). Leaders with positive moods have been found to be more creative in formulating a transcendent goal for the firm (Isen et al., 1987). Furthermore, positive mood results in flexible decision making that incorporates a broad expanse of options (Isen & Baron, 1991); it follows that developing an overarching goal for the firm will be facilitated by leaders in positive moods. Knowledge of followers' emotions permits the collectivization of vision in that such leaders influence them into accepting and supporting the vision and use emotional contagion (positive feeling about the shared vision) to communicate that commitment throughout the organization. Such leaders capitalize on meta-mood knowledge that positive affirmation of employee performance as improvements over prior conditions (Salovey & Mayer, 1990), regardless of whether the change is incremental or substantial, spurs employees to strive for progressively higher levels of achievement. EI promotes the prioritization of demands. Leaders, who realize emotions aroused by low priority demands, can effectively channel that energy to those of significant import. Positive moods promote flexibility in decision making. Leaders who employ meta-mood regulation become aware of negative moods causing overly pessimistic prognostications, which are then neutralized to open up a vein of hitherto unforeseen opportunity. Such flexibility in decision making, induced by EI, assists in establishing connections between divergent pieces of information thereby not only opening up new avenues of opportunity but permitting the simultaneous response to multiple demands. The identity of an organization is based upon its values, the embodiment of "symbols, language, narrative, and practices" (George, 2000, p. 1046). Values, fostered through the skillful management of symbols (e.g., parties, anniversaries, company songs, and stories) are emotion-driven; emotionally intelligent leaders are aware of the emotional basis of values as they use symbolic management to build loyalty and commitment.

Empirical validation for the above theory may be derived from a selected group of studies. Atwater and Yammarino (1992) found that self-awareness moderated transformational leadership and performance in military settings. Transformational leaders, with developed self-monitoring skills, are superior performers; however, their research was conducted in a military setting which may not be generalizable to the corporate environment. Accordingly, Sosik and Megerian (1999) extended their analysis to managers and subordinates of a business unit observing that for self-aware leaders, subordinate ratings of transformational leadership were directly related to purpose-in-life, personal efficacy, interpersonal control, and social self-confidence. This outcome suggests that self-awareness capability gives leaders control over incidents involving interpersonal relations. The instilling of self-confidence and feelings of self-efficacy among followers are valuable by-products of such self-awareness capability. Leaders whose self-ratings matched their ratings by subordinates were found to be superior performers in terms of their evaluations by superiors and subordinates. Self-monitoring was the foundation upon which interpersonal skills were built, so that self-aware leaders were more adept at managing emotions among superiors, leading to ratings of managerial effectiveness and subordinates who valued them for extra effort and satisfaction. The importance of self-awareness has been underscored by other studies of leadership success. In a survey of senior executives, Collins (2002) found that trait EI influenced the prediction of success through self-ratings. Emotionally intelligent nursing leaders, whose leadership skills are honed in the demanding environment of coordinating the delivery of health care by providers, demonstrated heightened emotional self-awareness in contrast to their low-scoring counterparts (Vitello-Cicciu, 2002).

Two other qualities of EI that have predicted leadership success include managing emotions in others and propensity for innovation and risk-taking. In the aforementioned nursing leadership study, leadership practices dubbed Modeling the Way and Encouraging the Heart were significantly associated with enhanced EI. Modeling the Way incorporates the creation of positive mood to permit the collectivization of vision to which the George (2000) theory alluded, while Encouraging the Heart is emotional regulation in others, or the management of emotional response in others. Campbell (2001) theorized that global competition, export of jobs overseas, and weak economy have mandated the need for constant innovation and responsible risk-taking. EI was significantly associated with both innovation and responsible risk taking behavior, with all facets of EI attributed to these outcomes.

12.4   WORKGROUP COHESION

Emotional intelligence leads to the harmonious sharing of competencies within groups whose performance surpasses those sharing only cognitive skills (Goleman, 1995). In experiments involving the comparison of groups involved in generating advertisements, it has been found that harmonious groups were able to benefit from the creativity of every group member in contrast with groups whose dominance by a single member fueled resentment and hostility (Williams & Sternberg, 1988). Peak performing groups have members who foster the development of consensus, using empathy, cooperation, and social competence skills (Kelley & Caplan, 1993). This study's investigation of group dynamics within the Bell Labs concluded that the social skills component of EI was vital in the creation and sustenance of informal networks. As knowledge for task completion was rarely within the domain of a single individual, superior performance could only be achieved through the formation of informal networks based on communication and trust (wherein members could freely express their opinions as they toiled together on tasks whose successful completion required the melding of diverse tasks of a highly specialized nature). Empirically, ingroup dynamics may be modeled by Schutte, Malouff, Simunek, McKenley, and Hollander's (2002) finding that EI was significantly associated with inter-personal skills. Specifically, only empathic perspective demonstrated significance among others including empathic fantasy, concern, and personal distress. They believed that these other forms of empathy were less emotionally adaptive; I would prefer to characterize empathic perspective as an understanding of the emotions of others that leads to the social skills needed to foster group harmony. Emotionally intelligent group members desire more cooperation, participation, and inclusion than others, the provision of which leads to the aforementioned highly effective networks.

Jordan, Ashkanasy, and Härtel (2003) tested the relationship between EI and two aspects of team performance, namely team process effectiveness and team goal focus. The ability to deal with others' emotions was found to contribute significantly to Acquisitive Self Monitoring, or by regulating and influencing emotional reactions in others, role senders were able to strengthen their own skills of self-awareness. Significant correlations of EI dimensions of Ability to Deal with Own Emotions, Ability to Deal with Others' Emotions, and Emotional Self-Control with intuitive, creative group process with no correlation with rational, logical process suggests that EI is related to creative group decision making with variance beyond that explained by mere rational cognitive processing capability. Partial support for the revised Salovey and Mayer model was obtained with Empathetic Control being weakly correlated with team performance as it is a predictor rather than a component of managing emotions.

Workgroup cohesion may depend on the ability of team members and team leaders to engage in successful conflict resolution. Organizations in which constructive conflict is the norm, whereby all parties express their opinions freely and then collaborate to achieve conflict resolution, are more capable of responding to change. EI was found to enhance the possibility of usage of constructive conflict with significant correlations between Collaboration and Awareness of Own Emotions, Discussion of Own Emotions, Control of Own Emotions, Recognition of Others' Emotions, and Management of Others' Emotions (Jordan & Troth, 2002). This preliminary result was explored further (using hierarchical regression) to determine which subscale of EI was related to collaboration. Ability to Deal with Own Emotions and Ability to Deal with Others' Emotions emerged as jointly contributing to a significant increase in variance in the criterion. Further analysis showed that Ability to Deal with Own Emotions, Discussion of Own Emotions, and Control of Own Emotions significantly predicted collaborative conflict resolution. It may be concluded that two facets of collaborative conflict resolution, the abilities to be assertive and cooperative, are directly related to the ability to discuss and control one's own emotions.

12.5   PERFORMANCE FEEDBACK

As empirical work in this area is nonexistent, we will summarize (Abraham, 1999) arguments theorizing that EI may moderate the relationship between self and supervisor ratings. Emotionally intelligent supervisors are more likely to provide ratings that correspond closely with self-ratings of subordinates. Optimism is a component of EI. Optimism rests on the premise that failure is not inherent in the individual; it may be attributed to circumstances that may be changed with a refocusing of effort. Emotionally intelligent criticism during annual performance reviews focuses on specific incidents that reveal deficiencies in performance and offers concrete solutions for rectifying them. The emotionally intelligent delivery of criticism provides valuable information to employees to take corrective action before problems escalate. Consequently, an empathic employee will be able to review weaknesses in his or her performance from the organization's perspective, perceiving them as detrimental to organizational success. Such an individual will be more receptive to suggestions for improvement and more willing to accept responsibility for failure and will perceive criticism as the opportunity to work with superiors and coworkers constructively to improve performance. EI on the part of both the superior and the subordinate will result in deeper understanding of each other, thereby increasing the correspondence between their performance appraisals. Not only does the greater congruence between superior and subordinate ratings stimulate development through greater acceptance of information provided during feedback, it also acts as a powerful reinforcer of the influence of self-assessment on motivation (Koresgaard, 1996) and promotes involvement in the appraisal process (Mohrmann, Resnick-West, & Lawler, 1990).

12.6 PERFORMANCE

Flow is the harnessing of emotions to achieve superior performance and learning (Goleman, 1995). Tasks that both challenge and permit an individual to draw on existing knowledge are most likely to send him or her into a state of flow. Post-It Notes, waterproof sandpaper, and Thinsulate were the products of instinctive feeling rather than rigorous scientific analysis. The ability to use emotional knowledge has been observed to be fundamental to successful decision making. When a novel problem arises, the decision maker draws on his or her knowledge base of relationships to arrive at workable solutions. Studies of traders at the stock exchange and generals in the field, both of whom belong to professions where split-second decision making is the norm, have found that they reject analytical problem solving in favor of a body of knowledge built through experience that provides successful solutions (Farnham, 1996).

Four empirical studies clarify the effect of EI on performance. Schutte, Schuettpelz, and Malouff (2000–2001) observed that emotionally intelligent undergraduates were more willing to complete both moderately and highly difficult tasks in an anagram experiment. However, they did not explore the dimensions of EI responsible for the additional variance in performance. Bachman, Stern, Campbell, and Sitarenios (2000) posited that self-awareness would prevent debt collectors from lapsing into excessive lenience caused by empathizing too closely with clients. At the other extreme, emotional self-control prevents belligerence on the part of the account officer so that the interaction does not degenerate into a shouting match. Empirical comparison of meritorious account officers, along with a control group, showed (as predicted) that the principal difference between the two groups was empathic skills. Meritorious account officers had less empathy and higher reality test scores indicating their capability to focus on the situation with clarity by distinguishing between subjective feeling and objective reality. Coupling this result with high scores on emotional self-control leads to the conclusion that successful debt collectors exhibit emotional self-control in their interactions with clients, which permits them to convey urgency. In a companion study, these authors found that superior performance rated highly on the EI competencies of independence, self-confidence, and optimism, which, in turn, resulted in enhanced time management, information processing, communications and negotiations leading to the formulation of mutually beneficial debt collection plans.

Fox and Spector (2000) related EI to interview outcomes, hypothesizing that empathy, self-regulation, mood, and positive self-presentation would enhance performance. Empathy assumes importance as the ability to prevent oneself from being trapped in difficult interview questions and depends on the ability to predict the reactions of other social actors (constituting the appraisal dimension of EI). Self-presentation skills, first articulated in Goffman's (1959) classic,

The Presentation of Self in Everyday Life, suggest that the focal person will be thoroughly prepared in creating a positive impression and controlling any nonverbal feelings conveying unfavorable impressions. The creation of positive mood in interviewers has been noted elsewhere, being clearly enunciated by Isen and Baron (1991) with reference to the job interview: "Such persons are evaluated more favorably in performance appraisals are more likely to be hired after a job interview, are more likely to obtain concessions from opponents in bargaining contexts, . . ." (p. 28). For a sample of 116 participants in a simulated job selection experience, trait affectivity emerged as the most powerful predictor of interview success making candidates appear more likable, and catalyzing emotional contagion or the induction of positive mood in the interviewer. The model was validated by significant prediction of the criterion by empathic concern, control of nonverbal behavior, and positive affect; each of which underlies the EI variables of empathy, presentation, and self-regulation.

In a direct test of the effects of EI on performance, Carmelli (2003) observed that emotionally intelligent managers in Israel displayed superior performance to their lower EQ peers both in terms of contextual (teamwork and cohesiveness) performance and task performance (quality of the job completed).

12.7   ORGANIZATIONAL COMMITMENT

Emotional intelligence incorporates the quality of emotional resilience, or flexible optimism, which gives the individual the ability to cope with interpersonal conflict. Instead of engaging in the disruptive activity of faultfinding, emotionally intelligent employees are flexibly optimistic enough to put difficulties behind them and redirect their attention to conflict resolution. They espouse a durable sense of success, despite setbacks and frustrations. Abraham (2000) found that EI was a powerful predictor of organizational commitment; 15% of the variance in organizational commitment was explained solely by EI.

A multidimensional approach to commitment argues that (a) the coalitional nature of the organization results in multiple commitments to top management, supervisors, work groups, and customers as distinct foci and that (b) commitments to these groups should be measured separately to determine whether they contribute to overall organizational commitment and, if so, to what extent (Reichers, 1985). Carmelli (2003) found that EI enhanced affective commitment or "positive feelings of identification with attachment to, and involvement in the work organization" (Meyer & Allen, 1984, p. 375) to the extent that high levels of EI depress withdrawal intentions. However, this attachment did not translate into increased career commitment, the ability to manage emotions to further career goals, a related measure of job involvement, or developing such strong emotional feeling for the job that one loses oneself in it. Clearly, both continuance commitment and job involvement have more complex relationships to EI than mere linear cause-and-effect. Such complexity is evident in EI's moderating effect on work-family conflict and continuance commitment, with EI weakening the harmful effects of such conflict on continuance commitment. For example, senior managers were more adept at managing the destructive emotional conflict that emanates from prolonged work-family conflict on their commitment to their careers; if such conflict escalated they reduced their commitment in a recognition of the supremacy of family commitment over their careers in sharp contrast to their less emotionally intelligent counterparts.

12.8   ORGANIZATIONAL CITIZENSHIP

Organizational Citizenship refers to prosocial behaviors whereby employees voluntarily assume the responsibility for intensive self-development, mentoring new employees, being spokespersons for the organization, and taking on projects that are novel, challenging, or futuristic. EI may stimulate such conduct by making employees more aware of the personal problems of others. Empathic skills permit the understanding of special problems including family matters or censure for failure to fulfill organizational responsibilities. Optimism may assist in the promotion of positive mood to offer counsel and support. Studies of mood have shown that positive moods, a characteristic of EI, promote organizational citizenship (see Brief & Motowidlo, 1986, for a review). Employees in positive moods remember positive information and dwell on positive experiences, making it more likely that they will perform acts that reinforce their positive moods such as volunteering to assist others (Isen, Shalker, Clarke, & Karp, 1978). As indicated earlier, the social- skills component of EI enhances work-group cohesion.

The initial empirical study of organizational citizenship as an outcome of EI is Charbonneau and Nicol's (2002) gender-based investigation of adolescents in a camp environment. Granted that camps for adolescents do not parallel modern organizations, the fact that this is the earliest empirical study in the field determines its worth. Providing partial support for my thesis of a significant association between EI and organizational citizenship, they found that among boys, EI correlated significantly with the altruism and civic virtue components of organizational citizenship, while for their female counterparts, altruism, conscientiousness, and civic virtue were significant outcomes of EI. The finding with conscientiousness supports my theory that emotionally intelligent employees are more aware of organizational requirements and therefore, more likely to conform to them in terms of punctuality, the meeting of deadlines, and attendance. Their surprise at finding that the Sportsmanship component of organizational citizenship had no relationship with EI may be explained by methodological artifact. Several of the items on the Sportsmanship subscale were self-rather than other-directed, while Martinez-Pons' (1998) path analysis showed that EI was more often associated with other-directed variables in the regulation of emotion in others. A more direct measure of the impact of EI on altruistic behavior was Carmelli (2003)'s investigation of senior managers in Israel, in which managers with high EI were found to exhibit higher levels of altruistic behavior.

12.9   JOB CONTROL

Salovey and Mayer (1990) identified "mood directed attention" as a facet of EI. Emotionally intelligent individuals are capable of setting priorities for tasks and attending to those of higher priority. As they pay attention to their own feelings, they permit themselves to be directed away from more trivial problems to those of greater importance. The freedom to set priorities, and, if necessary, redirect efforts to new goals, requires that employees have sufficient control over their jobs to allocate their time and efforts most appropriately. In the event that the organization permits the individual to have such control, job satisfaction and commitment are enhanced. In one of the few studies to examine EI within an organization, Cooper and Sawaf (1997) upheld the value of emotional honesty. They refer to the necessity to feelings of "inner truth" that arise partly from the link between EI and intuition and conscience. Emotional honesty rejects the repression of honesty feelings to take politically correct actions. However, in a repressive environment, the honest expression in feelings may result in censure by supervisors or even termination of employment. Consequently, job control with its provision of freedom of choice and expression is necessary for emotional honesty to flourish.

Cooper and Sawaf (1997) reviewed cases of highly emotionally intelligent firms in which the introduction of constructive discontent is viewed as an opportunity to tap creative energies that are often suppressed to maintain harmony. They cite examples of the "debate culture" at Motorola and the favoring of dissent over consensus at Sun Microsystems. Control over the job is necessary for the promotion of open dialogue. There is little merit in critically analyzing solutions and improvements of current procedures if the solutions or improvements cannot be implemented. Cooper and Sawaf (1997) represented this process in terms of the D (discontent) $\times$ D (direction) $\times$ M (movement) formula. Discontent about the current situation leads to a direction for change, which together with movement leads to the desired change. Movement is provided in part by job control, which grants the employee the freedom to take the steps needed to put change into action. Without it, only wishful thinking results. Open dialogue with the discretion to implement the necessary changes should lead both to increased job satisfaction and organizational commitment. Cooper and Sawaf (1997) and Ashkanasy and Jordan (1997) refer to the emotional resilience component of EI. The ability to monitor one's own and others' emotions gives the emotionally intelligent individual the insight to comprehend the causes of stress, to the extent that he or she may develop the ability to persevere in formulating strategies to deal with the negative consequences of stress or destructive conflict. Clearly, such perseverance is rewarded only in situations in which the decision maker has a reasonable expectation of achieving worthwhile results (e.g., an environment that offers the requisite decision-making control). EI and job control jointly explained a significant 26% of the variance in job satisfaction, $t(72) = 5.25, p < .001$. An even stronger moderator effect was observed for organizational commitment, with the EI-job control interaction explaining a significant 29% of the variance, $t(72) = 5.60, p < .001$.

12.10   SELF-ESTEEM

Self-esteem is the effective evaluation of the self occurring either as an innate characteristic (trait self-esteem) or a more transient state (state self-esteem). The association between EI and positive mood has been noted. Mood has been found to have both state and trait components (Watson & Clark, 1994; Watson, Clark, & Tellegen, 1988) with positive mood being characterized by enthusiasm, alertness, calmness, and serenity. The ability of the emotionally intelligent to understand and regulate emotion leads to the arousal of positive mood and higher self-esteem as the focal person can draw upon a reservoir of positive experience to sustain motivation. Schutte et al. (2002) present the example of a man who earned a high score on a test dwelling on that experience later in life, which, in turn, provided the motivation for future striving for excellence. The ability to understand emotions in others may result in the suppression of negative reaction to organizational trials. For instance, an employee whose composure is challenged by abusive supervisors and hostile coworkers may attribute their conduct to misbehavior or personality dysfunction without permitting it to affect his or her performance. In consecutive studies, Ciarrochi, Chan, and Caputi (2000) and Schutte et al. (2002) were able to observe correlations between EI and positive self-esteem. In a mood induction experiment, the former study showed a humorous film to participants; high EI participants responded with significantly higher positive mood. Probing the cause of higher positive mood, this study found a significant interaction effect of EI and mood perception followed by subgroup analysis showing EI associated with significantly higher recall of positive events to induce positive mood-states. The latter study induced varying moods in participants by making them read sets of positive and negative statements. Not only did they corroborate Ciarrochi et al.'s finding, but they extended it by observing that individuals with higher EI were able to maintain positive mood and self-esteem upon confrontation with a negative state induction and reinforce the positive mood induced by positive state intervention. Although not directly tested, self-esteem may be the culmination of a series of positive mood states generated by positive experience or the emotional ability to suppress negative stimuli over time; a longitudinal study is required to establish this relationship.

12.11   DISCUSSION

The principal conclusion from this review is that in order to develop meaningful relationships between EI and outcomes it is necessary to move beyond exploratory quasi-experimental correlational studies to sophisticated methodologies including structural equations and hierarchical regression. At present, relationships of EI with self-esteem, performance, and organizational citizenship are inconclusive as far as direction of causality is concerned; at best, they suggest a link between variables without any prediction of directional effects, that is, does EI lead to enhanced self-esteem, performance, and organizational citizenship? Early initiatives in this regard appear promising especially since they emphasize moderating effects either by EI or other variables. In Abraham's (2000) hierarchical regression of EI on job satisfaction and organizational commitment, more than twice the variance in the criteria was explained by the EI-job control interaction. Wong & Law (2002) obtained a similar result for the EI-emotional labor interaction on the same criteria. In other words, the effects of EI on organizational outcomes are much more powerful in the presence of moderators. Both autonomous environments (with job control) and those in which employees favorably manage their impressions (emotional labor) are more conducive for the emotionally intelligent to display positive affective outcomes. This result is supported by Boyatzis's (1982) model of the confluence of job characteristics; personality variables and organizational climate exert powerful influence on organizational outcomes. Future research should focus on developing theoretical propositions and empirically testing such three way interactions (see Abraham, 2004, for theoretical development).

The role of empathy in the relationship of EI with leadership warrants further investigation. Is empathy antecedent to or a component of EI? While much work has been undertaken to develop robust measures of EI, it would be worthwhile to examine the nature of this relationship. If it is antecedent, how does this explain direct relations between empathic perspective and interpersonal skills (Schutte et al., 2002)? Should empathic measures be divested of their less robust dimensions including empathic fantasy, concern, and personal distress?

The special role of self-awareness in leadership studies and in the fostering of work group cohesion is noteworthy with numerous studies attesting to the strength of this component of EI in affecting the criteria. Although global EI has proved to be the more powerful predictor for most organizational criteria, future work may reveal the predictive supremacy of certain aspects of EI.

Emotional intelligence showed a stronger relationship with organizational commitment than job satisfaction. Two components of EI are relevant in this regard. Ashkanasy and Jordan (1997) found that EI predicted the ability to endure job insecurity and periods of short-term unemployment. The underlying cause of such tenacity may have been higher organizational commitment based on emotional resilience, which confers on the individual the tenacity to "hang in there" and endure the vicissitudes of the workplace. The social skills component of EI may lead to the building of strong work networks with the workgroup and possibly with supervisors. Because this behavior is translated into organizational commitment, it is possible that emotionally intelligent employees view relationships with the organization as an extension of relationships at the work group level.

REFERENCES

Abraham, R. (1999). Emotional intelligence in organizations: A conceptualization. *Genetic, Social, and General Psychology Monographs, 125,* 209–224.

Abraham, R. (2000). The role of job control as a moderator of emotional dissonance and emotional intelligence-outcome relationships. *Journal of Psychology, 134,* 169–184.

Abraham, R. (2004). *Emotional intelligence as antecedent to performance: A contingency framework.* Manuscript submitted for publication.

Ashforth, B. E., & Humphrey, R. H. (1995). Emotion in the workplace: A reappraisal. *Human Relations, 48,* 97–125.

Ashkanasy, N. M., & Jordan, P. J. (1997, August). *Emotional intelligence: Is this the key to understanding the job insecurity-behavior link in organizational restructuring?* Paper presented at the meeting of the Academy of Management, Boston, MA.

Atwater, L. E., & Yammarino, F. J. (1992). Does self-other agreement on leadership perception moderate the validity of leadership and performance predictions? *Personnel Psychology, 45,* 141–164.

Aylward, J. (1985). Psychological testing and police selection. *Journal of Police Science and Administration, 13,* 201–210.

Bachman, J., Stern, S., Campbell, K., & Sitarenios, G. (2000). Emotional intelligence in the collection of debt. *International Journal of Collection and Assessment, 8,* 176–182.

Boyatzis, R. E. (1982). *The competent manager: A model for effective performance.* New York: Wiley.

Brief, A. P., & Motowidlo, S. J. (1986). Prosocial organizational behaviors. *Academy of Management Review, 11,* 701–725.

Brief, A. P., & Weiss, H. M. (2002). Organizational behavior: Affect in the workplace. *Annual Review of Psychology, 53,* 279–307.

Campbell, K. (2001). *Exploring the relationship between emotional intelligence, intuition, and responsible risk-taking in organizations.* Unpublished doctoral dissertation, California School of Professional Psychology, CA.

Carmelli, A. (2003). The relationship between emotional intelligence and work attitudes, behavior, and outcomes: An examination among senior managers. *Journal of Managerial Psychology, 18,* 788–813.

Charbonneau, D., & Nicol, A. M. (2002). Emotional intelligence and prosocial behaviors in adolescents. *Psychological Reports, 90,* 361–370.

Ciarrochi, J., Chan, A. Y. C., & Caputi, P. (2000). A critical evaluation of the emotional intelligence construct. *Personality and Individual Differences, 28,* 539–561.

Collins, V. L. (2002). *Emotional intelligence and leadership success.* Unpublished doctoral dissertation, University of Nebraska-Lincoln, Lincoln, NE.

Conger, J. A., & Kanungo, R. N. (1998). *Charismatic leadership in organizations.* Thousand Oaks, CA: Sage.

Cooper, R. K., & Sawaf, A. (1997). *Executive EQ: Emotional intelligence in leadership and organizations.* New York: Grosset/Putnam.

Csikszentmihalyi, M. (1990). *Flow: The psychology of optimal experience.* New York: Harper and Row.

Daft, R. L., & Weick, K. E. (1984). Toward a model of organizations as interpretation systems. *Academy of Management Review, 9*, 284–295.

Farnham, A. (1996). Are you smart enough to keep your job? *Fortune, 33*, 134–136.

Fisher, V. E., & Hanna, J. V. (1931). *The dissatisfied worker*. New York: MacMillan.

Fox, S., & Spector, P. E. (2000). Relations of emotional intelligence, practical intelligence, general intelligence, and trait affectivity with interview outcomes: It's not all "g". *Journal of Organizational Behavior, 21*, 203–220.

George, J. (2000). Emotions and leadership: The role of emotional intelligence. *Human Relations, 53*, 1027–1055.

Goffman, E. (1959). *The presentation of self in everyday life*. Garden City, NJ: Doubleday Anchor Books.

Goleman, D. (1995). *Emotional intelligence: Why it can matter more than IQ*. New York: Bantam Books.

Graves, J. G. (1999). *Emotional intelligence and cognitive ability: Predicting performance in job-simulated activities*. Unpublished doctoral dissertation, California School of Professional Psychology, CA.

Hatfield, E., Cacioppo, J. T., & Rapson, R. L. (1992). Primitive emotional contagion. In M. S. Clark (Ed.), *Review of personality and social psychology* (Vol. 14, pp. 151–177). Newbury Park, CA: Sage.

Hersey, R. B. (1932). *Workers' emotions in shop and home: A study of individual workers from the psychological and physiological standpoint*. Philadelphia: University of Pennsylvania Press.

Isen, A. M., & Baron, R. A. (1991). Positive affect as a factor in organizational behavior. *Research in Organizational Behavior, 13*, 1–54.

Isen, A. M., Daubman, K. A., & Nowicki, S. (1987). Positive affect facilitates creative problem solving. *Journal of Personality and Social Psychology, 52*, 1122–1131.

Isen, A. M., Shalker, T. E., Clarke, M., & Karp, L. (1978). Affect, accessibility of material in memory, and behavior: A cognitive loop? *Journal of Personality and Social Psychology, 36*, 1–12.

Jordan, P. J., Ashkanasy, N. M., & Härtel, C. E. J. (2003). The case for emotional intelligence in organizational research. *Academy of Management Review, 28*, 195–197.

Jordan, P. J., & Troth, A. C. (2002). Emotional intelligence and conflict resolution: Implications for human resource development. *Advances in Developing Human Resources, 4*, 62–79.

Kelley, R., & Caplan, J. (1993). How Bell Labs creates star performers. *Harvard Business Review, 81*, 128–139.

Koresgaard, M. A. (1996). The impact of self-appraisals on reactions to feedback from officers: The role of self-enhancement and self-consistency concerns. *Journal of Organizational Behavior, 17*, 301–311.

Locke, E. A. (1991). *The essence of leadership*. New York: Lexington Books.

Martinez-Pons, M. (1998). Parental inducement of emotional intelligence. *Imagination, Cognition and Personality, 18*, 5–23.

Mayer, J. D., & Gaschke, Y. N. (1988). The experience and meta-experience of mood. *Journal of Personality and Social Psychology, 55*, 102–111.

Meyer, J. P., & Allen, N. J. (1984). Testing the side-bet theory of organizational commitment: Some methodological considerations. *Organizational Behavior and Human Performance, 17,* 289–298.

Mohrmann, A. M., Jr., Resnick-West, S. M., & Lawler, E. E., III. (1990). *Designing performance appraisal systems: Aligning appraisals and organizational realities.* San Francisco: Jossey-Bass.

Reichers, A. E. (1985). A review and reconceptualization of organizational commitment. *Academy of Management Review, 10,* 465–476.

Roethlisberger, F. J., & Dickson, W. J. (1939). Core affect, prototypical emotional episodes, and other things called emotion: Dissecting the elephant. *Journal of Personality and Social Psychology, 76,* 805–819.

Salovey, P., & Mayer, J. D. (1990). Emotional intelligence. *Imagination, Cognition and Personality, 9,* 185–211.

Schutte, N. S., Malouff, J. M., Simunek, M., McKenley, J., & Hollander, S. (2002). Characteristic emotional intelligence and emotional well-being. *Cognition and Emotion, 16,* 769–785.

Schutte, N. S., Schuettpelz, E., & Malouff, J. M. (2000–2001). Emotional intelligence and task performance. *Imagination, Cognition and Personality, 20,* 347–354.

Sosik, J. J., & Megerian, L. E. (1999). Understanding leader emotional intelligence and performance: The role of self-other agreement on transformational leadership perceptions. *Group and Organization Management, 24,* 367–390.

Tesser, A. (1986). Some effects of self-evaluation maintenance on cognition and action. In R. M. Sorrentino & E. R. Higgins (Eds.), *The handbook of motivation and cognition* (pp. 1–31). Hillsdale, NJ: Erlbaum.

Van Rooy, D. L., & Viswesvaran, C. (2004). Emotional intelligence: A meta-analytic investigation of predictive validity and nomological net. *Journal of Vocational Behavior, 65,* 71–95.

Vitello-Cicciu, J. M. (2002). *Leadership practices and emotional intelligence of nursing leaders.* Unpublished doctoral dissertation, Fielding Graduate Institute, Santa Barbara, CA.

Wasielewski, P. L. (1985). The emotional basis of charisma. *Symbolic Interaction, 8,* 207–222.

Watson, D., & Clark, L. A. (1994). Emotions, moods, traits, and temperaments: Conceptual distinctions and empirical findings. In P. Ekman & R. J. Davidson (Eds.), *The nature of emotions* (pp. 89–93). New York: Oxford University Press.

Watson, D., Clark, L. A., & Tellegen, A. (1988). Development and validation of brief measures of positive and negative effect: the PANAS scales. *Journal of Personality and Social Psychology, 54,* 1063–1070.

Williams, N., & Sternberg, R. J. (1988). Group intelligence: Why some groups are better than others. *Intelligence, 12,* 351–377.

Wong, C.-S., & Law, K. S. (2002). The effects of leader and follower emotional intelligence on performance and attitude: An exploratory study. *The Leadership Quarterly, 13,* 243–274.

Zurcher, L. A. (1982). The staging of emotion: A dramaturgical analysis. *Symbolic Interaction, 5,* 1–22.

13

The Relevance of Emotional Intelligence for Clinical Psychology

James D. A. Parker
Trent University, Canada

Summary

This chapter examines the relevance of the emotional intelligence (EI) construct for clinical psychology. Although virtually no direct clinical research yet exists using the EI construct, several related constructs have generated a large clinical literature. Of particular relevance is the alexithymia construct. Although initially linked with individuals experiencing psychosomatic problems, alexithymia has come to be associated with a variety of clinical disorders, such as substance use disorders and eating disorders. Within various non-clinical populations, alexithymia has been associated with a variety of health, lifestyle, and interpersonal problems. Individuals who score high on measures of alexithymia are often unsuitable clients for many forms of insight-oriented psychotherapy. In response, several clinicians have developed therapeutic modifications for working with these individuals. As summarized in the chapter, these modifications attempt to increase client awareness of problems in the way they process and experience their emotions. Techniques particularly suited to the use of group intervention are also described.

13.1   INTRODUCTION

This chapter examines the relevance of the emotional intelligence (EI) construct for clinical psychology. To date, little clinical research exists related to EI. This is undoubtedly a result of the fact that reliable and valid measures for EI have only recently become available. Although there is little direct literature available on this topic, there are several constructs that overlap with EI that have generated a relatively large clinical literature. The first section of this chapter identifies several of these overlapping constructs (particularly the personality variable of alexithymia), along with summarizing some of the more important findings from the relevant clinical literature. The second part of this chapter describes a number of specialized psychotherapeutic techniques that may be helpful when working with individuals who have problematic levels of EI.

13.2   PRECURSORS TO THE EMOTIONAL INTELLIGENCE CONSTRUCT

Although various models have been proposed for the EI construct (Bar-On, 1997, 2002; Boyatzis, Goleman, & Rhee, 2000; Mayer, Caruso, & Salovey, 1999; Salovey & Mayer, 1990), implicit in all are important implications for clinical psychology. The ability to identify and communicate internal mental states, the ability to link particular mental events with specific situations and personal behaviors, the ability to use information about feelings and emotions to guide future behavior, as well as the ability to mentally regulate negative or extreme emotional states, constitute core abilities in most models of EI. The clinical implications of these types of abilities are vast, since they have been associated with a variety of clinical disorders, such as substance use disorders, somatoform disorders, eating disorders, and anxiety disorders; within various non-clinical populations, these abilities have been linked with a variety of health, lifestyle, and interpersonal problems (Taylor, Bagby, & Parker, 1997). These are also the type of basic abilities often linked with successful outcomes from various types of clinical interventions (Ackerman & Hilsenroth, 2003; Greenberg & Safran, 1987; Horowitz, 2002; Krystal, 1988; Taylor, 1987). For example, successful insight-oriented psychotherapy often depends on the client's "ability to see relationships among thoughts, feelings, and actions, with the goal of learning the meanings and causes of his experiences and behavior" (Applebaum, 1973, p. 36).

To date, little empirical literature exists on the implications of EI and clinical psychology. This state of affairs is likely a result of the lack of reliable and valid measures for the EI construct. However, if one broadens the search to include research on related constructs, a rather sizeable literature can be found. One of the oldest relevant literatures is associated with research trying to predict successful outcomes in psychotherapy. As is frequently noted in the clinical literature (Krystal, 1982; Silver, 1983; Taylor, 1977, 1984), many individuals respond quite poorly to insight-oriented psychotherapy. From the very start of treatment some individuals are more difficult to manage than others. These are often the same individuals who stop treatment after a few sessions, become quickly frustrated by the slow pace of therapy, and question the relevance of topics raised by the therapist (Beckham, 1992; Saltzman, Luetgert, Roth, Creaser, & Howard, 1976).

Taylor (1977) has noted that the patient is not the only one frustrated in these types of situations: "the therapist enters into a relationship expecting to be fed interesting fantasies and feelings only to encounter increasing frustration, dullness and boredom" (Taylor, 1977, p. 143). Not surprisingly, counter transference problems are a risk when working with these clients (Silver, 1983; Taylor, 1977). These types of difficulties (within the therapeutic process) have several important practical implications. One of the most obvious is the termination of therapy by the client. Depending on the populations being examined, an early study by Owen and Kohutek (1981) reported that drop out rates from psychotherapy can be as high as 80% to 90%, with almost half of the terminations occurring after the first few sessions (Baekeland & Lundwall, 1975; Pekarik, 1983; Reder & Tyson, 1980; Sue, McKinney, & Allen, 1976).

Given the potential for high termination rates among many clients, it is not surprising that the search for variables that might identify individuals less likely to benefit from psychotherapy has a long research history (see, e.g., Bachrach & Leaff, 1978; Barron, 1953; Tolor & Reznikoff, 1960). Knowing something about a potential client's level of emotional competency may be very useful to the therapist at the start of treatment. Although there are many reasons why individuals terminate psychotherapy (Luborsky, McLellan, Woody, O'Brien, & Auerbach, 1985), various emotional and social competencies appear to play an important role (Krystal, 1988; Mallinckrodt, King, & Coble, 1998; McCallum, Piper, & Joyce, 1992; Pierloot & Vinck, 1977; Piper, Joyce, McCallum, & Azim, 1998; Taylor et al., 1997). A rather sizeable literature has developed on the personality variables that predict successful outcomes with psychotherapy (Bachrach & Leaff, 1978). Some of the related constructs that have been identified include private self-consciousness (Fenigstein, Scheier, & Buss, 1975), self-awareness (Bloch, 1979), need for cognition (Cacioppo & Petty, 1982), ego strength (Lake, 1985), and levels of emotional awareness (Lane & Schwartz, 1987). Among these various overlapping constructs, psychological mindedness and mindfulness appear to have generated some of largest bodies of empirical literature (Langer, 1989; McCallum & Piper, 1997, 2000; see also Chapter 4 by Ciarrochi & Godsell).

There is considerable overlap between the constructs of psychological mindedness and EI. Silver (1983), in an early definition of psychological mindedness, suggested that it involved the individual's "desire to learn the possible meanings and causes of his internal and external experiences as well as the patient's ability to look inwards to psychical factors rather than only outwards to environmental factors" (p. 516). A more recent model suggests that psychological mindedness involves several basic mental abilities: having access to one's feelings, a willingness to talk about one's feelings and interpersonal problems to others, an active interest in the behaviors of others, and a capacity for behavioral change (Conte et al., 1990).

Not surprisingly, individuals with limited psychological mindedness often experience psychotherapy as a confusing and frustrating experience (Piper et al., 1998) and this personality variable has been consistently linked with negative outcomes in psychotherapy (McCallum et al., 1992; McCallum, Piper, Ogrodniczuk, & Joyce, 2003; Piper et al., 1998; Piper, McCallum, Joyce, Rosie, & Ogrodniczuk, 2001). According to Piper et al. (1998), psychological mindedness (PM) "may reflect a useful general ability to analyze conflicts and solve problems, whether the conflicts are internal or external. Thus, PM may be of value to a variety of individual therapies, even those of different theoretical and technical orientations (e.g., cognitive-behavioral therapy)" (p. 565). Clinicians may want to consider assessing their client's level of psychological mindedness at the start of treatment.

13.3   ALEXITHYMIA

Alexithymia is another construct with considerable clinical relevance to EI (Parker, Taylor, & Bagby, 2001; Taylor, 2000; Taylor et al., 1997). Compared to other related constructs, however, alexithymia has generated a vast literature. The abstract database maintained by PsycINFO is a useful tool for tracking the growth of work on alexithymia. Although the concept was not formally introduced until the mid-1970s (Sifneos, 1973), over 1200 papers and chapters (using the words alexithymia or alexithymic in the abstract or title) were included in the database at the end of 2003.

The concept of alexithymia evolved from clinical observations of individuals who responded poorly to psychotherapy. Writing over half a century ago, Ruesch (1948) identified a cluster of personality variables in a subset of his patients who were experiencing various psychosomatic health problems. Many of these individuals seemed to be quite immature and unimaginative in their thinking and had a tendency to use direct physical action for emotional expression. Another contemporary, Karen Horney (1952), described a similar set of characteristics in many of her patients who responded poorly to psychoanalytic intervention: they had a profound lack of emotional awareness, minimal interest in fantasies and dreams, and a very concrete (externalized) style of thinking. Drawing on this early clinical work, as well as his own research on the personality of individuals experiencing various classic psychosomatic diseases (Nemiah & Sifneos, 1970; Sifneos, 1967), Sifneos (1973) coined the word *alexithymia* (from the Greek: a = lack, lexis = word, thymos = emotion) to identify the cognitive and affective characteristics of many of his patients. Over the past three decades alexithymia has come to be defined by the following core features: difficulty identifying feelings and distinguishing between these feelings and the bodily sensations of emotional arousal; difficulty describing feelings to others; constricted imaginal processes; and a stimulus-bound, externally-orientated, cognitive style (see Taylor, 1984, 2000; Taylor et al., 1997).

In addition to these core parts of the definition, several other common characteristics have been observed in alexithymic individuals that have important clinical implications. Alexithymia has been linked with a limited capacity for empathy (Guttman & Laporte, 2002; McDougall, 1989; Taylor, 1987), problems in processing emotionally-toned or charged information (Stone & Nielson, 2001; Suslow & Junghanns, 2002), as well as difficulties identifying emotions from the facial expressions of others (Lane et al., 1996; Parker, Taylor, & Bagby, 1993). The relationship between dreams and alexithymia has also been of interest to researchers. An early work by Krystal (1979) reported that it was very difficult to work dreams into psychotherapy when treating alexithymic patients. Several different research teams have found empirical evidence that alexithymic individuals have difficulty remembering or recalling dreams (De Gennaro et al., 2003; Krystal, 1979; Nemiah, Freyberger, & Sifneos, 1976). A study by Parker, Bauermann, and Smith (2000) found evidence that the quality of the dreams was also associated with alexithymia. When alexithymic individuals were awakened during REM periods their dream reports were significantly less bizarre and strange than the reports of non-alexithymic individuals.

Since alexithymic individuals often have problems identifying and understanding their emotions, as well as communicating these experiences to others, they are less likely to turn to other people for emotional support. Their limited range of healthy affect regulating abilities also limits the likelihood that alexithymic individuals will regulate emotional distress via daydreams or other imaginative mental activities (Mayes & Cohen, 1992; Taylor et al., 1997). The end result is that these individuals are at an elevated risk for developing a number of clinical disorders:

> It is not surprising that alexithymia has been conceptualized as one of several possible personality risk factors for a variety of medical and psychiatric disorders involving problems in affect regulation. For example, hypochondriasis and somatization disorder might be viewed as resulting, at least in part, from the alexithymic individual's limited subjective awareness and cognitive processing of emotions, which leads both to a focusing on, and amplification and misinterpretation of, the somatic sensations that accompany emotional arousal. (Taylor et al., 1997, p. 31)

Although alexithymia was initially linked with individuals experiencing psychosomatic problems (for a review of this literature see De Gucht & Heiser, 2003), it has become quite evident in the clinical literature that the core features of alexithymia can be observed among patients experiencing a number of psychiatric disorders, such as posttraumatic stress disorder (Badura, 2003; Zlotnick, Mattia, & Zimmerman, 2001), substance use disorders (Cecero & Holmstrom, 1997; Rybakowski, Ziólkowski, Zasadzka, & Brzezinski, 1988), eating disorders (Zonnevijlle-Bender, van Goozen, Cohen-Kettenis, van Elburg, & van Engeland, 2002), and problem gambling (Parker, Wood, Bond, & Shaughnessy, 2005).

For health care professionals, the presence of alexithymia features in their clients has other implications (apart from an increased vulnerability for various psychological disorders). These individuals may be at an increased risk for unnecessary medical consultation and procedures. A recent Finnish study found that alexithymic adults used significantly more health care resources during a 1-year period than non-alexithymic adults (Jyvaesjaervi et al., 1999). The poor communication style of alexithymic individuals, combined with the tendency to somatize their distress (Taylor et al., 1997), may be a contributing factor to this finding. When it comes to medical or psychological health problems, alexithymia may have an important mediating role inhibiting effective diagnosis and patient-physician communication (Tacon, 2001; Williams et al., 2001). Health care professionals generally respond to somatic problems in their patients with tests and interventions. The subsequent failure of these interventions to provide symptom relief often leads to additional tests and interventions being prescribed. The overall effect is that alexithymic individuals are at risk for medical complications or other iatrogenic problems.

Given the widespread health care implications associated with alexithymia, the dramatic increase in empirical work on the construct in the past few decades is not surprising. Another reason for the rapid growth of research must also rest with the proliferation of measures that quickly developed for the construct. Since the mid-1970s a wide assortment of alexithymia measures have been developed: observer-rated questionnaires and interviews (Haviland, Warren, Riggs, & Nitch, 2002; Sifneos, 1973, 1986; Taylor et al., 1997), self-report scales (Apfel & Sifneos, 1979; Bagby, Parker, & Taylor, 1994; Bermond, Vorst, Vingerhoets, & Gerritsen, 1999; Kleiger & Kinsman, 1980; Parker, Taylor, & Bagby, 2003; Sifneos, 1986; Taylor, Ryan, & Bagby, 1986), projective techniques (Acklin & Alexander, 1988; Cohen, Auld, Demers, & Catchlove, 1985), and Q-sort measures (Haviland & Reise, 1996). Although the psychometric properties of these measures vary greatly (for detailed reviews on alexithymia measures, see Taylor, Bagby, & Luminet, 2000; Taylor et al., 1997), researchers interested in alexithymia have been able to choose from a wide range of potential measures (depending on their populations and research questions).

Recent empirical evidence, using different self-report measures for the constructs, indicates that alexithymic individuals score low on measures of EI. Schutte et al. (1998) developed a 33-item self-report scale for EI derived from an early model proposed by Salovey and Mayer (1990). Using the 26-item Toronto Alexithymia Scale (TAS; Taylor et al., 1986), they found a correlation of $-.65$ in a small sample ($N = 25$). More recently, using the same measure of EI, Saklofske, Austin, and Minski (2003) found a similar moderate negative association ($-.52$) between the EI measure and alexithymia using the psychometrically superior 20-item TAS (Bagby et al., 1994). Palmer, Donaldson, and Stough (2002), using the Trait Meta-Mood Scale (TMMS; Salovey, Mayer, Goldman, Turvey, & Palfai, 1995) to measure EI, found a correlation of $-.42$ in a sample of adults using the TAS-20. Using the BarOn Emotional Quotient Inventory (EQ-i; Bar-On, 1997), Dawda and Hart report a correlation of $-.49$ for men and $-.55$ for women between the total EI scale and the TAS-20. Parker et al. (2001), using a larger sample of adults (N = 734), report a correlation of $-.72$ between the same two measures. Parker, Hogan, Majeski, and Bond (2004) report a similar high correlation ($-.68$) between the TAS-20 and the total EI scale on the short form of the EQ-i (i.e., EQ-i: Short, Bar-On, 2002). This consistent pattern of moderate to high correlations is quite remarkable given the different models for EI used in these various studies.

It should be noted, however, that most of the existing empirical work on the relationship between EI and alexithymia has utilized self-report measures. This state of affairs is not surprising, since alternatives to a self-report methodology have only recently been available for the EI construct. Mayer et al. (1999), for example, developed a performance-based measure of EI that asks respondents to solve a variety of different emotion-related problems (Multi-Factor Emotional Intelligence Scale; MEIS). Mayer, Salovey, and Caruso (2002) have since revised the MEIS (now called the Mayer-Salovey-Caruso Emotional Intelligence Test; MSCEIT). Future research needs to explore the empirical relationship between alexithymia and EI using a variety of measurement approaches for both constructs. However, two unpublished studies using the MSCEIT and the TAS-20 provide additional evidence for conceptual overlap between the two constructs (Lumley et al., 2002; Parker, Bagby, & Taylor, 2003). Both studies, using samples of undergraduate students, found moderate negative associations between total scores on the two instruments.

The consistent negative association that has been found between self-report measures of alexithymia and EI is consistent with theoretical work on both constructs. A comparison of the definitions of alexithymia and EI suggests that the two constructs are closely related (Parker et al., 2001; Taylor, Parker, & Bagby, 1999). In an early paper describing their model of EI (see Chapter 2 by Neubauer & Freudenthaler), Salovey, Hsee, and Mayer (1993) conceptualized alexithymia as the extreme lower end of the EI continuum. Thus, while few clinical studies have directly examined the clinical implications of EI, clinicians interested in these implications can turn to the vast literature on alexithymia (given the conceptual and empirical overlap between these two concepts).

As several writers have noted (Krystal, 1982; Taylor, 1987), individuals with high levels of alexithymia, while they may be at risk for developing a variety of physical and mental health problems, are often unsuitable clients for many forms of insight-oriented psychotherapy: Alexithymia may be "the most important single factor diminishing the success of psychoanalysis and psychodynamic psychotherapy" (Krystal, 1982, p. 364). Consistent with Horney's (1952) clinical observations over half a century ago, the psychological problems experienced by many of these individuals may actually be made worse by traditional forms of psychotherapy (Krystal, 1982; Sifneos, 1975; Taylor, 1987; Taylor et al., 1997).

Faced with the problem that conventional forms of psychotherapy might not work, or might make some clients worse, some clinicians have developed a number of therapeutic modifications for working with alexithymic individuals. These modifications contrast with traditional psychotherapy because they attempt

> ...to elevate emotions from a level of perceptually bound experience (a world of sensation and action) to a conceptual representational level (a world of feelings and thoughts) where they can be used as signals of information, thought about, and sometimes communicated to others. (Taylor et al., 1997, p. 252)

In general, these modifications attempt to increase client awareness of problems in the way they process and experience their emotions. The following section describes a number of these therapeutic interventions, as well as some of the empirical literature exploring the clinical benefits.

13.4   PSYCHOTHERAPY AND ALEXITHYMIA

Krystal (1979, 1988) has written some of the most detailed accounts yet on the attempt to modify or adapt traditional forms of psychotherapy for use with alexithymic clients. An important first step in the clinical process, according to Krystal (1979, 1988), is to try and make the client aware that a major cause of their problems is a deficiency in the way he/she understands and communicates emotion. This may prove to be a difficult step to achieve, since many alexithymic individuals give little importance to emotions; many alexithymic patients initially find discussions about emotions and feelings boring and frustrating (Taylor, 1995). A second step in the clinical process, according to Krystal (1979, 1988) is often quite basic and educational. The therapist works to improve basic emotional skills in the client: helping the individual to recognize and correctly label specific emotions, learning to differentiate among different emotional experiences, and learning to better communicate these feelings to others.

This type of modified psychotherapy is often a slow and tedious process (Taylor, 1995). One of the first difficulties the therapist must try to overcome is the alexithymic client's often poor inter-personal skills. These individuals often find close attachments quite difficult (Taylor et al., 1997). With a limited capacity to share personally significant feelings and experiences with others (Fischer & Good, 1997; Mallinckrodt et al., 1998), they are often quite fearful of intimacy. Not surprisingly, alexithymic clients often prevent close emotional relationships from developing with their therapist (Brown, 1985; Taylor, 1987). Although they are quick to assume a dependent patient role, alexithymic individuals often expect that their problems can be "cured" with specific medical interventions. When a quick "fix" is not forthcoming, the client's initial feelings of boredom from individual therapy sessions can quickly escalate to frustration and anger, with an increased risk of treatment being terminated (Taylor, 1995).

13.4.1   Individual Therapy

Using the type of techniques and ideas described in this section, a number of clinicians have written about being able to reduce alexithymic symptoms in their patients (Krystal, 1988; Taylor et al., 1997). Individuals with problematic levels of alexithymia have learned to have a better understanding of their feelings, a better ability to differentiate between different emotional experiences, and developed a larger repertoire of skills for communicating information about their emotions and feelings. For some individuals it has also been found useful to start the intervention process by combining psychotherapy with behavioral techniques, such as relaxation training or biofeedback (Taylor, 1987; Taylor et al., 1997). These types of behavioral techniques may improve introceptive awareness in alexithymic clients, especially the ability to self-regulate different physiological states. Greenberg and Safran (1987, 1989) have also suggested that the therapist might want to pay more attention to non-verbal expressions of emotion (e.g., body movements, gestures, and sighs) than is usually done during specific therapy sessions. These behavioral events can become important information sources in the process of teaching the client to better communicate their feelings (and to better interpret the internal states in others).

There is also evidence that teaching alexithymic individuals to pay attention to their dreams may improve the progress of psychotherapy (Cartwright, 1993). As tangible mental events, dreams provide the therapist with convenient material for getting the alexithymic individual to focus on inner feelings and experiences. The therapist can also increase the likelihood of developing better emotional skills in alexithymic clients by using their own emotional experiences (generated in specific therapeutic sessions) more than is usually done in traditional insight-oriented psychotherapy (Krystal, 1982; McDougall, 1989; Taylor, 1987). If counter transference problems arise, which often happens with alexithymic clients (Krystal, 1979; Taylor, 1977), the therapist might want to talk about his/her feelings of boredom and frustration with the client. The therapist might also want to share humor and daydreams during individual sessions. All of these forms of communications help the client associate specific interpersonal situations with particular inner experiences.

One of the first studies to examine the benefits of different types of psychotherapy for clients with alexithymia was conducted by Pierloot and Vinck (1977). Outpatients experiencing a variety of different anxiety problems were randomly assigned to one of two different interventions: short-term psychodynamic psychotherapy versus behavior therapy (i.e., systematic desensitization). These authors found that "patients with more alexithymia characteristics are more likely to drop out from psychodynamic therapies, but in systematic desensitization they persist as well as those without alexithymic characteristics" (Pierloot & Vinck, 1977, p. 162). Keller, Carroll, Nich, and Rounsaville (1995) examined responses to different forms of psychotherapy in cocaine abusers who were alexithymic or nonalexithymic. Participants were randomly assigned to four different treatment groups: 1) cognitive-behavioral treatment plus a drug placebo; 2) cognitive-behavioral treatment combined with the tricyclic antidepressant desipramine; 3) clinical management plus a drug placebo; and 4) clinical management combined with the tricyclic antidepressant. The type of clinical management used in the two groups required little internal focusing on the part of the participant. Individual sessions gave the researchers an opportunity to monitor the individual's clinical status and response to treatment, as well as provide a supportive relationship. The type of cognitive-behavioral therapy used in the study asked participants to identify and communicate internal mental states associated with their drug use, as well as encouraging these individuals to identify, monitor, and analyze their drug cravings. After 12 weeks of treatment the alexithymic and nonalexithymic clients were found to have responded differently to the two types of psychotherapy: nonalexithymic participants had better outcomes with the cognitive-behavioral approach, while the alexithymic participants responded better when treated with clinical management.

13.4.2   Group Therapy

Group therapy has also been suggested as a useful and practical form of intervention for alexithymic clients (Swiller, 1988; Taylor et al., 1997). While individual sessions may be particularly suited for educating alexithymic clients about basic emotional abilities, there are a number of emotional and social competencies that are particularly suited to the use of group intervention. As noted elsewhere:

> While it is essential that the alexithymic patients experience the group as a safe and supportive setting, candid feedback from other group members should be encouraged, to the extent that it does not threaten the patients' self-esteem, as this can help them learn about the impact of their lack of empathy on other people. At the same time, the group therapist can direct an alexithymic patient's attention to communications between other group members that demonstrate more successful and sensitive ways of relating. (Taylor et al., 1997, p. 253-254)

There are, however, some practical issues and concerns that arise when using group therapy with alexithymic individuals. As noted by Swiller (1988), the poor inter-personal skills of alexithymic individuals often generate feelings of boredom and frustration in other group members. Since these negative experiences increase the likelihood that members will drop out of the group, therapists should take care to limit the number of alexithymic individuals included in a group. Swiller (1988) suggests that when there has to be more than one alexithymic client in the group they be selected to be at different stages in their treatment.

Several different groups of researchers have examined the effectiveness of group therapy for reducing alexithymic symptoms. A form of family psychotherapy with a group of alcohol abusers was used by Fukunishi, Ichikawa, Ichikawa, and Matsuzawa (1994). Adults in the study met in small groups (4 to 5 participants) once a week for two hour sessions. After six months of intervention alexithymia levels were significantly lower among family members. Beresnevaite (2000), using a sample of post-myocardial infarction patients, also examined the effectiveness of group therapy for reducing alexithymic symptoms. Participants in the study attended the group therapy session once a week for 90 minutes. Several different therapeutic techniques were employed over the 4 months of treatment. For example, patients were taught relaxation techniques, as well as being required to participate in various role-playing and nonverbal communication activities. Participants listened to music while in a relaxed state, and were encouraged to write down dreams and fantasies. Alexithymia levels were assessed at several time-points: before the start of treatment, at the end of treatment, six months after treatment, 12 months after treatment, and 24 months after treatment. There was a significant reduction in alexithymia scores following group therapy, which was maintained over the two year follow-up period.

A recent study by Ciano, Rocco, Angarano, Biasin, and Balestrieri (2002) compared the efficacy of two different types of group therapy on reduction of alexithymic characteristics in a small group of patients with binge-eating disorder. One group of patients participated in 14 group psychoanalytic sessions over a 28-week period; the second group participated in 10 psychoeducational sessions over a 10-week period (that focused on providing nutritional information as well as improving the client's communication abilities). When alexithymia levels were compared before and after treatment, there was a significant reduction of alexithymic symptoms only in the group of patients who had received the psychoeducational intervention.

13.5   CONCLUSION

This chapter has described a number of important clinical and therapeutic implications for EI based on the literature related to several overlapping constructs. Several related models have been proposed for the EI construct (e.g., Bar-On, 1997; Mayer et al., 1999), and while this construct has obvious relevance to clinical psychology, it is important to emphasize that virtually all of the existent published research on the construct has examined non-clinical populations. Researchers need to examine the direct relationship between EI and relevant clinical disorders (particularly those that have been found to be associated with alexithymia). There is also the need for clinicians and researchers to explicitly investigate the relationship between EI and various psychotherapy outcome variables, as well as the effectiveness of specific therapeutic interventions for improving specific emotional and social competencies. Of particular importance is that this new research utilizes diverse measurement approaches for the EI construct, rather than focus exclusively on a single approach (e.g., self-report measures). One can expect that many of the EI measures that have only recently been developed will stimulate this new clinical research (e.g., Bar-On, 1997, 2002; Bar-On & Parker, 2000; Mayer, Salovey, Caruso, & Sitarenios, 2003). These new measures may also help in the process of matching clients with appropriate therapeutic interventions, as well as in monitoring the progress of clients during treatment.

Author Note

The writing of this chapter was supported by research grants from the Social Sciences and Humanities Research Council of Canada (SSHRC), the Ontario Government's Premier's Research Excellence Award program, and the Canadian Foundation for Innovation (CFI). The author would like to thank Jennifer Eastabrook and Laura Wood for their help with this chapter.

REFERENCES

Ackerman, S. J., & Hilsenroth, M. J. (2003). A review of therapist characteristics and techniques positively impacting the therapeutic alliance. *Clinical Psychology Review, 23*, 1–33.

Acklin, M. W., & Alexander, G. (1988). Alexithymia and somatization: A Rorschach study of four psychosomatic groups. *Journal of Nervous and Mental Disease, 176*, 343–350.

Apfel, R. J., & Sifneos, P. E. (1979). Alexithymia: Concept and measurement. *Psychotherapy and Psychosomatics, 32*, 180–190.

Applebaum, S. A. (1973). Psychological-mindedness: Word, concept, and essence. *International Journal of Psychoanalysis, 54*, 35–45.

Bachrach, H. M., & Leaff, L. A. (1978). "Analyzability": A systematic review of the clinical and quantitative literature. *Journal of the American Psychoanalytical Association, 26*, 881–920.

Badura, A. S. (2003). Theoretical and empirical exploration of the similarities between emotional numbing in posttraumatic stress disorder and alexithymia. *Journal of Anxiety Disorders, 17*, 349–360.

Baekeland, F., & Lundwall, L. (1975). Dropping out of treatment: A critical review. *Psychological Bulletin, 82*, 738–783.

Bagby, R. M., Parker, J. D. A., & Taylor, G. J. (1994). The Twenty-Item Toronto Alexithymia Scale-I: Item selection and cross-validation of the factor structure. *Journal of Psychosomatic Research, 38*, 23–32.

Bar-On, R. (1997). *BarOn Emotional Quotient Inventory (EQ–i): Technical manual.* Toronto, Canada: Multi-Health Systems.

Bar-On, R. (2002). *BarOn Emotional Quotient Inventory: Short (EQ-i: S): Technical manual.* Toronto, Canada: Multi-Health Systems.

Bar-On, R., & Parker, J. D. A. (2000). *BarOn Emotional Quotient Inventory: Youth version (EQ-i: YV): Technical manual.* Toronto, Canada: Multi-Health Systems.

Barron, F. (1953). An ego-strength scale which predicts response to psychotherapy. *Journal of Consulting Psychology, 17*, 327–333.

Beckham, E. (1992). Predicting patient dropout in psychotherapy. *Psychotherapy, 29*, 177–182.

Beresnevaite, M. (2000). Exploring the benefits of group psychotherapy in reducing alexithymia in coronary heart disease patients: A preliminary study. *Psychotherapy and Psychosomatics, 69*, 117–122.

Bermond, B., Vorst, H. C. M., Vingerhoets, A. J., & Gerritsen, W. (1999). The Amsterdam Alexithymia scale: Its psychometric values and correlations with other personality traits. *Psychotherapy and Psychosomatics, 68*, 241–251.

Bloch, S. (1979). Assessment of patients for psychotherapy. *British Journal of Psychiatry,* *135,* 193–208.

Boyatzis, R. E., Goleman, D., & Rhee, K. S. (2000). Clustering competence in emotional intelligence: Insights from the Emotional Competence Inventory. In R. Bar-On & J. D. A. Parker (Eds.), *The handbook of emotional intelligence: Theory, development, assessment, and application at home, school, and in the workplace* (pp. 343–362). San Francisco: Jossey-Bass.

Brown, L. J. (1985). On concreteness. *Psychoanalytic Review, 72,* 379–402.

Cacioppo, J. T., & Petty, R. E. (1982). The need for cognition. *Journal of Personality and Social Psychology, 42,* 116–131.

Cartwright, R. D. (1993). Who needs their dreams? The usefulness of dreams in psychotherapy. *Journal of the American Academy of Psychoanalysis, 21,* 539–547.

Cecero, J. J., & Holmstrom, R. W. (1997). Alexithymia and affect pathology among adult male alcoholics. *Journal of Clinical Psychology, 53,* 201–208.

Ciano, R., Rocco, P. L., Angarano, A., Biasin, E., & Balestrieri, M. (2002). Group-analytic and psychoeducational therapies for binge-eating disorder: An exploratory study on efficacy and persistence of effects. *Psychotherapy Research, 12,* 231–239.

Cohen, K. R., Auld, F., Demers, L. A., & Catchlove, R. F. H. (1985). Alexithymia: The development of a valid and reliable projective measure (the objectively scored archetypal 9 test). *Journal of Nervous and Mental Disease, 173,* 621–627.

Conte, H. R., Plutchik, R., Jung, B. B., Picard, S., Karasu, T. B., & Lotterman, A. (1990). Psychological mindedness as a predictor of psychotherapy outcome: A preliminary report. *Comprehensive Psychiatry, 31,* 426–431.

De Gennaro, L., Ferrara, M., Cristiani, R., Curcio, G., Martiradonna, V., & Bertini, M. (2003). Alexithymia and dream recall upon spontaneous morning awakening. *Psychosomatic Medicine, 65,* 301–306.

De Gucht, V., & Heiser, W. (2003). Alexithymia and somatisation: A quantitative review of the literature. *Journal of Psychosomatic Research, 54,* 425–434.

Fenigstein, A., Scheier, M. F., & Buss, A. H. (1975). Public and private self consciousness: Assessment and theory. *Journal of Consulting and Clinical Psychology, 43,* 522–527.

Fischer, A. R., & Good, G. E. (1997). Men and psychotherapy: An investigation of alexithymia, intimacy, and masculine gender roles. *Psychotherapy, 34,* 160–170.

Fukunishi, I., Ichikawa, M., Ichikawa, T., & Matsuzawa, K. (1994). Effect of family group psychotherapy on alcoholic families. *Psychological Reports, 74,* 568–570.

Greenberg, L. S., & Safran, J. D. (1987). *Emotions in psychotherapy.* New York: Guilford Press.

Greenberg, L. S., & Safran, J. D. (1989). Emotion in psychotherapy. *American Psychologist, 44,* 19–29.

Guttman, H., & Laporte, L. (2002). Alexithymia, empathy, and psychological symptoms in a family context. *Comprehensive Psychiatry, 43,* 448–455.

Haviland, M. G., & Reise, S. P. (1996). A California Q-set alexithymia prototype and its relationship to ego-control and ego-resiliency. *Journal of Psychosomatic Research, 41,* 597–608.

Haviland, M. G., Warren, W. L., Riggs, M. L., & Nitch, S. (2002). Concurrent validity of two observer-rated alexithymia measures. *Psychosomatics, 43*, 472–477.

Horney, K. (1952). The paucity of inner experiences. *American Journal of Psychoanalysis, 12*, 3–9.

Horowitz, M. J. (2002). Self- and relational observation. *Journal of Psychotherapy Integration, 12*, 115–127.

Jyvaesjaervi, S., Joukamaa, M., Vaeisaenen, E., Larivaara, P., Kivelae, S., & Keinaenen-Kiukaanniemi, S. (1999). Alexithymia, hypochondriacal beliefs, and psychological distress among frequent attenders in primary health care. *Comprehensive Psychiatry, 40*, 292–298.

Keller, D. S., Carroll, K. M., Nich, C., & Rounsaville, B. J. (1995). Alexithymia in cocaine abusers: Response to psychotherapy and pharmacotherapy. *American Journal on Addictions, 4*, 234–244.

Kleiger, J. H., & Kinsman, R. A. (1980). The development of an MMPI alexithymia scale. *Psychotherapy and Psychosomatics, 34*, 17–24.

Krystal, H. (1979). Alexithymia and psychotherapy. *American Journal of Psychotherapy, 33*, 17–31.

Krystal, H. (1982). Alexithymia and the effectiveness of psychoanalytic treatment. *International Journal of Psychoanalysis and Psychotherapy, 9*, 353–388.

Krystal, H. (1988). *Integration and self-healing: Affect, trauma, alexithymia.* Hillsdale, NJ: Analytic Press.

Lake, B. (1985). Concept of ego strength in psychotherapy. *British Journal of Psychiatry, 147*, 471–478.

Lane, R., & Schwartz, G. E. (1987). Levels of emotional awareness: A cognitive-developmental theory and its application to psychopathology. *American Journal of Psychiatry, 144*, 133–143.

Lane, R., Sechrest, L., Reidel, R., Weldon, V., Kaszniak, A., & Schwartz, G. E. (1996). Impaired verbal and nonverbal emotion recognition in alexithymia. *Psychosomatic Medicine, 58*, 203–210.

Langer, E. (1989). *Mindfulness.* New York: Addison-Wesley.

Luborsky, L., McLellan, A., Woody, G., O'Brien, C., & Auerbach, A. (1985). Therapist success and its determinants. *Archives of General Psychiatry, 42*, 602–611.

Lumley, M. A., Davis, M., Labouvie-Vief, G., Gustavson, B., Clement, R., Barry, R., et al. (2002, March). *Multiple measures of emotional abilities: Their interrelationships and associations with physical symptoms.* Presentation at the annual meeting of the American Psychosomatic Society, Barcelona, Spain.

Mallinckrodt, B., King, J. L., & Coble, H. M. (1998). Family dysfunction, alexithymia, and client attachment to therapist. *Journal of Counseling Psychology, 45*, 497–504.

Mayer, J. D., Caruso, D. R., & Salovey, P. (1999). Emotional intelligence meets traditional standards for an intelligence. *Intelligence, 27*, 267–298.

Mayer, J. D., Salovey, P., & Caruso, D. R. (2002). *The Mayer-Salovey-Caruso Emotional Intelligence Test (MSCEIT): User's manual.* Toronto: Multi-Health Systems.

Mayer, J. D., Salovey, P., Caruso, D. R., & Sitarenios, G. (2003). Measuring emotional intelligence with the MSCEIT V2.0. *Emotion, 3*, 97–105.

Mayes, L. C., & Cohen, D. J. (1992). The development of a capacity for imagination in early childhood. *Psychoanalytic Study of the Child, 47*, 23–47.

McCallum, M., & Piper, W. E. (1997). *Psychological mindedness: A contemporary under-standing*. Mahwah, NJ: Lawrence Erlbaum.

McCallum, M., & Piper, W. E. (2000). Pychological mindedness and emotional intelligence. In R. Bar-On & J. D. A. Parker (Eds.), *The handbook of emotional intelligence: Theory, development, assessment, and application at home, school, and in the workplace* (pp. 118–135). San Francisco: Jossey-Bass.

McCallum, M., Piper, W. E., & Joyce, A. S. (1992). Dropping out from short-term group therapy. *Psychotherapy, 29*, 206–215.

McCallum, M., Piper, W. E., Ogrodniczuk, J. S., & Joyce, A. S. (2003). Relationships among psychological mindedness, alexithymia, and outcome in four forms of short-term psychotherapy. *Psychology and Psychotherapy: Theory, Research and Practice, 76*, 133–144.

McDougall, J. (1989). *Theatres of the body: A psychoanalytic approach to psychosomatic illness*. New York: Norton.

Nemiah, J. C., Freyberger, H., & Sifneos, P. E. (1976). Alexithymia: A view of the psychosomatic process. In O. W. Hill (Ed.), *Modern trends in psychosomatic medicine* (Vol. 3, pp. 430–439). London: Butterworths.

Nemiah, J. C., & Sifneos, P. E. (1970). Affect and fantasy in patients with psychosomatic disorders. In O. W. Hill (Ed.), *Modern trends in psychosomatic medicine* (Vol. 2, pp. 26–34). London: Butterworths.

Owen, P., & Kohutek, K. (1981). The rural mental health dropout. *Journal of Rural Community Psychology, 2*, 38–41.

Palmer, B. R., Donaldson, C., & Stough, C. (2002). Emotional intelligence and life satisfaction. *Personality and Individual Differences, 33*, 1091–1100.

Parker, J. D. A., Bagby, R. M., & Taylor, G. J. (2003, August). *Twenty-Item Toronto Alexithymia Scale: Is it distinct from basic personality?* Presentation at the annual meeting of the American Psychological Association, Toronto, Canada.

Parker, J. D. A., Bauermann, T. M., & Smith, C. T. (2000). Alexithymia and impoverished dream content: Evidence from REM sleep awakenings. *Psychosomatic Medicine, 62*, 486–491.

Parker, J. D. A., Hogan, M. J., Majeski, S. A., & Bond, B. J. (2004). *Assessing emotional intelligence: Reliability and validity of the short form for the Emotional Quotient Inventory*. Manuscript submitted for publication.

Parker, J. D. A., Taylor, G. J., & Bagby, R. M. (1993). Alexithymia and the recognition of facial expressions of emotion. *Psychotherapy and Psychosomatics, 59*, 197–202.

Parker, J. D. A., Taylor, G. J., & Bagby, R. M. (2001). The relationship between emotional intelligence and alexithymia. *Personality and Individual Differences, 30*, 107–115.

Parker, J. D. A., Taylor, G. J., & Bagby, R. M. (2003). The Twenty-Item Toronto Alexithymia Scale–III. Reliability and factorial validity in a community population. *Journal of Psychosomatic Research, 55*, 269–275.

Parker, J. D. A., Wood, L. M., Bond, B. J., & Shaughnessy, P. (2005). Alexithymia in young adulthood: A risk-factor for pathological gambling. *Psychotherapy and Psychosomatics, 74*, 51–55.

Pekarik, G. (1983). Follow-up adjustment of outpatient dropouts. *American Journal of Orthopsychiatry, 53*, 501–511.

Pierloot, R., & Vinck, J. (1977). A pragmatic approach to the concept of alexithymia. *Psychotherapy and Psychosomatics, 28,* 156–166.

Piper, W. E., Joyce, A. S., McCallum, M., & Azim, H. F. (1998). Interpretive and supportive forms of psychotherapy and patient personality variables. *Journal of Consulting and Clinical Psychology, 66,* 558–567.

Piper, W. E., McCallum, M., Joyce, A. S., Rosie, J. S., & Ogrodniczuk, J. S. (2001). Patient personality and time-limited group psychotherapy for complicated grief. *International Journal of Group Psychotherapy, 51,* 525–552.

Reder, P., & Tyson, R. (1980). Patient dropout from individual psychotherapy. *Bulletin of the Menninger Clinic, 44,* 229–252.

Ruesch, J. (1948). The infantile personality. *Psychosomatic Medicine, 10,* 134–144.

Rybakowski, J., Ziólkowski, M., Zasadzka, T., & Brzezinski, R. (1988). High prevalence of alexithymia in male patients with alcohol dependence. *Drug and Alcohol Dependence, 21,* 133–136.

Saklofske, D. H., Austin, E. J., & Minski, P. S. (2003). Factor structure and validity of a trait emotional intelligence measure. *Personality and Individual Differences, 34,* 707–721.

Salovey, P., Hsee, C. K., & Mayer, J. D. (1993). Emotional intelligence and the self-regulation of affect. In D. M. Wegner & J. W. Pennebaker (Eds.), *Handbook of mental control* (pp. 258–277). Englewood Cliffs, NJ: Prentice Hall.

Salovey, P., & Mayer, J. D. (1990). Emotional intelligence. *Imagination, Cognition and Personality, 9,* 185–211.

Salovey, P., Mayer, J. D., Goldman, S., Turvey, C., & Palfai, T. (1995). Emotional attention, clarity, and repair: Exploring emotional intelligence using the Trait Meta-Mood Scale. In J. W. Pennebaker (Ed.), *Emotion, disclosure, and health* (pp. 125–154). Washington, DC: American Psychological Association.

Saltzman, C., Luetgert, M. J., Roth, C. H., Creaser, J., & Howard, L. (1976). Formation of a therapeutic relationship: Experiences during the initial phase of psychotherapy as predictors of treatment duration and outcome. *Journal of Consulting and Clinical Psychology, 44,* 546–555.

Schutte, N. S., Malouff, J. M., Hall, L. E., Haggerty, D. J., Cooper, J. T., Golden, C. J., et al. (1998). Development and validation of a measure of emotional intelligence. *Personality and Individual Differences, 25,* 167–177.

Sifneos, P. E. (1967). Clinical observations on some patients suffering from a variety of psychosomatic diseases. *Acta Medicina Psychosomatica, 7,* 1–10.

Sifneos, P. E. (1973). The prevalence of "alexithymic" characteristics in psychosomatic patients. *Psychotherapy and Psychosomatics, 22,* 255–262.

Sifneos, P. E. (1975). Problems of psychotherapy of patients with alexithymic characteristics and physical disease. *Psychotherapy and Psychosomatics, 26,* 65–70.

Sifneos, P. E. (1986). The Schalling-Sifneos Personality Scale-Revised. *Psychotherapy and Psychosomatics, 45,* 161–165.

Silver, D. (1983). Psychotherapy of the characterologically difficult patient. *Canadian Journal of Psychiatry, 28,* 513–521.

Stone, L., & Nielson, K. A. (2001). Intact physiological responses to arousal with impaired emotional recognition in alexithymia. *Psychotherapy and Psychosomatics, 70,* 92–102.

Sue, S., McKinney, H., & Allen, D. (1976). Predictors of the duration of therapy for clients in the community mental health system. *Community Mental Health Journal, 12*, 365–375.

Suslow, T., & Junghanns, K. (2002). Impairments of emotion situation priming in alexithymia. *Personality and Individual Differences, 32*, 541–550.

Swiller, H. I. (1988). Alexithymia: Treatment utilizing combined individual and group psychotherapy. *International Journal of Group Psychotherapy, 38*, 47–61.

Tacon, A. (2001). Alexithymia: A challenge for mental health nursing practice. *Australian and New Zealand Journal of Mental Health Nursing, 10*, 229–235.

Taylor, G. J. (1977). Alexithymia and the counter-transference. *Psychotherapy and Psychosomatics, 28*, 141–147.

Taylor, G. J. (1984). Alexithymia: Concept, measurement, and implications for treatment. *American Journal of Psychiatry, 141*, 725–732.

Taylor, G. J. (1987). *Psychosomatic medicine and contemporary psychoanalysis.* Madison, CT: International Universities Press.

Taylor, G. J. (1995). Psychoanalysis and empirical research: The example of patients who lack psychological mindedness. *Journal of the American Academy of Psychoanalysis and Dynamic Psychiatry, 23*, 263–281.

Taylor, G. J. (2000). Recent developments in alexithymia theory and research. *Canadian Journal of Psychiatry, 45*, 134–142.

Taylor, G. J., Bagby, R. M., & Luminet, O. (2000). Assessment of alexithymia: Self-report and observer-rated measures. In R. Bar-On & J. D. A. Parker (Eds.), *The handbook of emotional intelligence: Theory, development, assessment, and application at home, school, and in the workplace* (pp. 301–319). San Francisco: Jossey-Bass.

Taylor, G. J., Bagby, R. M., & Parker, J. D. A. (1997). *Disorders of affect regulation.* Cambridge, UK: Cambridge University Press.

Taylor, G. J., Parker, J. D. A., & Bagby, R. M. (1999). Emotional intelligence and the emotional brain: Points of convergence and implications for psychoanalysis. *Journal of the American Academy of Psychoanalysis, 27*, 339–354.

Taylor, G. J., Ryan, D., & Bagby, R. M. (1986). Toward the development of a new self-report alexithymia scale. *Psychotherapy and Psychosomatics, 44*, 191–199.

Tolor, A., & Reznikoff, M. (1960). A new approach to insight: A preliminary report. *Journal of Nervous and Mental Disease, 130*, 286–296.

Williams, K. R., Galas, J., Light, D., Pepper, C., Ryan, C., Kleinmann, A. E., et al. (2001). Head injury and alexithymia: Implications for family practice care. *Brain Injury, 15*, 349–356.

Zlotnick, C., Mattia, J. I., & Zimmerman, M. (2001). The relationship between post-traumatic stress disorder, childhood trauma, and alexithymia in an outpatient sample. *Journal of Traumatic Stress, 14*, 177–188.

Zonnevijlle-Bender, M. J. S., van Goozen, S. H. M., Cohen-Kettenis, P. T., van Elburg, A., & van Engeland, H. (2002). Do adolescent anorexia nervosa patients have deficits in emotional functioning? *European Child and Adolescent Psychiatry, 11*, 38–42.

14

Emotional Intelligence and Inter-Personal Skills

Elisabeth Engelberg and Lennart Sjöberg
Stockholm School of Economics, Sweden

Summary

Although emotionally intelligent individuals are assumed to be socially effective, there has been little exploration of the concept in this respect. In the present chapter, we argue that emotion-based abilities, as outlined by Mayer and colleagues (Mayer, Salovey, Caruso, & Sitarenios, 2001), provide a framework for the assessment of inter-personal skills. It is our contention that research on emotional intelligence (EI) may involve attempts to delineate emotional processes underlying skills to promote social interactions and relationships. We present empirical support for the notion that emotional competence characteristic of high EI confers advantages for social adaptation. Our premise is consistent with much current work building on the assumption that there are emotional skills with a high degree of generality, and it supports, in particular, the original idea of measuring EI by means of performance measures.

14.1   INTRODUCTION

Emotional Intelligence (EI) has become popular to the extent that it flourishes in the test market and is probably seen as a major individual difference construct of the twentieth century. In spite of this, claims that EI is far more important than traditional intelligence have not yet been empirically supported. Traditional intelligence remains as the main dimension in the prediction of achievement and adjustment (Austin et al., 2002; Schmidt & Hunter, 1998). This does not preclude EI from adding an important piece of information, particularly since the appeal of the concept seems to lie in its social implications. Emotionally intelligent individuals are perceived as ideal employees in jobs that require communication skills and social competence, which almost all jobs do, more or less (see, e.g., Slaski & Cartwright, 2002). The enthusiasm over EI may in fact reflect the lack of an appropriate standard to assess social skills, or social intelligence (Sternberg, 1985). Although social intelligence has been notoriously difficult to measure (Kihlstrom & Cantor, 2000), the current interest in EI may perhaps contribute to the long overdue revival of this field.

Contrary to what might be expected, our aim for the present chapter is not to present possible avenues to reconcile the two concepts of EI and social intelligence. Comparable aspects between the two concepts are already dealt with elsewhere in the present volume (see Chapter 5 by Kang, Day, and Meara as well as Chapter 10 by Weis and Süß). We merely contend that emotion-based abilities as outlined in the work by Mayer and Salovey (Salovey & Mayer, 1990; Mayer, Salovey, Caruso, & Sitarenios, 2001) provide a framework for the assessment of inter-personal skills.

The concept of EI was launched along with the view that emotions are embedded within ongoing social interactions (e.g., Averill, 1980; Lazarus, 1991). Research on EI may therefore be seen as involving attempts to delineate emotional processes underlying skills to promote social interactions and relationships. Although emotionally intelligent individuals are assumed to be socially effective (Caruso, Mayer, & Salovey, 2002), there has been little exploration of the concept in this respect. Other emergent conceptualizations of EI more clearly emphasize social functioning, especially those based on traits discerned in cross-situational consistencies in behavior (e.g., Bar-On, 2000; Goleman, 1995; Petrides & Furnham, 2001; Schutte et al., 1998). Yet, emergent formulations do not specifically deal with social or inter-personal skills as a product of emotion-related abilities.

Our assumption of EI as a basis for inter-personal skills is grounded in different theories of the function of emotions. Functional approaches vary across levels of analysis that may be linked and inter-related (Keltner & Gross, 1999; Keltner & Haidt, 1999). However, all of them emanate from the premise that people are social by nature, as articulated by Brian Parkinson (1996) in a very compelling manner. In the present chapter we base our overall argument on two major points that will be elaborated in detail. First, perceptual and cognitive abilities are prerequisites for social functioning, since they provide us with the ability to perceive and process emotion information. Second, individual variation in apprehending and responding to emotional cues in others constitutes a meaningful platform for an analysis of emotion as a social-adaptive function.

14.2 PERCEPTION AND COGNITION IN THE PROCESSING OF EMOTIONS

Early emotion theorists espoused a functionalism consistent with evolutionary theory in the sense that emotional expressions were selected on the basis of their potential to enhance communication and subsequent coordination of social interactions (Ekman, 1992; Izard, 1971; Öhman, 1986; Plutchik, 1980). Contemporary theorists, who focus on the evolution of the human mind for solving adaptive problems, posit that the majority of our psychological processes have probably evolved to deal with inter-personal contacts (Bereczki, 2000). Inter-personal skills have assumedly evolved from simply processing emotion-laden, perceptual stimuli to elaborating upon the social significance of this type of cues by means of our aptitude to think, reason, and organize knowledge. As a result of evolution, it is believed that emotion information is processed through perceptual and cognitive systems that are hierarchically organized (see, e.g., LeDoux, 1996).

Findings pointing to a hierarchic architecture for emotion processing map neatly onto the model of EI as sub-divisible into different branches (Mayer, Caruso, & Salovey, 2000). The first, apparently most basic branch involves the perception of emotion cues conveyed through non-verbal signals as, for instance, appears through facial expressions and gestures. In this respect, the concept of EI bears resemblance to the notion that our emotions serve as a primordial form of communication (Darwin, 1872/1998). The non-verbal information inherent in expressions of joy, for example, most likely signals social acceptance, and that of disgust, disapproval.

Vocal communication is believed to have taken place through a system of instinctive calls that were expressive of emotional states, such as distress or elation. Language itself is assumed to have arisen late in human evolution (see, e.g., Bradshaw & Rogers, 1993). Therefore, differences in the two forms of communication—non-verbal and verbal—are probably a result of differences in their neural foundation (Buck, 1984). Non-verbal communication evolved on the basis of mainly sub-cortical brain structures of the right hemisphere. Semantic processes underlying verbal communication evolved, more or less superimposed upon existing brain structures, in association with the more recently developed neo-cortex and in the left hemisphere. Research supports the idea that emotion information is processed in different systems of the brain, and that these are hierarchically organized as a result of evolution (see Gainotti, Caltagirone, & Zoccolotti, 1993, for an overview).

This conclusion raises the issue as to what extent modern day humans use non-verbal, emotional cues as social signals to and from other people in the environment. In studies of EI, processing of such cues is studied, for example, by means of tests of the ability to perceive emotions as expressed through facial expressions . The model of EI proposed by Mayer et al. (2000) also includes a branch involved with the cognitive processing of emotion information. The task is to judge the emotions experienced by each of two actors involved in a scenario depicting social problems. This procedure provides a measure of the ability to discern emotion information from the depicted context, and it requires knowledge about emotions and the situations in which they are likely to arise. More precisely, the ability to judge social episodes reflects verbal and cognitive skills in dealing with emotion information, as well as the degree of insight into cultural conventions pertinent to emotional reactions. Knowledge of this kind should be useful in discerning the nature of expressions performed by the same facial muscles, such as disappointment and regret (see Ekman, 1993). It should be equally useful for interpreting emotions as expressed by a combination of facial expressions, such as awe, which has been suggested to be a blend of expressions for fear and surprise (Plutchik, 1980).

Research within appraisal theory, originating from Magda Arnold (1960), can be seen as a pioneering attempt to study the cognitive nature of emotion knowledge. Basically, findings within this research tradition suggest that the essence of an emotional reaction can be best predicted on the basis of the appraisal of an antecedent situation or event (e.g., Roseman, 1984). A crude form of emotion knowledge thus consists of criteria such as perceived situational control and predictability of the consequences, which determine the emotion elicited as a result of given circumstances. Studies in this tradition have been criticized for reducing emotion to a static phenomenon (Scherer, 1999), whereas emotions are assumed to reflect relational processes that coordinate the dynamics of human interaction. Although emotional experiences may generally be understood according to common ways to appraise situations, many emotions may not be differentiated in a standard fashion. Jealousy or envy, for instance, would require a more comprehensive assessment of the individual context since these emotion terms encompass a range of behavioral tendencies and social circumstances (East & Watts, 1999). That is, in order to anticipate how a person is going to react, we often need to get a sense of his or her expectations and goals with regard to the situation. The former only takes on meaning in the context of the latter, as specific emotions arise out of the personal meanings that people bring to situations that have relevance to their intentions and aspirations (Mesquitas & Frijda, 1992; Lazarus, 1991).

Perceptual and cognitive abilities as outlined within the framework of Mayer and colleagues, in particular Branches 1 and 3 (see Chapter 2 by Neubauer and Freudenthaler), are prerequisites for social functioning as they enable proper understanding of emotional signals. The value of EI-related abilities in this respect is implied in findings that some individuals may differ markedly from the rest of the population in their ability to grasp emotion information. There is a wealth of research suggesting that dysfunctional appraisal styles (Lazarus, 1966) and thought patterns (Beck, Rush, Shaw, & Emery, 1979) are causes of social maladjustment. As people with affective disorders process information differently from others (Beck, Emery, & Greenberg, 1985), it is reasonable to assume that cognitive impairments entail a decrement in the ability to appropriately process emotion information. In addition, affective disorders, particularly depression, are often also associated with a lack of emotional expressiveness (Gotlib & Lee, 1989). Depressed persons typically engage in less eye contact with their interaction partners, and they exhibit facial expressions of happiness, sadness, fear, surprise, and interest less frequently (e.g., Fossi, Faravelli, & Paoli, 1984). The common assumption that depression eventually causes social dysfunction has been challenged by the argument that deficient social skills play a part in the etiology and maintenance of depression. According to Segrin and Abramson (1994), there may be an increased risk for developing symptoms of depression among individuals with poor social skills simply because their behavior elicits negative reactions from other people. The onset of depression may exacerbate a behavior that is already dysfunctional from a social-adaptive point of view.

Adaptation to the social world not only seems to necessitate abilities to construe meaning on what we perceive, but also aptitude to reciprocate in a fairly predictable manner. Social skills hence seem to be contingent upon our emotional functioning that develops and is shaped in interaction with the outside world.

14.3   THE SOCIAL-ADAPTIVE FUNCTION OF EMOTION

The contention that EI is related to social skills draws on theory and findings on the role of emotion in coordinating interaction between the individual and his or her environment. Theorists attribute the quality of providing the individual with both a sense of self, and a means to define social relationships, to emotion. According to Zajonc (1980), affective reactions implicate the self and affective responses are hence self-referential by definition. Lazarus (1991) similarly postulates that emotions are self-referential to the extent that they provide information on what is consistent with our goals in relation to others. Emotions are in this sense social since they typically arise in inter-personal contexts. The respective positions on emotion as merely affect, as opposed to elaborate meaning structures, correspond to the notion of emotions as basic or complex phenomena.

Basic emotions, such as surprise, fear, and joy, emerge early in life. They mostly arise by triggering emotion that essentially bypasses cognitive processing. As development progresses, emotional functioning becomes more dependent on social learning. The ability to symbolize or label emotions involves inferential or interpretive processes that depend on cognitive development (Izard, 2001). A more evolved cognitive ability enables the experience of complex emotions, such as shame, guilt, pride, or embarrassment by virtue of awareness of self as independent of others. The importance of self-concept in developing more sophisticated emotional function has been documented through observations which reveal that children who do not recognize their own self in one situation, do not show embarrassment in another context

(Lewis, Sullivan, Stanger, & Weiss, 1989). Complex emotions are therefore re-ferred to as "self-conscious" because they require a consciousness of self as an actor whose behavior has the potential to influence others' feelings, thoughts, and actions. For instance, the induction of guilt is almost entirely confined to close relationships, and the motive to induce guilt may be understood as a means to signal disturbances in interpersonal attachments (Baumeister, Still-well, & Heatherton, 1994).

The emergence of a self-concept eventually enables the taking of another person's perspective. Many theorists have in fact argued that perspective tak-ing (which may be viewed as an ability) is responsible for much of human social capacity (e.g., Piaget, 1932/1997). The importance of both self-concept and perspective taking is implied in findings that we tend to organize percep-tion and represent the social world in reference to the mental category of rela-tionships (Sedikides, Olsen, & Reis, 1993). Information about others is stored in memory within social contexts that have implications for our individual sense of self, presumably because emotions structure relationships as between members of a family (e.g., Dunn & Munn, 1985), and during play, courtship, and romance (Andersen, Eloy, Guerrero, & Spitzberg, 1995; Feeney, 1995; Gar-ner, Robertson, & Smith, 1997). These findings suggest that there are inter-personal features of particularly self-conscious emotions. They are, according to Tangney (1999), "not only intimately connected to the self. They are also intimately connected to our relationships to others" (p. 543). Emotions in this sense have a bearing on the notion of collective self (Markus & Kitayama, 1991; Pratkanis & Greenwald, 1985). That is, in collective or communal contexts, self-identity is embedded in the larger network of relationships with impor-tant group members.

The instrumentality of emotions for the differentiation of the self as a way of assimilating to the social environment is particularly discernable in stud-ies on gender differences in emotion and gender roles. Women are believed to feel emotions more frequently than men (Grossman & Wood, 1993) and are typically reported to display happiness, nervousness, fear, shame, and guilt (see Brody & Hall, 1993, for an overview). These are emotions that should be functional when rearing children and caring for social relations. The female tendency to display more of a variety of non-verbal behaviors such as smiling and gesturing (Barr & Kleck, 1995) might also be seen as functional for tradi-tional female tasks. Men have been found to report more pride in the self than do women (Tangney, 1990), along with less embarrassment, shame, and guilt (Stapley & Haviland, 1989). Greater male pride and contempt presumably cor-respond with the traditional male role of entering in competition with others and managing valuable resources. There seems to be an adaptive advantage of gender differences in emotion when taking on the different roles that males and females are expected to play in Western culture (Brody, 1997). Findings of this kind also imply that EI-related abilities are important when adjusting to roles that will benefit the overall purpose of different social contexts and task-oriented groups.

It has, however, been found that gender differences of this kind are less likely to appear when self-reports concern emotional experience as opposed to emotional expression, and when they are related to impersonal circumstances as opposed to interpersonal context. In other words, gender differences do not appear in self-reports when data are collected concurrently with ongoing experiences (e.g., Shields, 1991). Findings pointing to disparities between global and specific self-reports of emotion have lead Robinson, Johnson, and Shields (2001) to propose that there is a *gender heuristic*. It is plausible that we rely on gender stereotypes as a rule of thumb in judging emotions of self and others when we lack easy access to target- and situation-specific information. The notion of a gender heuristic implies that emotion knowledge contains stereotypes about emotion. If this is indeed the case, it would appear that emotion knowledge may occasionally lead us astray in our perception of the social world. Emotion knowledge as such should provide necessary aspects of social skills to adapt to most situations, but there seem nonetheless to be some shortcomings when challenged with more subtle aspects of human behavior.

14.4   EI AS A SOCIAL-ADAPTIVE ABILITY: RESEARCH FINDINGS

Social skills merely involve the ability to interpret emotional expressions and to draw on emotion knowledge that will enable the individual to blend into social contexts of different kinds. Inter-personal skills additionally involve the ability to enter into the bi-directional exchange of emotion information; more precisely, the ability, on the one hand, to apprehend the genuine meaning of social cues in others' behavior, and on the other hand, to calibrate one's own emotional behavior. With this definition, inter-personal skills involve different ways that people affect each other's moods and emotions, as evident through research on emotional contagion, non-verbal cues, and behavior; with clear implications for social functioning.

In short, emotional contagion can be conceived of as a transfer of feelings between persons through a three-stage-process involving mimicry, feedback, and contagion (Hatfield, Cacioppo, & Rapson, 1994). It has been observed that during interaction, people automatically mimic and synchronize their movements with the facial expressions, voices, postures, and movements of other people. It has even been found between people who are unfamiliar to each other that smiles and mannerisms are capable of automatically eliciting the same behavior in the observer (Chartrand & Bargh, 1999). According to theory, subjective emotional experience arises through the activation and feedback from facial, vocal, postural, and movement mimicry. As a result, there is a contagion of feelings from emitter to observer. Other studies suggest, however, that the peripheral activation and feedback as elicited by mimicry are not a necessary condition for contagion to occur (Hess & Blairy, 2001; Neumann & Strack, 2000). The empirical study of the emotional contagion hypothesis suggests that there are individual variations in the susceptibility to emotional contagion (e.g., Doherty, Orimoto, Singelis, & Hatfield, 1995; LeBlanc, Bakker, Peeters, van Heesch, & Schaufeli, 2001). When explored in a sales context, emotions via facial cues during a conversation were monitored in a study by Verbeke (1997). The data on emotions were analyzed in relation to sales performance that was taken as a measure of social efficacy. Results showed that performance was better among salespersons with, on the one hand, a high ability to transfer emotions, and on the other hand, a great sensitivity to the emotions of the customer. Performance was worse among salespersons with less of an ability to transfer emotions, although they showed high sensitivity to their interacting partners' emotions.

Prior research has revealed that behavioral cues are a source of information that people use to assess the nature of ongoing social interaction (Scheflen, 1964) and, furthermore, that the coordination of inter-personal behavior promotes a sense of social rapport. Work on posture mirroring shows that ratings of involvement, togetherness, and liking, tend to be positively correlated with the display of the same postural configuration on the part of the interaction partner (Chartrand & Bargh, 1999). Emotional state is usually reflected in the behavioral configuration of people in general and it should therefore follow that a match in mood (or feeling states) should be part of the overall influence toward a smoother interaction.

On the basis of this assumption, we formulated a hypothesis that sensitivity to others' mood is related to common EI-performance measures. In other words, we assumed that susceptibility to emotional contagion is part of inter-personal skills grounded in EI-related abilities to perceive and process emotion information.

We were able to test this hypothesis when administrating an entrance test to the Stockholm School of Economics. The group of participants consisted of 191 applicants (102 men, 88 women), average age 20.5 years (range 18–34). We used methods (Sjöberg, 2001a, 2001b) that briefly consist of the following two measures:

- performance measures developed according to the model underlying the Mayer-Salovey-Caruso Emotional Intelligence Test (MSCEIT), mainly to investigate the ability to identify emotions,

- an instrument to measure the ability to assess others' mood, as developed by the second author.

Emotion identification was measured by two tests. Twelve pictures from the Lightfoot series of facial expressions (Engen, Levy, & Schlosberg, 1957). measured the ability to identify emotions from facial expressions. Participants rated each picture on eight unipolar three-category scales: happiness, anger, sadness, shame, guilt, contempt, surprise, and fear. The "correct" response in this test was the most common response given by the present group of test takers. This scoring method is thus based on the principle of consensus (see Chapter 8 by Legree, Psotka, Tremble, & Bourne), which was also applied in the next test. Emotion identification was measured with the help of written

Table 14.1   Correlations between Traditional Performance Measures of EI, Accuracy in the Perception of Others' Mood, and Deviance of Own Mood Relative That of Others

	1	2	3	4
1. Facial Expressions	1.00			
2. Social Episodes	.78**	1.00		
3. Mood Perception	−.32*	−.35*	1.00	
4. Mood Deviance	−.51**	−.58**	.39*	1.00

Notes. * $p < .05$, ** $p < .01$.

descriptions of brief social problem episodes involving two actors. The task was to rate the extent to which each of the actors felt each of ten different emotions, using unipolar three category scales: happy, angry, sad, ashamed, proud, afraid, relieved, disappointed, surprised, and guilty.

The instrument to measure mood perception is based on a 71-item scale (Sjöberg, Svensson, & Persson, 1979) measuring six factors (i.e., happiness, tension, fatigue, confidence, extraversion, and social orientation). Respondents were instructed to rate their own current feeling state, as well as that of fellow participants. As every individual was assumed to be an expert on their own mood, a "correct" assessment of others' mood corresponds to the mean rating of own mood in the whole group of test takers. An individual score on perception of others' mood was thus obtained by taking the difference between the participant's rating of others' mood and the mean rating of their own mood state *as they actually rated it*. This score, termed *mood perception*, thus provides a measure of how well judges assess the authentic experience of a specific target, as opposed to the principle of consensus scoring (which produces a measure of how well judges perform in relation to each other). The correlations of the performance measures are presented in Table 14.1.

As expected, the measure for mood perception was inversely related to traditional EI performance measures, that is, facial expressions and social episodes. This result indicates that persons who are less accurate in their assessment of others' mood in the concurrent situation tend to deviate from the general consensus on how to perceive and interpret emotion information from facial expressions and narratives describing social problems. However, the objection could be raised concerning the source of information used in generating a more accurate assessment of others' mood. Were accurate judges ignorant of emotional cues and simply assessed the implications of the situation, as such, in relation to more fine-tuned emotion knowledge? This could be the case and would curtail our assumption that emotion knowledge enters into the computation to make sense of emotional cues as observed in others' behavior.

In view of this ambiguity, we performed another calculation on the mood data to strengthen our case that greater susceptibility to mood contagion enables a more accurate assessment of others' mood. Results would be more convincing on this point if they were to show that accurate judges tended to converge towards the mood of those they observe in their immediate vicinity. Another score was therefore obtained by forming the difference between the ratings of own mood of each participant and the mean rating of own mood as actually rated by all test takers. This measure, termed *mood deviance* presented in Table 14.1, gives the extent to which the respondent differs in own mood from that of other test takers. The negative correlations between mood deviance and EI performance measures suggest that individuals of high EI tended to converge with others in feeling state that was generally prevailing in that particular situation. In addition to the positive correlation between mood deviance and mood perception, there seems to be support for the assumption that susceptibility to mood contagion enhances the perception of others' feelings.

In another study, we found that affect intensity (or heightened reactivity to emotional stimuli) was associated with greater accuracy in the perception of others' mood as assessed in a concurrent situation (Engelberg & Sjöberg, 2004). Additionally, results strongly suggested that accurate emotion perception was linked to indices of social adjustment.

Building on these results, it is plausible to assume that social functioning should be facilitated by a propensity to converge with others in the judgment of emotion information. In sharing very similar emotion knowledge, interaction partners will be more efficient in understanding others' intentions and orientations to different relationships, and also to adjust accordingly. In this sense, emotion knowledge could be viewed as encompassing cognition of cultural display rules (Ekman & Friesen, 1975) that are basically norms of interaction on how to conform to the expectations of a social situation (cf. Grandey, 2000; Totterdell & Holman, 2003).

Additional skills of an inter-personal character seem, however, to consist of an ability to converge in emotional composure. Convergence of this kind seems to consist of susceptibility to emotional signals in order to reciprocate with appropriate behaviors. The exact nature of such behavior may only be guided to an approximate extent by cultural display rules. Whether a matter of susceptibility to emotional contagion or emotional reactivity, it seems to be instrumental for tailoring one's behavior in accordance with the specifics of a situation. Rather than merely sharing similar emotion knowledge, inter-personal skills are about emotional sharing through corresponding behavior and feeling states.

Faking Social Skills: Performance Measures Versus Self-Report Scales

In line with our reasoning so far, it should be possible to fake social skills when drawing on emotion knowledge of more sophisticated kinds. This would especially be true in situations where EI is measured with self-report instruments, since these provide some leeway to the respondent to embellish his or her actual qualities and abilities. Studies suggest that performance measures of EI are more adequate in this respect than self-report instruments (Geher, Warner,

& Brown, 2001; Otto, Döring-Seipel, Grebe, & Lantermann, 2001, a conclusion also drawn by Mayer et al. 2000).

Hence, there are good reasons to believe that effects of social desirability influence self-report measures and this would, of course, warrant more extensive development of performance measures (Morand, 2001). In our studies, we have therefore included measures of social desirability and, in order to estimate the effect of faking, we have carried out a special study in which we compared two different groups.

One of these groups consisted of 41 participants who were recruited among students at the Stockholm School of Economics (SSE). All testing was anonymous, a fact stressed to the participants. The other group consisted of the same 191 participants as mentioned above, and who had taken the same tests about 11 months earlier, as part of a process for assessing applicants to the SSE. As participants in the latter group had been invited to take part in the test on the basis of high school grades or a test of intellectual ability similar to the SAT, they were comparable to the group of 41 participants. Admission to the school is highly competitive and very desirable for many of these applicants. Instructions stressed that they should give honest and frank answers.

Did the respondents who performed in the testing session, which had real consequences, (called *real testing* in the following) differ from those who were tested anonymously? We first investigated three common response bias variables, as well as a combined faking index.

The well-known scale of social desirability by Crowne and Marlowe (1960) was used, as was the Paulhus scales of impression management and self deception (Paulhus, 1991, 1998; Paulhus & Reid, 1991). In addition, we constructed a scale based on data collected under the instruction to give faked answers that would likely contribute to a positive admission decision regarding the test taker. A score under explicit faking instructions (that was close to the score on the same dimension obtained under non-faking instructions) was taken as a measure of the extent of faking under instructions to give honest answers[1].

The results obtained from this study are encouraging because they show that the response bias variables all worked as expected (see Table 14.2). Note that the last variable, the faking score, should be related in the opposite direction from the other three scores.

The next question concerns to what extent the various EI measures and other variables were affected by tactical answering (see Table 14.3 for performance measures and Table 14.4 for self-report measures). Self-report measures consisted of the scale developed by Schutte et al. (1998) as a direct measure of EI, different scales commonly considered as facets of EI, and a five-factor model of personality. Table 14.4 also contains the results of adjusting the dif-

---

[1]Tactical responses to the instruction to fake explicitly may have endangered the validity of this measure. Some test-takers may have realized the way their responses were going to be scored, and adjusted them accordingly. However, results supported strongly the approach we used.

Table 14.2   Response Bias Scores in Two Groups

Response Bias Variable	Mean, Real Testing	Mean, Anonymous Testing	t	df	p
Crown-Marlowe Social Desirability	0.20	−0.93	7.29	229	< .0005
Paulhus Impression Management	0.15	−0.70	5.23	229	< .0005
Paulhus Self Deception	0.15	−0.68	5.04	229	< .0005
Combined Faking Score on Instructions to Fake	−0.29	1.32	11.83	229	< .0005

Notes. All measures are standardized (i.e., $M = 0$ and $SD = 1$) in the combined group.

Table 14.3   Test Scores in Two Groups: Performance Scales

Test variable	Mean, Real Testing	Mean, Anonymous Testing	t	df	p
Facial Expressions	−0.01	0.04	ns		
Social Episodes	−0.19	0.87	6.69	227	< .0005
Mood/Expert	−0.02	0.11	ns		

Notes. ns = not significant at level $\alpha = .05$. All measures are standardized (i.e., $M = 0$ and $SD = 1$) in the combined group.

ferences between real testing and anonymous testing for impression management and faking.

Note that the test-takers in the high-stakes situation did not differ significantly from the anonymous participants in two of the three performance measures. Test-takers performed significantly *worse* than the anonymous group with regard to social episodes. There is hence no indication in these data that the performance measures could be successfully faked.

Turning to Table 14.4, the picture is very different. The results suggest that the respondents in the high-stakes situation faked a positive image of themselves, because the comparable group that took the test under anonymity gave a much less rosy picture of themselves. All these differences, with the exception of empathy, are quite large. This result agrees well with the fact that the two groups also differed—even more strongly—on measures of impression management, faking, and self-deception.

In all cases, with one exception, statistical control for impression management and faking removed virtually all of the mean difference between the two

Table 14.4   Test Scores in Two Groups: Self-Report Measures

Test variable	Mean, Real Testing	Mean, Anon. Testing	t	df	p	adj. diff.	t of adj. diff.
Schutte et al. EQ	0.16	−0.73	5.43	229	< .0005	0.02	ns
Alexithymia	−0.17	0.80	6.09	229	< .0005	0.07	ns
Self actualization	0.18	−0.82	6.32	229	< .0005	−0.05	ns
Machiavellianism	−0.14	0.67	4.96	229	< .0005	0.12	ns
Empathy	0.00	−0.02			ns	0.07	ns
Big 5: Agreeableness	0.13	−0.62	4.55	229	< .0005	−0.17	ns
Big 5: Emotional stability	0.19	−0.86	6.65	229	< .0005	−0.03	ns
Big 5: Extraversion/ Introversion	0.15	−0.71	5.30	229	< .0005	0.13	ns
Big 5: Intellectual Openness	0.21	−0.99	7.90	229	< .0005	−0.18	ns
Big 5: Conscientiousness	0.18	−0.82	6.24	229	< .0005	−0.47	2.78**

Notes. Anon. = Anonymous, ns = not significant at level $\alpha = .05$, adj. diff. = adjusted difference. Differences between mean residuals when the four impression management and faking variables have been controlled for by linear regressions. All measures are standardized (i.e., $M = 0$ and $SD = 1$) in the combined group.
** $p < .01$

groups. In other words, statistical control was sufficiently powerful to remove the motivational effects of the high-stakes testing situation. The only test variable for which this was not true was the five-factor model measure of conscientiousness. However, even in that case about half of the effect of the high-stakes situation as compared to the anonymous situation was removed. The reason for the relative failure of this particular variable, as distinguished from all others tested for the influence of impression management, may be related to the fact that the measure of faking did not include conscientiousness.

Hence, statistical control for tactical responses that was made possible by our design was successful. Of the two approaches to measuring EI, performance scales showed considerably more promise in two ways. The two most important performance measures showed strong convergence. They were unaffected by tactics of responding in a high-stakes selection context, while self-report measures, as expected, were found to be excessively distorted by such tactics. Extensive coverage of impression management and faking tendencies, and separate measurement of such tendencies, made it possible to exert statistical control over faking and to remove virtually all of its effects. This finding supports the conclusions and the interpretations of results we have given. EI performance measures and mood knowledge scores converged, strengthening the notion of a dimension of individual differences in EI. The performance measures were not affected by faking. On the other hand, self-report measures were clearly strongly affected, a factor which could be removed in almost all cases by means of statistical control based on social desirability scales.

14.5 CONCLUDING REMARKS

The pattern of results that has emerged in our research supports the notion that the emotional competence characteristic of high EI confers advantages for adaptation to the social environment. As pointed out by Roberts, Zeidner, and Matthews (2001), the pervasive use of consensus scoring in studies on EI presumes that a match between responses of an individual and the group as a whole indicates a better adjustment. It is interesting to note that one of the few strong and replicable findings in Rorschach research concerns "good form", that is, conventional answers. Conventional answers tend to be related to a higher degree of social adjustment on the part of the respondent (Dawes, 1999). This type of finding not only provides some additional support for the consensual scoring of EI performance measures, it also provides an input to the conceptual underpinnings of EI as a construct to encompass the ability for adaptation (cf. Izard, 2001), conformity being one aspect of social adaptation (Chan, 2003).

In view of the results concerning statistical control, self-report measures might still be quite useful in situations where the test takers are highly motivated to give many tactical responses. This is, of course, under the assumption that they are not all equally tactical. People always differ. Yet, many practitioners would probably prefer to avoid the psychometric niceties of measuring tactical behavior and use them for statistical control of impression management and instead go for performance measures. We believe that there are good reasons for doing so. Most probably, performance cannot be faked, certainly not without expending considerable effort.

In our theoretical analysis, we argued that skill in understanding and managing emotions constitute an important part of social intelligence, and that emotional skills therefore should be related to social adaptation. This argument presumes that there are emotional skills with a high degree of generality, and that they can be measured. The results of our empirical work support these assumptions. Our work is consistent with much current work in these respects, and it supports, in particular the original idea of measuring EI by means of performance tasks.

Self-report measures have been more popular in practical work, in spite of the problems of faking. Ones and Viswesvaran (1998) acknowledge that faking is prevalent in self-report measures of personality, but they also argue that extensive empirical research shows that the validity of such personality scales is not compromised by faking (Ones & Viswesvaran, 1998; Viswesvaran & Ones, 1999). This is a surprising finding and it may show that faking skills and willingness to fake have, by themselves, a component of validity. Maybe people who fake on personality tests are clever manipulators also in other contexts. Be that as it may, we find it worrisome that tests should be contaminated with unwanted components of this kind and procedures which avoid them altogether (for ethical reasons) are to be preferred.

REFERENCES

Andersen, P. A., Eloy, S. V., Guerrero, L. K., & Spitzberg, B. H. (1995). Romantic jealousy and relational satisfaction: A look at the impact of jealousy experience and expression. *Communication Reports, 8,* 77–85.

Arnold, M. B. (1960). *Emotion and personality* (Vol. 1). New York: Columbia University Press.

Austin, E. J., Deary, I. J., Whiteman, M. C., Fowkes, F. G. R., Pedersen, N. L., Rabbit, P., et al. (2002). Relationships between ability and personality: Does intelligence contribute positively to personal and social adjustment? *Personality and Individual Differences, 32,* 1391–1411.

Averill, J. R. (1980). A constructivist view of emotion. In R. Plutchik & H. Kellerman (Eds.), *Emotion: Theory, research, and experience. Vol. 1. Theories of emotion* (pp. 305–339). New York: Academic Press.

Bar-On, R. (2000). Emotional and social intelligence: Insights from the Emotional Quotient Inventory. In R. Bar-On & J. D. A. Parker (Eds.), *The handbook of emotional intelligence: Theory, development, assessment, and application at home, school, and in the workplace* (pp. 363–388). San Francisco: Jossey-Bass.

Barr, C. L., & Kleck, R. E. (1995). Self-other perception of the intensity of facial expressions of emotion: Do we know what we show? *Journal of Personality and Social Psychology, 68,* 608–618.

Baumeister, R. F., Stillwell, A. M., & Heatherton, T. F. (1994). Guilt: An interpersonal approach. *Psychological Bulletin, 115,* 243–267.

Beck, A. T., Emery, G., & Greenberg, R. C. (1985). *Anxiety disorders and phobias: A cognitive perspective.* New York: Basic Books.

Beck, A. T., Rush, A. J., Shaw, B. F., & Emery, G. (1979). *Cognitive therapy of depression.* New York: Guilford Press.

Bereczki, T. (2000). Evolutionary psychology: A new perspective in the behavioral sciences. *European Psychologist, 5,* 175–190.

Bradshaw, J. L., & Rogers, L. J. (1993). *The evolution of lateral asymmetries, language, tool use, and intellect.* San Diego, CA: Basic Books.

Brody, L. R. (1997). Gender and emotion: Beyond stereotypes. *Journal of Social Issues, 53,* 369–393.

Brody, L. R., & Hall, J. A. (1993). Gender and emotion. In M. Lewis & J. M. Haviland-Jones (Eds.), *Handbook of emotions* (pp. 447–460). New York: Guilford Press.

Buck, R. (1984). *The communication of emotion.* New York: Guilford Press.

Caruso, D. R., Mayer, J. D., & Salovey, P. (2002). Relation of an ability measure of emotional intelligence to personality. *Journal of Personality Assessment, 79,* 306–320.

Chan, D. W. (2003). Dimensions of emotional intelligence and their relationships with social coping among gifted adolescents in Hong Kong. *Journal of Youth and Adolescence, 32*, 409–418.

Chartrand, T. L., & Bargh, J. A. (1999). The chameleon effect: The perception-behavior link and social interaction. *Journal of Personality and Social Psychology, 76*, 893–910.

Crowne, D. P., & Marlowe, D. (1960). A new scale of social desirability independent of psychopathology. *Journal of Consulting and Clinical Psychology, 24*, 349–354.

Darwin, C. (1998). *The expression of the emotions in man and animals.* New York: Oxford University Press. (Original work published 1872)

Dawes, R. M. (1999). Two methods for studying the incremental validity of the Rorschach test. *Psychological Assessment, 11*, 297–302.

Doherty, R. W., Orimoto, L., Singelis, T. M., & Hatfield, E. (1995). Emotional contagion: Gender and occupational differences. *Psychology of Women Quarterly, 19*, 355–371.

Dunn, J. F., & Munn, P. (1985). Becoming a family member: Family conflict and the development of social understanding in the second year. *Child Development, 56*, 480–492.

East, M. P., & Watts, F. N. (1999). Jealousy and envy. In T. Dalgleish & M. Power (Eds.), *The handbook of cognition and emotion* (pp. 569–590). Chichester, UK: John Wiley.

Ekman, P. (1992). Facial expression of emotion: New findings, new questions. *Psychological Science, 6*, 34–38.

Ekman, P. (1993). Facial expression and emotion. *American Psychologist, 48*, 384–392.

Ekman, P., & Friesen, W. V. (1975). *Unmasking the face: A guide to recognizing emotions from facial clues.* Englewood Cliffs, NJ: Prentice-Hall.

Engelberg, E., & Sjöberg, L. (2004). Emotional intelligence, affect intensity, and social adjustment. *Personality and Individual Differences, 37*, 533–542.

Engen, T., Levy, N., & Schlosberg, H. (1957). A new series of facial expressions. *American Psychologist, 12*, 264–266.

Feeney, J. A. (1995). Adult attachment and emotional control. *Personal Relationships, 2*, 143–159.

Fossi, L., Faravelli, C., & Paoli, M. (1984). The ethological approach to the assessment of depressive disorders. *Journal of Nervous and Mental Disease, 172*, 332–341.

Gainotti, G., Caltagirone, C., & Zoccolotti, P. (1993). Left/right and cortical/subcortical dichotomies in the neuropsychological study of human emotions. *Cognition and Emotion, 7*, 71–93.

Garner, P. W., Robertson, S., & Smith, G. (1997). Preschool children's emotional expressions with peers: The roles of gender and emotion socialization. *Sex Roles, 36*, 675–691.

Geher, G., Warner, R. M., & Brown, A. S. (2001). Predictive validity of the emotional accuracy research scale. *Intelligence, 29*, 373–388.

Goleman, D. (1995). *Emotional intelligence: Why it can matter more than IQ.* New York: Bantam Books.

Gotlib, I. H., & Lee, C. M. (1989). The social functioning of depressed patients: A longitudinal assessment. *Journal of Social and Clinical Psychology, 8*, 223–237.

Grandey, A. A. (2000). Emotional regulation in the workplace: A new way to conceptualize emotional labor. *Journal of Occupational Health Psychology, 5,* 95–110.

Grossman, M., & Wood, W. (1993). Sex differences in intensity in emotional expression: A social role interpretation. *Journal of Personality and Social Psychology, 65,* 1010–1022.

Hatfield, E., Cacioppo, J. T., & Rapson, R. L. (1994). *Emotional contagion.* Cambridge, UK: Cambridge University Press.

Hess, U., & Blairy, S. (2001). Facial mimicry and emotional contagion to dynamic facial expressions and their influence on decoding accuracy. *International Journal of Psychophysiology, 40,* 129–141.

Izard, C. E. (1971). *The face of emotion.* New York: Appleton-Century-Crofts.

Izard, C. E. (2001). Emotional intelligence or adaptive emotions? *Emotion, 1,* 249–257.

Keltner, D., & Gross, J. J. (1999). Functional accounts of emotions. *Cognition and Emotion, 13,* 467–480.

Keltner, D., & Haidt, J. (1999). Social functions of emotions at four levels of analysis. *Cognition and Emotion, 13,* 505–521.

Kihlstrom, J. F., & Cantor, N. (2000). Social intelligence. In R. J. Sternberg (Ed.), *Handbook of intelligence* (pp. 359–379). New York: Cambridge University Press.

Lazarus, R. S. (1966). *Psychological stress and the coping process.* New York: McGraw-Hill.

Lazarus, R. S. (1991). *Emotion and adaptation.* New York: Oxford University Press.

LeBlanc, P. M., Bakker, A. B., Peeters, M. C., van Heesch, N., & Schaufeli, W. B. (2001). Emotional job demands and burnout among oncology care providers. *Anxiety, Stress, & Coping: An International Journal, 14,* 243–263.

LeDoux, J. E. (1996). *The emotional brain: The mysterious underpinnings of emotional life.* New York: Simon and Schuster.

Lewis, M., Sullivan, M., Stanger, C., & Weiss, M. (1989). Self-development and self-conscious emotions. *Child Development, 60,* 146–156.

Markus, H. R., & Kitayama, S. (1991). Culture and the self: Implications for cognition, emotion, and motivation. *Psychological Review, 98,* 224–253.

Mayer, J. D., Caruso, D. R., & Salovey, P. (2000). Selecting a measure of emotional intelligence: The case for ability testing. In R. Bar-On & J. D. A. Parker (Eds.), *The handbook of emotional intelligence: Theory, development, assessment, and application at home, school, and in the workplace* (pp. 320–342). San Francisco: Jossey-Bass.

Mayer, J. D., Salovey, P., Caruso, D. R., & Sitarenios, G. (2001). Emotional intelligence as a standard intelligence. *Emotion, 1,* 232–242.

Mesquitas, B., & Frijda, N. H. (1992). Cultural variations in emotions: A review. *Psychological Bulletin, 112,* 179–204.

Morand, D. A. (2001). The emotional intelligence of managers: Assessing the construct validity of a nonverbal measure of "people skills". *Journal of Business and Psychology, 16,* 21–33.

Neumann, R., & Strack, F. (2000). "Mood contagion": The automatic transfer of mood between persons. *Journal of Personality and Social Psychology, 79,* 211–223.

Öhman, A. (1986). Face the beast and fear the face: Animal and social fears as prototypes for evolutionary analysis of emotion. *Psychophysiology, 23,* 123–145.

Ones, D. S., & Viswesvaran, C. (1998). The effects of social desirability and faking on personality and integrity assessment for personnel selection. *Human Performance, 11,* 245–269.

Otto, J. H., Döring-Seipel, E., Grebe, M., & Lantermann, E.-D. (2001). Entwicklung eines Fragebogens zur Erfassung der wahrgenommenen emotionalen Intelligenz. Aufmerksamkeit auf Klarheit und Beeinflussbarkeit von Emotionen [Development of a questionnaire for measuring perceived emotional intelligence: Attention to, clarity , and repair of emotions]. *Diagnostica, 47,* 178–187.

Parkinson, B. (1996). Emotions are social. *British Journal of Psychology, 87,* 663–683.

Paulhus, D. L. (1991). Measurement and control of response bias. In J. P. Robinson, P. R. Shaver, & L. S. Wrightsman (Eds.), *Measures of personality and social-psychological attitudes* (pp. 17–59). San Diego, CA: Academic Press.

Paulhus, D. L. (1998). Interpersonal and intrapsychic adaptiveness and trait self-enhancement: A mixed blessing? *Journal of Personality and Social Psychology, 74,* 1197–1208.

Paulhus, D. L., & Reid, D. (1991). Enhancement and denial in socially desirable responding. *Journal of Personality and Social Psychology,* 307–317.

Petrides, K. V., & Furnham, A. (2001). Trait emotional intelligence: Psychometric investigation with reference to established trait taxonomies. *European Journal of Personality, 15,* 425–448.

Piaget, J. (1997). *The moral judgment of the child.* New York: Free Press Paperbacks. (Original work published 1932)

Plutchik, R. (1980). A general psychoevolutionary theory of emotion. In R. Plutchik & H. Kellerman (Eds.), *Emotion: Theory, research and experience. Vol. 1. Theories of emotion* (pp. 3–33). New York: Academic Press.

Pratkanis, A. R., & Greenwald, A. G. (1985). How shall the self be perceived? *Journal for the Theory of Social Behaviour, 15,* 311–329.

Roberts, R. D., Zeidner, M., & Matthews, G. (2001). Does emotional intelligence meet traditional standards for an intelligence? Some new data and conclusions. *Emotion, 1,* 196–231.

Robinson, M. D., Johnson, J. T., & Shields, S. A. (2001). The gender heuristic and the database: Factors affecting the perception of gender-related differences in the experience and display of emotions. In G. W. Parrott (Ed.), *Emotions in social psychology: Essential readings* (pp. 157–169). Philadelphia: Psychology Press.

Roseman, I. J. (1984). Cognitive determinants of emotion: A structural theory. In I. P. Shaver (Ed.), *Review of personality and social psychology* (Vol. 5, pp. 11–36). Beverly Hills, CA: Sage.

Salovey, P., & Mayer, J. D. (1990). Emotional intelligence. *Imagination, Cognition and Personality, 9,* 185–211.

Scheflen, A. E. (1964). The significance of posture in communication systems. *Psychiatry, 27,* 316–331.

Scherer, K. R. (1999). Appraisal theory. In T. Dalgleish & M. Power (Eds.), *The handbook of cognition and emotion* (pp. 637–663). Chichester, UK: John Wiley.

Schmidt, F. L., & Hunter, J. E. (1998). The validity and utility of selection methods in personnel psychology: Practical and theoretical implications of 85 years of research findings. *Psychological Bulletin, 124,* 262–274.

Schutte, N. S., Malouff, J. M., Hall, L. E., Haggerty, D. J., Cooper, J. T., Golden, C. J., et al. (1998). Development and validation of a measure of emotional intelligence. *Personality and Individual Differences, 25,* 167–177.

Sedikides, C., Olsen, N., & Reis, H. T. (1993). Relationships as natural categories. *Journal of Personality and Social Psychology, 64,* 71–82.

Segrin, C., & Abramson, L. Y. (1994). Negative reactions to depressive behaviors: A communication theories analysis. *Journal of Abnormal Psychology, 103,* 655–668.

Shields, S. A. (1991). Gender in the psychology of emotion: A selective research review. In K. T. Strongman (Ed.), *International review of studies on emotion* (Vol. 1, pp. 227–245). New York: John Wiley.

Sjöberg, L. (2001a). Emotional intelligence: A psychometric analysis. *European Psychologist, 6,* 79–95.

Sjöberg, L. (2001b). *Emotional intelligence measured in a highly competitive testing situation* (SSE/EFI Working Paper Series in Business Administration No. 2001:13). Stockholm, Sweden: Stockholm School of Economics.

Sjöberg, L., Svensson, E., & Persson, L.-O. (1979). The measurement of mood. *Scandinavian Journal of Psychology, 20,* 1–18.

Slaski, M., & Cartwright, S. (2002). Health, performance and emotional intelligence: An exploratory study of retail managers. *Stress & Health, 18,* 63–68.

Stapley, J. C., & Haviland, J. M. (1989). Beyond depression: Gender differences in normal adolescents' emotional experiences. *Sex Roles, 20,* 295–308.

Sternberg, R. J. (1985). *Beyond IQ: A triarchic theory of human intelligence.* New York: Cambridge University Press.

Tangney, J. P. (1990). Assessing individual differences in proneness to shame and guilt: Development of the self-conscious affect and attribution inventory. *Journal of Personality and Social Psychology, 59,* 102–111.

Tangney, J. P. (1999). The self-conscious emotions: Shame, guilt, embarrassment and pride. In T. Dalgleish & M. Power (Eds.), *The handbook of cognition and emotion* (pp. 541–568). Chichester, UK: John Wiley and Sons.

Totterdell, P., & Holman, D. (2003). Emotion regulation in customer service roles: Testing a model of emotional labor. *Journal of Occupational Health Psychology, 8,* 55–73.

Verbeke, W. (1997). Individual differences in emotional contagion of salespersons: Its effect on performance and burnout. *Psychology and Marketing, 14,* 617–636.

Viswesvaran, C., & Ones, D. S. (1999). Meta-analysis of fakability estimates: Implications for personality measurement. *Educational and Psychological Measurement, 59,* 197–210.

Zajonc, R. B. (1980). Feeling and thinking—Preferences need no inferences. *American Psychologist, 35,* 151–175.

Part IV

Conclusion

15

Understanding, Measuring, and Applying Emotional Intelligence: What Have We Learned? What Have We Missed?

Richard D. Roberts
Educational Testing Service, USA
University of Sydney, Australia

Ralf Schulze
Educational Testing Service, USA
Westfälische Wilhelms-Universität Münster, Germany

Moshe Zeidner
University of Haifa, Israel

Gerald Matthews
University of Cincinnati, USA

Summary

This chapter provides a synthesis of the theory, research, and applications surrounding emotional intelligence (EI) that are presented throughout the current volume. We note, for example, the breadth of the theoretical models that have been offered in discussing the concept of EI. Providing definitional issues are resolved and efforts towards demarcation of the subject domain are made, this may be a more healthy state-of-affairs than previously suggested. Measurement issues provide one of the more intractable problems currently facing the field, particularly disjunctions between performance-based and self-report approaches to assessment. Some considerable space is given to describing a possible rapprochement between these measurement approaches, along with some paradigms that we have recently developed. Applications of EI in the fields of education, organizational, and clinical psychology hold much promise, particularly if theory and measurement issues are satisfactorily resolved. This commentary ends with discussion of two additional areas that EI might find ready application—gerontology and affective computing—wherein we provide ideas for future research that might be profitably explored.

15.1   INTRODUCTION

In this concluding commentary, we set about the task of reconciling the various chapters. This is by no means an easy task as the authors often represent conflicting views and perspectives on the nature of emotional intelligence (EI). Nevertheless, we point out how each chapter contributes to the current state-of-the art in theory, assessment, and applications. We also highlight some areas that seemingly need to be considered in order to enhance current knowledge and understanding of EI.

One point of consensus emerging throughout this volume is that populist accounts of EI should find a firmer scientific foundation. The extent to which popular accounts have embraced the concept (or its various derivatives) is perhaps not surprising. Peddling the virtues of new, emerging intelligences— moral, sexual, promotional, naturalistic, entrepreneurial, political, cultural, spiritual; the list seems boundless—appears part of effective, twenty-first century marketing strategies by business-people, journalists, and media-savvy scientists alike.[1]   In turn, these groups feed into the laypersons interest in self-help issues, often without the care required of emergent, scientific constructs. Equally, interest in EI owes much to sober attempts to develop and validate tests of EI (and other measures of affective processes), which, potentially, may be as important for psychological assessment as measures of academic, cognitive performance. Indeed, as commentators throughout the book attest, the concept of EI appears among the more promising of the new constructs emerging from psychological science that are directed towards improving the human condition. Moreover, the construct resonates with a popular zeitgeist that emphasizes personal growth, the minimization of psychological harm (to both self and to others), and an appreciation of elevated levels of self-esteem (Matthews, Zeidner, & Roberts, 2005, in press-a, in press-b; Salovey, Mayer, & Caruso, 2002).

---

[1]The phenomenon may not be as recent as we perhaps think. In a recent historical review, Landy (in press) notes that for various reasons, eminent psychologist like Thorndike (1920) might have done something similar in order to promote the virtues of early psychological research and differentiate it from its less scientific ancestors like phrenology.

Reviewed throughout the current volume, in almost every chapter, are a large number of tests that appear to meet conventional standards for reliability. Several of these tests of EI also possess at least some properties supporting their validity. At the same time, difficulties remain apparent with current approaches to understanding the concept of EI (see also Matthews, Zeidner, & Roberts, 2002). Conceivably, in being just over a decade old, the field is too new for definitive judgments, and in several instances the contributors to this volume go to great extremes to try and remedy the status quo. One feature emerging from these various commentaries is that the term *emotional intelligence* refers to multiple constructs, a sample of which may not represent forms of intelligence at all. Equally, since some of these constructs may already be encapsulated by existing theories of personality it appears problematic to develop new models around them. At the same time, individual differences in affective processes had received short shrift until recently; EI has focused scientific research on this doubtless important topic (MacCann, Matthews, Zeidner, & Roberts, 2004; Zeidner, Matthews, & Roberts, in press).

In the remainder of this concluding exposition, we recapitulate the promises offered throughout the present volume for the study of EI, while also suggesting domains of this emerging subdiscipline where there might be a need for more balanced discourse. In this commentary, we also alert the reader to certain pitfalls that may impede proper scientific progress if due caution is not exercised. In addition, we offer some suggestions for a more unified, scientific framework, discussing both a measurement and developmental model we have developed with this goal in mind. It is pivotal that EI also find meaningful applications and real life consequences; we review further evidence supporting the calls made by commentators in that section. Finally, we suggest some additional domains of applied psychology where we believe the construct of EI might be profitably explored.

15.2 THEORETICAL ISSUES

15.2.1 What We Have Learned

The range of theories of EI actually covered in this volume may be construed as daunting. First, there exists a great divide between so-called ability and mixed model approaches, with the latter, if the review by Pérez, Petrides, and Furnham (Chapter 9) is any guide, yielding over a dozen idiosyncratic theories tied to specific self-report measures. Second, even the well-known performance-based Mayer-Salovey-Caruso model, as noted by Neubauer and Freudenthaler (Chapter 2), has noteworthy differences between early and later versions, such that the reader should be circumspect in assuming that they have the same conceptual underpinnings. Further still, in this volume, an account is made outside of these approaches (doubtless not for the last time), with Ciarrochi and Godsell's (Chapter 4) attempt to mesh a theory from clinical psychology with EI concepts. Finally, we note from various commentators that there exists a possible rapprochement between social, emotional, and practical intelligence that might not only add in definitional clarity across these various domains, but also the assessment of EI itself (see Austin & Saklofske, Chapter 6; Kang, Day, & Meara, Chapter 5; Weis & Süß, Chapter 10).

The question that springs to mind is whether this is a healthy state-of-affairs. The answer to this question is by no means straightforward. In intelligence research, which appears further advanced there appears a great deal of tolerance for alternative perspectives. Thus, some researchers favor a view of a single, important construct—psychometric g—while others talk of multiple cognitive abilities (see Roberts, Markham, Zeidner, & Matthews, 2005, for a recent review). Within these approaches there are also noticeable disjunctions. For example, the theory proposed by Gardner (e.g., 1993) assumes seven to ten multiple intelligences, determined largely on the basis of neurological, computational, evolutionary, and developmental criteria, and often a weak empirical base. By contrast, the theory of fluid and crystallized intelligence is steeped in psychometric evidence, test construction, and gerontological research, yet posits different constructs, albeit a similar number to Gardner (see, e.g., Carroll, 1993; Horn & Noll, 1997; Roberts & Stankov, 1999). Sternberg (e.g., 1985) provides a still different perspective. His triarchic theory encapsulates analytic intelligence, creativity, and practical intelligence.

Given this precedent, it is perhaps appropriate that there are so many different models of EI. However, consider several important facts. First, principles for measuring intelligence constructs are largely undisputed. Individual differences in cognitive ability can be determined on the basis of the responses to tasks scored correct/incorrect or determined as response per unit of time (see, e.g., Carroll, 1993; Guttman & Levy, 1991). Self-reports of intellectual ability have been utilized, but in general these are thought to provide different information from the actual test scores; notably, the term *intelligence* is generally not reserved for such measures (see Wilhelm, Chapter 7). Furthermore, taxonomic models have been posited, by which it is possible to locate both the universe of ability constructs and measures. Moreover, models underlying test performance have been linked to developmental, neurophysiological, cognitive, biological, and evolutionary concomitants. These ubiquitous and important features of ability models stand in stark contrast to the current state of play in EI research, which raises the possibility of researchers talking at cross-purposes (Matthews, Roberts, & Zeidner, 2004).

Fortunately, the contributors to the present volume, where possible, attempt to bridge these gaps. For example, Schultz, Izard, and Abe (Chapter 3) provide a much needed call to consider developmental models. Notably their arguments combine neurophysiological concepts, developmental evidence, emerging principles from educational practice, and measurement models. Wilhelm's (Chapter 7) appeal to consider the modeling of EI concepts and to suggest that some of these might be arranged in similar fashion to cognitive constructs is consistent with our contention that taxonomic models are needed to guide EI research. Legree, Psotka, Tremble, and Bourne's (Chapter 8) discussion of models of consensual scoring suggest too that it is possible to develop promising psychometric analyses for non-veridical responses (i.e., those not having a clearly defined right or wrong answer). Chapters of this kind provide a much needed impetus towards a sounder theoretical basis for the conceptualization and measurement of EI, offering the potential to take it to a similar plateau to academic intelligence measures in rapid time. They also provide a number of noteworthy suggestions for principled, systematic research.

Perhaps more important, however, when it comes to evaluating the impetus of research in the domain of academic abilities, is the societal value given by the intelligence test. Many proponents of these instruments, rightly or wrongly, see this as the most practical contribution made to humanity by all of psychology (e.g., Anastasi & Urbina, 1997). Several lines of converging evidence support the pragmatic usefulness of intelligence tests. First, standardized tests of intelligence, multiple aptitudes, and academic achievement are widespread across the Western world, influencing individual life decisions en masse (Campbell & Knapp, 2001). Second, various meta-analyses indicate that measures of intelligence predict job and academic performance particularly well, in the process saving national economies billions of dollars (Roberts et al., 2005). Indeed, these instruments appear better suited for this purpose than any other measure of psychological, sociological, or demographic significance (see, e.g., Schmidt & Hunter, 1998). Finally, scores on intelligence tests have been implicated with physical and psychological well-being and quality of life constructs (Neisser et al., 1996), with studies also demonstrating that it is an important predictor of mortality (e.g., Deary & Derr, 2005).

The question that perhaps will be become most pertinent in any long-term evaluation of the importance of EI research might also be those psychological, sociological, and demographic factors that it consistently predicts. This possibility is certainly acknowledged in, and arguably may even be at the crux of, many of the chapters comprising the present volume. Thus, besides each of the chapters focusing on educational, organizational, and clinical applications (i.e., Goetz, Frenzel, Pekrun, & Hall, Chapter 11; Abraham, Chapter, 12; Parker, Chapter 13), where prediction is clearly vital, we are presented with data that are suggestive of the predictive validity of EI measures in a variety of domains (sometimes for the first time). For example, Schultz et al. (Chapter 3) review several studies in their own laboratory where emotion expression, emotional, and situational knowledge predict teacher ratings of social skills, behavioral problems, and objective measures of academic competence in first- and third-grade children. The studies reviewed by Engelberg and Sjöberg (Chapter 14) suggest relations between measures of emotion perception and various indices of social adjustment in adult samples. Indeed, proposed relations between EI and factors like social skills, social support, and other indices of social adaptation, as they define it, are further buttressed by the studies examined by Austin and Saklofske (Chapter 6), as well as studies conducted by Lopes, Salovey, and Strauss (e.g., 2003).

The onus will be on researchers to replicate and extend these findings and, providing a corpus of knowledge is reached, undertake the kind of principled meta-analyses advocated by Schulze (2004).[2] Careful demarcation of the criterion space will also need to be undertaken; simply correlating self-report measures against other self-report measures runs the risk of criterion contamination. Moreover, those criteria that are most important, are more likely to be variables that are outside the traditional criterion space (i.e., number of widgets, worker output derived from supervisor ratings, etc.), though certainly those it might predict are clearly vital (e.g., life satisfaction, lowered absenteeism, citizenship behaviors). Furthermore, EI may be useful for the prediction of certain job clusters (e.g., those in the health and service industries) and not others. As evidenced in the discussions by Austin and Saklofske (Chapter 6), Kang et al. (Chapter 5), and Weis and Süß (Chapter 10), it will be necessary to not only show the extent that EI provides incremental validity over personality and academic intelligence but also exhibit how EI measures differ from the related constructs of social and practical intelligence. Nevertheless, the fact that data on the predictive validity of EI constructs is accruing stands as testament to the potential of the field.

15.2.2   What We Have Missed

Each of the commentators dealing with theoretical issues highlight the need for greater conceptual coherence, positing models that offer a rapprochement between developmental (Schultz et al., Chapter 3) and evolutionary (Ciarrochi & Godsell, Chapter 4) antecedents of EI, or else offering a compelling case as to why one approach to the conceptualization of EI—often in terms of performance components—is superior to others (e.g., Neubauer & Freudenthaler, Chapter 2). The missing ingredient, arguably, is how each of these disparate aspects might coalesce, in a similar fashion to what has happened with cognitive abilities, to move the field forward. Integrating each of these features is no trivial undertaking, yet the onus to do so rests with the current authors. In the passages that follow, we attempt to provide an integrative summary of the preceding chapters, which also encapsulates features that may have been overlooked by the contributors.

Implicit in virtually every chapter is the prospect that EI refers to multiple constructs that are weakly, though meaningfully, related to one another. For example, measures of self-reported EI, like the SEIS correlate around .30 with performance-based measures like the MSCEIT (e.g., Wilhelm, Chapter 7). Similarly, as Austin and Saklofske (Chapter 6) demonstrate, a cognitive measure of emotional processing based on the inspection time methodology correlates around −.30 with self-reported EI. The correlations between self-report EI also tend to vary considerably, seemingly because some such as the BarOn EQ-i are largely proxies for personality measures (see Neubauer & Freudenthaler, Chapter 2), while tests like the TEIque tend to be based more on a concep-

---

[2]We note that at least one meta-analysis has already been conducted with EI measures (Van Rooy & Viswesvaran, 2004), though as we suggest later in this chapter, there are several problematic features associated with it.

tual match to the Mayer-Salovey-Caruso model, and hence may act more like self-reports of intelligence than proxies for personality (Pérez et al., Chapter 9). There is also evidence from performance-based measures that emotion perception and assimilating emotions form a separate higher-order construct (i.e., Experiential EI) that is moderately correlated with a second-order factor comprising the understanding and managing branches (i.e., Strategic EI) (Wilhelm, Chapter 7; also Mayer, Salovey, Caruso, & Sitarenios, 2003). Of note, this latter set of distinctions parallels that offered by Kang et al. (Chapter 5) when they suggest it might be judicious to consider separate forms of fluid and crystallized social-emotional intelligence.

Toward a unified measurement framework: The four-source model. It appears feasible that there are discrete sets of constructs discussed throughout these chapters that may be differentiated psychometrically, in terms of processing concomitants, and in terms of adaptive significance. In Table 15.1 we list four of these constructs, while drawing parallels with similar constructs from the literature on intelligence, as well as some comments on developmental influences that likely operate in each instance.

It is worth noting that several commentators, among them Schultz et al. (Chapter 3), Kang et al. (Chapter 5), and Wilhelm (Chapter 7) explicitly make reference to the need for multiple constructs (which they variously refer to as *emotion systems, declarative emotion knowledge, fluid emotional intelligence,* and the like). In the passages that follow, we discuss our proposed integrative, working model in more depth, and highlight some potentially important research issues that need to be resolved in terms of it (see also MacCann, Matthews, et al., 2004). We suggest this framework as a comprehensive way to categorize the domain of EI (including its constructs, assessments, and underlying processes). To date, research has only focused on the measurement of EI and its relations to other constructs, but has not tried to create an overarching framework for the field. This framework, which draws ready parallels to the approach that Weis and Süß (Chapter 10) advocate for social intelligence (SI), was developed to circumvent this limitation.

Temperament. The dimensions of childhood temperament (Schultz et al., Chapter 3) map onto adult personality dimensions such as neuroticism, extraversion, and conscientiousness that, in turn, are highly correlated with many EI questionnaires. Complexes of various biological and cognitive processes support such dimensions, the adaptive consequences of which are not easily traced since intricate and multifaceted (Matthews, Emo, Funke, Zeidner, & Roberts, 2003; Matthews et al., 2005; Matthews, Zeidner, & Roberts, in press-a). For example, although distress-prone children may have difficulties in interacting with the caregiver, vulnerability to distress may also attract the caregiver's attention, and promote risk-avoidance. Much is known of temperamental qualities (e.g., Rothbart & Bates, 1998), though as we note in subsequent discussion, this appears an important aspect of EI certainly in any attempt to develop a comprehensive developmental model.

Table 15.1   Multiple Types of Construct That May Contribute to Emotional Intelligence

Construct	Possible measure in chapters	Equivalent in IQ research	Key processes	Adaptive significance	Developmental influences
Emotionality-Temperament	Scales for Big Five personality EQ-i ECI	None that are direct, though links to Openness	Neural and cognitive processes controlling arousal, attention, and reinforcement sensitivity	Mixed: most temperamental factors confer a mixture of costs and benefits	Genetics and early learning
Emotional Self-Confidence	SEIS sub-components TEIque subscales	Self-assessed intelligence	Self-concept and self-regulation	Predominantly, but not exclusively positive: presumed similar to self-esteem	Learning and social-ization: for example, mastery experiences, modeling, etc.
Emotional Information Processing	Lightfoot Facial Expressions, Emotional Inspection Time, Emotional Stroop	Choice Reaction Time, Inspection Time, working memory	Specific processing modules	Uncertain: Is speed of processing necessarily adaptive?	Genetics and early learning
Emotional knowledge and skills	MSCEIT, LEAS, SJTs	Crystallized intelligence (and related aptitudes)	Multiple acquired procedural and declarative skills	Adaptive within context for learning; may be irrelevant or counter-productive in certain other contexts	Learning, social-ization and training of specific skills and knowledge

Note. EQ-i = Emotional Quotient inventory, ECI = Emotional Competence Inventory, SEIS = Schutte Emotional Intelligence Scales, TEIque = Trait Emotional Intelligence Questionnaire, MSCEIT = Mayer-Salovey-Caruso Emotional Intelligence Test, LEAS = Levels of Emotional Awareness Scale, SJT = Situational Judgment Test.

Emotional self-confidence. A novel aspect of EI research is that it provides assessments of an individual's belief of the extent that they can manage emotions and interpersonal encounters (e.g., self-reported confidence in understanding emotional states). Emotional self-confidence may be at the core of questionnaires such as the TEIque (see Pérez et al., Chapter 9). This construct is akin to self-rated intelligence and at the process level might compare favorably with self-knowledge. That is, self-confidence may depend on the content of the self-schema shaped by social learning (Bandura, 1999). As such, it is likely to be more dependent on learning within specific contexts than is temperament. Like self-esteem, high emotional self-confidence may be predominantly adaptive, but with a dark side, taking the form of narcissism, denial of problems, and excessive self-enhancement (Baumeister, Smart, & Boden, 1996). We note, in passing, that alternative means, other than self-assessment, exist for measuring self-confidence (e.g., having participants make confidence judgments after responding to cognitive test items; see e.g., Pallier et al., 2002).

Emotional information processing. Individual differences in processing stimuli of positive or negative valence are best known from personality research. For example, extraversion and neuroticism may relate to small biases towards prioritizing positive and negative stimuli, respectively (Rusting & Larsen, 1998). It is unclear whether factors for processing emotive stimuli exist (e.g., whether some individuals are quick to recognize negative stimuli). However, factors that define aptitudes for processing emotional stimuli appear an aspect of EI. Austin and Saklofske's (Chapter 6) findings with the Emotional Inspection Time paradigm are important here, as is our own recent work with the Emotional Stroop paradigm (O'Brien, MacCann, Reid, Schulze, & Roberts, 2005). There also appears to be a factor for accurate emotion perception, discussed for example by Engelberg and Sjöberg (Chapter 14), which may share relations with the Experiential EI component of the MSCEIT (Matthews, Zeidner, & Roberts, in press-a). If factors of this kind exist, they would appear to constitute abilities. A general factor for such abilities might correspond to fluid intelligence (Gf) in the abilities domain, especially given similar measures of cognitive processing from the intelligence domain correlate highest with Gf (Roberts & Stankov, 1999). However, the adaptive value of such factors remains to be explored; it is unclear that rapid processing of positive stimuli and slow processing of negative stimuli (or various permutations thereof) is necessarily beneficial. Plausibly such a factor might improve over the course of schooling and decline in the later years of life.

Emotional knowledge. EI also appears related to acquired, contextualized skills for handling specific encounters, such as calming an upset friend. Conceivably, such skills have similar properties to cognitive skills. Thus, although emotional self-confidence may facilitate acquisition and execution of skills, skills are numerous, and specialized for specific problems. Similarly, depending on levels of practice and the stimulus-response mapping (consistent or varied), skills will likely vary on an explicit-implicit continuum. Implicit skills

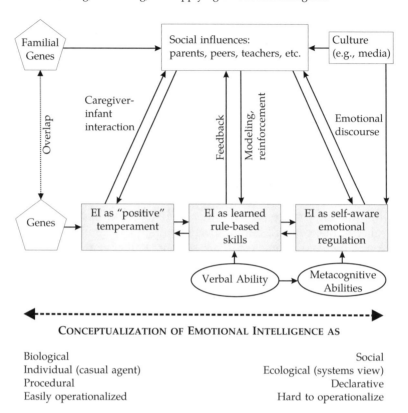

Figure 15.1   An investment model of emotional intelligence (see also Zeidner et al., 2003).

perhaps resemble crystallized intelligence, while explicit skills might correspond to declarative knowledge of emotions (Ackerman, 1996). It is likely that the understanding and management branches of the MSCEIT involve explicit skills, with implicit skills important to perception and assimilation (Neubauer & Freudenthaler, Chapter 2). By and large, increased knowledge is adaptive, but it may transfer poorly across different situations. The fact that these various types of emotional components are related to knowledge, suggests that they are likely to improve over the school years, perhaps late into life, and be susceptible to various forms of intervention.

A developmental framework: The investment model.   Consistent with ideas contained in Schultz et al. (Chapter 3), Zeidner, Matthews, Roberts, and Mac-Cann (2003) have suggested that the multiple constructs discussed above may be linked developmentally rather than structurally. Their investment model, akin to that proposed for cognitive abilities, is shown in Figure 15.1.

    The model describes how developmental processes may generate associations between different components of EI, such that lower levels (e.g., positive temperament) are invested through experience into the development of higher levels of EI (e.g., emotion management). In particular, a child's positive temperament, when invested in interactions conducive to the acquisition of emotional knowledge, produces returns of declarative, rule-based knowledge about emotions. This knowledge, when invested in interactions in emotional situations, produces returns of self-aware emotion regulation, social skills, and the like. The model describes how basic temperamental qualities influence the acquisition of emotional skills and self-understanding. For instance, temperament appears to interact with situational factors to influence rule-based skills. Much of this learning is verbal in nature, such that verbal ability also facilitates skill acquisition. However, aspects of temperament (e.g., being excessively distress-prone) may disrupt the child's conversations with the caregiver, delaying emotional skill learning. The older child acquires skills that are more dependent on insight into self and others, allowing a more flexible response to interpersonal situations. Both temperament and rule-based competence may moderate insight-based learning. In addition, metacognitive awareness and regulation of personal thoughts and feelings become increasingly important. The adult thus possesses a varied repertoire of emotional responses, ranging from low-level emotional modulation (temperament), through simple rule-based skills, to more complex competencies based on insight (emotional knowledge).

The investment model is suggestive both of long-term macro developmental processes (continuing into adulthood), and the short-term micro processes that govern responses within a specific interpersonal encounter or emotive event (Zeidner et al., 2003). Personality research identifies various developmental patterns of person-situation interaction. One developmental pattern is that distress-prone temperament (linked to adult trait anxiety and neuroticism) leads to hypervigilance for threat, avoidance of feared social situations, and diversion of attentional resources to process internal worries rather than the environment. This configuration of response reduces exposure to emotional stimuli, meaning fewer opportunities to develop emotion recognition skills (e.g., Wells & Matthews, 1994). The resultant skills deficits lead to further avoidance, and maladaptive self-beliefs and metacognitions that typically lead to further withdrawal. Similarly, temperamental activity and impulsivity (corresponding to adult extraversion) lead to engagement with challenging situations, and hence greater opportunities for learning skills for handling exciting (but potentially risky) encounters. Thus, temperamental traits may influence emotional development both directly, via individual differences in emotion and attention, and indirectly, through exposure to emotional situations and opportunities for practicing and learning skills for specific emotional challenges.

It is also possible to look at a micro-process for the interaction between the individual's traits, skills, and the environment to determine how the different EI constructs relate to the cognitive processes that mediate adaptation to situational challenges. The leading theory of the adaptational process is Lazarus's (1999) transactional model, which includes several sub-processes.

Appraisal refers to the evaluation of the personal significance of an event, and the likelihood of successfully coping. Appraisal depends on multiple information processing components, including fast, unconscious evaluations and consciously accessible processing that is more flexible and context-sensitive (Scherer, 2001). Coping includes efforts to manage demands appraised as threatening, overtaxing, or challenging (e.g., Shimazu & Kosugi, 2003). Coping strategies are varied; they differ in the extent to which the skills required are well-learned and routine, or require controlled processing in order to formulate a new strategy for dealing with exigent or unfamiliar demands (Matthews & Wells, 1999). Thus, both appraisal and coping may recruit different levels of processing depending on the nature of external demands, and the person's repertoire of skills for understanding and managing the situation concerned.

The idea of relating EI to individual differences in these cognitive stress processes is appealing. There is some conceptual overlap between the literatures on stress and on EI, and indeed each of the four different conceptualizations discussed previously may play some role in adaptation. Emotionally intelligent individuals might, for example, have more accurate appraisals or be better able to focus attention on the stimuli critical for resolving a difficult social encounter. Information processing may also influence some of the more automatic, less consciously accessible aspects of appraisal, influencing speed of making emotional judgments. EI might also relate to the subset of coping strategies that are directed towards adaptive emotion-management and processing, such as emotion repair and emotional disclosure (Salovey, Bedell, Detweiler, & Mayer, 1999). In a recent review, however, we suggested that existing research literature does not support the notion of a continuum of adaptive competence, though we also welcomed future efforts directed towards resolving this issue (Zeidner et al., in press). To fulfill this objective, we also proposed that research linking EI, coping with stress, and adaptation would be need to be guided by the following principles: (1) clearer conceptual and psychometric discrimination of the multiple constructs related to EI; (2) a stronger focus on mediating mechanisms; (3) a stronger focus on situational moderators of EI constructs; and (4) a greater emphasis on building causal models using data from experimental and longitudinal studies.

15.3   MEASUREMENT ISSUES

15.3.1   What We Have Learned

Almost all of the chapters comprising the current edited volume, whether they be theoretically focused or slated towards discussing applications, have also at their core some additional concern with measurement issues. The number of assessment instruments discussed in this volume is large and, in light of our preceding commentary, touch on disparate constructs that collectively fall under the broad umbrella of *emotional intelligence*. Also included, is fairly detailed discussion of social and practical intelligence measures. The lessons learned, from each of these chapters, are many and varied. In this section, we offer a distillation of core perspectives, some potential promises, and a series of conceivable pitfalls that should be avoided.

Pérez et al.'s (Chapter 9) account is worth noting, most especially in light of the large number of self-report measures that propagate the field. A similar array of instruments populates the field of personality assessment, and it is worth drawing to the reader's attention that these have been the subject of detailed comparisons and cross-tabulation. For example, Goldberg (in press) has formed the International Personality Item Pool (IPIP) website[3] that essentially references all known personality instruments with respect to the Five Factor Model of personality. Conceivably, it may be in the best interests of EI researchers to at least show the extent that self-report measures map onto each other. Currently, it appears that there is a notable disjunction between these measures, rendering them talking at cross-purposes and creating a virtual Tower of Babel (MacCann, Matthews, et al., 2004). If our previous account is correct, the divide between these measures may indeed be extreme—some relate to temperament, others to self-rated EI, while still others might represent an amalgam of these two domains. While Pérez et al. (Chapter 9) have admirably isolated a number of self-report measures they fall short in drawing commonalities and divergences between them. This is no fault of these authors; the vast majority of researchers working with self-report measures seem content to suggest that their new instrument is superior to all others, without requisite attention to empirical instantiation.[4] Landy (in press) has recently attributed a similar state-of-affairs at early attempts to measure SI, which has arguably left that field short of reaching its full potential.

Wilhelm's (Chapter 7) account of measurement issues is thought provoking. While we feel the criticisms of self-report measures per se are certainly pertinent, we suspect too that there may be something more to them. Indeed, the notions of typical intellectual engagement and need for cognition have been at the core of Wilhelm's own research interests, with some remarkable evidence for incremental validity (Wilhelm, Schulze, Schmiedek, & Süß, 2003; see also Ackerman, 1996; Cacioppo, Petty, Feinstein, & Jarvis, 1996). We suspect that there may be a dimension of self-motivated cognition to emotionally relevant stimuli that, to our knowledge, no EI researcher has attempted to fully develop (see, however, Epstein, 1998). Notwithstanding, the type of structural models that Wilhelm proposes appears an urgent research issue, worthy of empirical investigation. Moreover, his suggestion to consider paradigms like the Levels of Emotional Awareness Scale (LEAS; Lane, Quinlan, Schwartz, Walker, & Zeitlin, 1990) is one that finds resonance among the current commentators as well as several contributors to this volume. Clearly, the more objective such indices, the more resemblance they will share with traditional intelligence measures, though commensurate with this, such tests run the risk of becoming

[3]http://ipip.ori.org/
[4]We note that such criticisms cannot be leveled at the actual co-authors of this chapter; Petrides and Furnham have been particularly active in studies that included various self-report EI measures in large multivariate designs (see e.g., Petrides & Furnham, 2001).

proxies for academic intelligence (more so given Spearman's [1927] concept of the indifference of the indicator). Even so, in later passages, we discuss potential objective measures of EI not considered elsewhere in this volume.

Legree et al.'s (Chapter 8) account of situational judgment tests (SJTs) and the methods that might be used to scores these are also in the spirit of finding new and innovative ways of assessing dimensions of social-emotional behavior. It is non-incidental that the consensual scoring paradigm advocated in the MSCEIT and MEIS was derived from Legree's (1995) original research examining measures of SI for military personnel. Elsewhere, we have drawn certain problems to consensual scoring procedures (Zeidner, Matthews, & Roberts, 2001), as well as some psychometric techniques that might increase both their reliability and validity (MacCann, Roberts, Matthews, & Zeidner, 2004). Leaving this issue aside, Legree et al.'s (Chapter 8) account is the first to lay out the full-blown rationale supporting this scoring technique, which we believe, with sufficient development, might lead to important advances in measuring EI and related constructs. Interestingly, as early as Thorndike (1920), so-called *in situ* tasks were advocated for assessing SI; why there has not been more concerted test development using SJTs is puzzling (Landy, in press).

The chapter by Weis and Süß (Chapter 10), albeit focusing largely on SI, is, in many ways, highly similar to our earlier exposition highlighting the need for multiple assessment techniques, and a means of classifying these appropriately, in the domain of EI. Multitrait multimethod (MTMM) designs have so far received relatively short shrift in the literature, and their call to consider this methodology (along with that made by Kang et al., Chapter 5) is well taken (more so given the success that they appear to have had in using such techniques). Indeed, Carroll (1993), among others, has advocated the usefulness of MTMM designs incorporating objective, self-, and peer-reports, with respect to SI research. We contend (like many of the issues raised in this section on measurement) that this approach is requisite in developing a more fully developed science of EI.

15.3.2   What We May Have Missed

The preceding discussion, as well as our exposition of the four-source measurement model, offers some interesting suggestions for forms of assessment that were not necessarily covered by any of the contributors. Some of these have been used elsewhere, particularly in emotions research, while others have a track record in personality research and industrial-organizational psychology. Still others have been developed in our own laboratories, largely as a result of our reviews and critiques in the area. Indeed, we are in the midst of developing a series of EI instruments, comparing these with tests like the MSCEIT and other emotion measures and collecting predictive validity in various countries (USA, Germany, Norway, and Australia) with different populations (young, elderly, community college, and university students). In the passages below, we briefly describe a selection of the measures we are examining in these studies, along with findings where available, or speculations as to what they might actually assess. Our focus in these passages (as in this program of research) is on measures of self-confidence, information processing, and emotional knowledge, since we contend that measures of temperament have saturated the field.

Assessing emotional self-confidence.   We have recently developed the Personal Introspection of Emotional State (PIES), a self-report measure that requires participants to rate the extent to which they agree or disagree with statements about their emotions in specific contexts. In the underlying model, it is hypothesized that emotional self-confidence involves different skills when directed towards the self versus when directed at others, and when the emotions involved are positive versus negative in terms of emotional-salience. In addition, the questionnaire is designed to measure all four facets of EI proposed by Mayer et al. (2003). Thus, through the complete cross of all of these dimensions, some 16 sub-scales have been designed, with 7–8 items per scale. To give the reader some impression of these scales, we present sample items in Table 15.2. Data are currently being collected on the instrument, which we intend to examine using confirmatory factor analytic techniques.

Assessing emotional processing.   Of note, tests measuring the ability to recognize emotion in various stimuli (i.e., tests of emotion recognition ability; ERA) have not generally been conceptualized as measures of EI. Indeed, the disjuncture between experimental and individual differences psychology is apparent here (see Cronbach, 1957), though the former is tied more directly to theory and could with psychometric development more fully meet the demands imposed by the latter subdiscipline. Indeed, conceptual correspondence with branches of the Mayer-Salovey-Caruso model (especially, emotion perception) makes many of these tasks feasible candidates for assessing EI (see Wilhelm, Chapter 7). In Table 15.3 we list a selection of these, along with source references, and a brief description.

Consideration of these experimental paradigms might plausibly lead to a model of EI more closely resembling taxonomies common to the intelligence domain (see MacCann, Matthews, et al., 2004). With this fact in mind, we recently had 138 first-year university students complete the MSCEIT, two measures of ERA (JACBART and RAFL), and measures of fluid (Gf) and crystallized (Gc) intelligence (O'Brien et al., 2005). Exploratory and confirmatory factor analysis recovered the two MSCEIT higher-order factors (Experiential and Strategic EI) and Gc; however, there was also evidence for a third factor that combined Gf and the ERA measures. The study suggests that the relation between performance-based EI and ERA is not substantial and that ERA is more strongly related to Gf than the MSCEIT, a finding we preempted in our previous discussion of emotional processing.

Aside from measures of ERA, future experimental paradigms assessing emotional processing components might include: the emotional Stroop and derivatives thereof (e.g., taboo Stroop); variants of the Wisconsin card-sorting task utilizing emotional stimuli; and variations on search tasks utilizing emo-

Table 15.2   A Faceted Framework for Self-Assessment of Emotional Skills

	Self		Others	
	Positive	Negative	Positive	Negative
Emotion Perception	I can tell when I am happy	I feel flushed when embarrassed	I can tell if people are happy or not	I can tell when others are in a bad mood
Emotion Facilitation	I play happy music when doing boring tasks	When I am angry, solving problems is easy for me	I generate a positive mood in others when coming up with new ideas in a group	When I'm in a position of authority, I find that generating fear in others will make them more productive
Emotion Understanding	When I'm in a good mood I can usually tell people why	It is unusual for me to be unhappy without knowing why	When people are in good mood it's easy for me to see why	When people are glum it's easy for me to understand what caused it
Emotion Management	When I am happy, I feel like I have more control over my emotions	When I am in a bad mood, I feel like I have more control over my emotions	I can easily put another person in a good mood	If I wanted to, I could easily make someone feel angry

Table 15.3   Test, Sampling Domain, and Scoring Methodology for Tests of Emotion Recognition Ability

Test	Sampling Domain	Test composition	Scoring
JACBART	Emotion recognition for faces varying	56 items, one score	According to veridical criteria from FACS
ERT	Emotion recognition (in verbal labels, faces and simple contexts)	8 × 4-part item	Multiple choice with 1 correct alternative from among 4 choices
DANVA2-AF	Emotion recognition of facial expressions	24 items	Multiple choice with 1 correct alternative from among 4 choices
DANVA2-AP	Emotion recognition in tone and voice	24 items	Multiple choice with 1 correct alternative from among 4 choices
RAFL	Emotion recognition (for tone and voice)	30 items, one score	According to veridical criteria from acoustic research

Note. JACBART = Japanese and Caucasian Brief Affect Recognition Test (Matsumoto et al., 2000), FACS = Facial Affect Coding System, ERT = Emotion Recognition Test (Shimokawa et al., 2000), DANVA2-AF = Diagnostic Assessment of Non Verbal Affect—Adult Facial Expressions (Nowicki & Carton, 1993), DANVA2-AP = Diagnostic Assessment of Non Verbal Affect—Adult Paralanguage (Baum & Nowicki, 1998), RAFL = Recognition of Affect in a Foreign Language (Scherer, Banse, & Wallbott, 2001).

tional stimuli (e.g., finding and circling sad faces among an array of sad, scared, and angry faces) (MacCann, Matthews, et al., 2004). Indeed, there are several possibilities for constructing such tasks from cognitive and differential psychology; a principled selection of such measures included in a large-scale multivariate design might result in an empirically founded taxonomy of emotional ability. Indeed, resolving the dimensionality of emotional processing arguably appears a necessary step for theoretically enriching EI models.

Assessing explicit emotional knowledge. Of note, virtually all measures of emotional knowledge constructed thus far make use of consensual scoring techniques. Notwithstanding the advantages of this approach highlighted by Legree et al. in this volume, various commentators have expressed concern about the ease with which such rubrics might be coached, their legal and ethical soundness, and/or various other features that would make them unlikely to be used in high-stakes assessment (Kyllonen & Lee, 2005). For this reason, we have embarked on developing measures of emotional knowledge that have a response that may be scored objectively. One of these is the Affective Quote Completion Test (AQCT), which assesses the ability to label emotions and recognize the relationships between them, the ability to understand complex feelings, and the transitions that can take place between them. A 20-item test, AQCT essentially measures emotional understanding using a veridical scoring procedure; that is, selected quotes on human emotions, uttered by famous philosophers, scientists, or literary figures, which have responses that may be scored as right or wrong. The measure uses a cloze procedure, in which key emotion-relevant words have been removed from these quotations. One's ability level is reflected in one's understanding of the words related to emotions and the relations among the words and the emotions themselves. Data are currently being collected on this new measure; one issue we are targeting is the extent to which this measure overlaps with crystallized intelligence.

Assessing implicit emotional knowledge. Most individuals can be thought of as having at least functional EI. For example, they can be considered to be respectful toward others, to abide by the rules of society, to accept legitimate authority, and to attempt to lead productive lives. In contrast, a small proportion of people may be thought of as emotionally illiterate (Goleman, 1995). These individuals are undependable and untrustworthy, frequently aggressive, and defiant of social norms. One form of emotional illiteracy appears to be aggression. James and colleagues (e.g., James, 1998; James et al., 2005; James, McIntyre, Glisson, Bowler, & Mitchell, in press) have spent the last ten years developing a new technique to break through aggressive individuals' attempts to mask their true dispositions.

Justification mechanisms are reasoning biases that operate below the level of consciousness of the reasoner. Unconscious or implicit biases in reasoning can be measured using indirect and objective procedures. On the surface, these problems appear to be basic reasoning tasks, which in fact they are. However, the real purpose of these problems, which is not apparent, is to draw out aggressive respondents' reliance on reasoning biases—that is, justification mechanisms—to determine what they believe is logical. What consciously appears to be rational versus implausible reasoning is determined not by reasoning skills, but by whether reasoning is (or is not) guided by unconscious justification mechanisms. These mechanism bear close correspondence to the management components of the Mayer-Salovey-Caruso model; hence, we consider this may serve as a measure of this component (notably distinct from expert- or consensus-scoring per se).

Based on the preceding rationale, James (1998) has developed the Conditional Reasoning Test for Aggression (CRT-A). This instrument has been shown to have acceptable psychometric properties and an average, uncorrected validity of .44 against behavioral indicators of aggression (James et al., 2005, in press). These results are consistent with prior conditional reasoning studies on achievement motivation, and indicate that it is possible to make reasonably accurate assessments of aggressive tendencies that people often attempt to deny or conceal. The results suggest further that it is possible to increase, perhaps substantially, the ability to predict whether people will behave aggressively in the future. We are currently collecting data on this instrument, along with measures of self-report and performance-based EI, and a range of criteria (biographical data, social support, mental health, and emotional well-being).

15.4   APPLICATIONS

15.4.1   What We Have Learned

As we noted in discussion of theoretical issues, at least part of the importance of traditional intelligence research derives from demonstration of its ecological validity and practical utility. Claims for the relevance of EI to school, work, and family life appear part of its initial appeal, not only in popular instantiations (e.g., Goleman, 1995, 1998), but also in the titles (and content) of at least two previous edited volumes with a clearer academic focus (Bar-On & Parker, 2000; Ciarrochi, Forgas, & Mayer, 2001). Indeed, much of our own previous research has discussed the extent that EI may contribute to handling challenging events successfully in a wide array of domains, including the workplace (see Zeidner, Matthews, & Roberts, 2004), clinical intervention (Matthews et al., 2002), education (Zeidner, Roberts, & Matthews, 2002), and in social interaction, more generally (Aicher et al., 2005). The chapters by Abraham, Parker, Goetz et al., Engelberg and Sjöberg are thus in domains we have special interest in and appear recurring themes for showing the value-added of studying EI.

Organizational applications of EI.   Abraham (Chapter 12) rightfully pays homage to the fact that many workplaces now acknowledge the importance of overall emotional climate and both team and individual levels of EI. Thus, corporations are currently selecting incumbents on the basis of EI assessment or else using these for succession planning, while seminars promising to increase EI have become the standard fare of staff-in-service. However, contrary to some of the data Abraham cites, her admirable attempts to develop a model of EI that is relevant in organizational settings, and a focus on showing how EI relates to organizational commitment, we suggest that the scientific evidence supporting workplace applications is often equivocal.

Thus, in reviewing research on the validity of EI in occupational settings, Zeidner et al. (2004) concluded that the various scales for EI are, at best, weak predictors of job performance. For example, in a study of customer service teams, Feyerherm and Rice (2002) found that, at the team level, the MEIS predicted some subjective performance criteria, including customer service but not productivity. Moreover, contrary to expectation, several significant negative correlations were found between the EI of the team leader and team performance. A more recent study conducted by Donaldson-Feilder and Bond (2004) showed that with psychological acceptance and job-control statistically controlled, EI did not significantly predict any major workplace outcomes, including job satisfaction.

Abraham (Chapter 12) cites the meta-analysis reported by Van Rooy and Viswesvaran (2004) as supporting associations between EI and occupational criteria. Importantly, many of these studies, even now, have not appeared in the peer-reviewed literature. Another concern that we have with this meta-analysis is that occupational studies typically use supervisor ratings; given that EI scales typically correlate with social involvement and desirable personality characteristics, such ratings may be confounded by a halo effect. Another serious problem is that studies have typically ignored the personality and ability confounds of EI tests, which might be responsible for the typically modest validity coefficients that have been reported. On the flip side, as we suggested earlier, the criterion that EI might need to predict in work settings remains poorly operationalized and in urgent need of attention. Abraham's (Chapter 12) insights into studies of organizational commitment are in the spirit of this call, as is her contention that more sophisticated methodologies are required other than quasi-experimental correlational studies.

We note, in closing this section, that the benefits of training EI in the workplace have also yet to be demonstrated satisfactorily. For example, Slaski and Cartwright (2002) found that a training program improved self-reported EI scores (as measured by the EQ-i), but had no effect on ratings of managerial performance. Training studies using objective measures to assess interventions would arguably be more compelling, with the interventions perhaps tailored to each of the dimensions provided by the four-branch model or perhaps even specific information processes. There is clearly a need to conduct these types of studies, as well as suitably designed longitudinal investigations, which would ultimately give measures of EI (if suggestive) greater impact in the occupational context.

Educational applications of EI.   Goetz et al.'s (Chapter 11) insightful chapter on educational applications of EI contains a number of suggestions for instructional techniques (both for student use and teacher implementation) that promote social emotional learning (SEL; see Zins, Weissberg, Wang, & Walberg, 2004) and other closely related constructs. Consistent with this body of work, they emphasize that person-centered approaches are insufficient; the learning environment (including teachers, administrators, the family, and community) must also support SEL.

Programs instantiating these principles have a good record of success, with beneficial outcomes reported for mental health, antisocial behaviors, and academic performance (e.g., Greenberg et al., 2003). One issue of some concern though, not necessarily addressed by Goetz et al., is that of scalability. Thus, it is unclear whether these programs can be applied across a whole nation or in locales with weaker infrastructure than those where these programs are presently implemented. It is also unclear what recent conceptions of EI add to the research described by Goetz et al. Although educational programs capitalize on enthusiasm for EI, interventions are actually tailored towards specific skills (e.g., conflict-resolution) rather than a general factor (Zeidner, Matthews, & Roberts, 2002). It is also unclear whether training general EI would be more cost-effective than focusing on the specific skills discussed by Goetz et al. (a point they certainly acknowledge).

Supposing a general factor of EI is found, the practical techniques of choice in many educational interventions will also depend on the conception adopted. Conceptions of EI can be divided into those primarily dependent on gene-environment interaction in early childhood (e.g., temperament) and those that are most directly influenced by learning and socialization (e.g., specific knowledge). In principle, temperament and information processing competencies might be altered in infancy and early childhood, within the range of reaction set by the child's genotype. However, without an adaptive analysis, there is little basis for choosing to do so (Matthews, Emo, Zeidner, & Roberts, in press).

An alternate strategy rests in exploring aptitude-by-treatment interactions, leading to recommendations that would allow the person to make best use of their emotional dispositions (Matthews, Emo, et al., in press). By contrast, providing the learner actively cooperates, emotional self-confidence, declarative knowledge, and procedural skills may be trained at any stage of life. Emotional self-confidence might be trained by assisting the person through learning experiences that build a sense of mastery. Generally, although a worthy goal, there is also a danger of building narcissism and indifference to personal limitations, commensurate with the growing awareness in psychology of the limited benefits of high self-esteem (Baumeister, Campbell, Krueger, & Vohs, 2003). Training declarative emotional knowledge appears less contentious, although, as with any skill, the person requires insight into its applicability.

These caveats notwithstanding, the Collaborative of Academic, Social, and Emotional Learning (CASEL) states that one of the main questions educators ask is how they can measure student social skills and how they can evaluate the quality and effects of SEL practices (Greenberg et al., 2003; Zins et al., 2004). To address this concern, CASEL plans to compile and create tools that (a) educators can use to assess SEL-related student outcomes and (b) schools and districts can use to assess implementation of SEL programs. Given their attempt to develop a theoretical model around educational interventions, we contend that many of the recommendations made by Goetz et al. (Chapter 11) might be of benefit to this initiative. It is hoped too that our four-source model might guide considerations related to the development of a scientifically sound assessment system for measuring the effects of SEL programs.

Clinical applications of EI.   Direct applications of EI in clinical psychology have been more cursory than in the two previous applied areas discussed, though there are a series of studies that have emerged since Parker (Chapter 13) completed the writing of his chapter and this book going to press. These include studies showing EQ-i scores to be lower in an offender population (Hemmati, Mills, & Kroner, 2004), the TMMS to be related to borderline personality disorders (Leible & Snell, 2004), and the TEIque predicting deviant behavior at school (Petrides, Frederickson, & Furnham, 2004). Various reasons might be offered for the relatively slow transition of EI to clinical applications. Related concepts like psychological mindedness have been in clinical psychology almost since its inception and may explain why the field has not so readily embraced EI; why invest resources studying an emergent construct when another with a considerable background literature, which it closely resembles, already exists? Moreover, as we noted earlier, up until the present point in time, applications of EI to understanding human behavior seem to have been directed more strongly towards positive psychology and that part of clinical psychology dealing with normal individuals: life skills coaching.

Parker (Chapter 13) does, however, provide an excellent exposition of alexithymia, a concept thought to be on the opposite end of a continuum anchored by high EI. The means for measuring alexithymia extend beyond self-report to include structured behavioral interviews and peer-ratings, with an impressive body of evidence supporting its biological, developmental, and other psychological concomitants. The fact that this concept shares moderate negative relations between self-report and performance-based measures of EI is suggestive; perhaps as with academic intelligence there is less differentiation at the lower end of the EI continuum. Even so, as with other applications, different implications for applied clinical psychology may derive from the particular form of EI assessed; how to intervene at the information processing level is less clear than how one might develop targeted clinical approaches for changing self-confidence and explicit knowledge. Parker's (Chapter 13) remarks concerning tailoring different forms of therapy (e.g., group versus individual) for individuals with alexithymia also appears worthy of consideration by those engaged in professional practice.

Social adaptation and EI.   Closing this edited volume with a chapter on the relations between EI and social adaptation is non-accidental; the sorts of criteria discussed by Engelberg and Sjöberg (Chapter 14) are precisely those that may prove essential to establishing the study of EI as a legitimate scientific discipline. As with many of the other applied areas discussed, the significance of EI to a variety of socially relevant phenomena may, however, depend on the manner that EI is assessed. Relations between performance-based measures of EI and self-reported social support do constitute one of the more impressive findings in the field to date, more so given that shared method variance (and/or criterion contamination) can not explain the observed results (see Aicher et al., 2005; Lopes et al., 2003). We are currently exploring whether these findings are replicable with some of the new measures of EI that we have developed (e.g., the AQCT) or borrowed from other disciplines (e.g., information processing measures like the Emotional Stroop).

15.4.2 What We May Have Missed

There appear a number of applied fields where we might have spent more detailed time considering the status of EI by inviting specialists in a core domain. For example, as Ciarrochi and Godsell (Chapter 4) allude, the issue of physical health and well-being may be at the core of successfully managing emotional states (see also, e.g., Pennebaker, 1997). An entire chapter devoted to that topic would not have seemed unreasonable. While Abraham (Chapter 12) covers organizational applications, there has also been a recent spate of articles devoted to specific applications of EI in medical (e.g., Bellack, Morjikian, & Barger, 2001), legal (e.g., Silver, 1999), and engineering (e.g., Marshall, 2001) professional practice. Further, as we have outlined elsewhere, there are pertinent human factors issues that research on EI might address (Matthews et al., 2003; Matthews, Emo, et al., in press). In the interests of space and time, we will outline two domains where EI is, or could readily be, applied beyond those domains of interest that we have already mentioned in this brief account. The first is gerontology, and the second, affective computing.

Aging and EI.   Having found various practical applications, as well as being considered as part of the modeling of early human development, the time would appear ripe to consider EI across the adult lifespan. Thus far, information on this relationship is scant, though there are various studies that have linked both emotional regulation and memory for emotionally salient events to chronological aging (see, e.g., Carstensen, Pasupathi, Mayr, & Nesselroade, 2000; Charles, Mather, & Carstensen, 2003; Isaacowitz, Charles, & Carstensen, 2000). Four questions related to the conceptualization, measurement, and lifespan trajectory of EI appear pertinent to a detailed investigation. These are:

1. *Are there age-related differences in EI?* No studies have determined empirically how EI might rise or fall as a function of chronological age when assessed by various methodologies or their ensuing constructs (i.e., temperament, self-confidence, processing, or knowledge measures). Conceivably, some perceptual and lower level processing components of EI change in similar function to those linked to more pure, sensory and/or cognitive processes (i.e., visual perception, Gf), while higher-order measures, requiring the investment of language, emotional understanding, and metacognitive components change in similar fashion to knowledge components (i.e., crystallized intelligence).

2. *How do age-related differences in EI compare to age-related differences in ability and personality?* Processing measures of EI are poorly understood. Because they may simply represent common processes tied to different media (i.e., emotional stimuli versus stimuli containing verbal, spatial, or numeric material), it is important to include traditional measures of fluid intelligence and processing speed, in particular, when considering the developmental trajectory of emotional processes.

3. *What does EI predict across the lifespan?* Almost all previous predictive studies have focused on adolescent or workforce samples; the outcomes predicted by EI remain poorly specified with respect to to older adults. We contend that there are several that appear theoretically justified and practically important, including quality of life, loneliness, ability to cope with stress, and physical and mental health and well-being.

4. *Are there race and gender differences in EI, and if so, do they change across the lifespan?* One of the most appealing features of EI, especially in its var-

ious popular instantiations, has been the suggestion that it counters the pessimism contained in various academic treatises that cognitive ability is destiny (e.g., Herrnstein & Murray, 1994). Being on the one hand noncognitive (because of its emotional constituents) and on the other, cognitive (because information, reasoning, and metacognitive processes are simultaneously implicated), another appeal of the EI construct appears its promise in redressing issues associated with adverse impact (see, e.g., Sackett, Schmitt, Ellingson, & Kabin, 2001). In short, EI offers hope for a more utopian, classless society, less constrained by biological heritage and conditions where assessment of it does not presuppose "destiny" (Goleman, 1995). Despite these claims, the data on group differences in EI are scant. Norms for at least one published instrument, the EQ-i (Bar-On, 1997) show substantial cross-national differences in mean EI, but no corroborative evidence has been offered to show that such differences are in any way meaningful.

We have planned a large-scale, cross-sectional multivariate study investigating these four issues. Participants, from various ethnical backgrounds and age cohorts, will be administered many of the measures previously explicated in discussion of EI measures. Using structural equation modeling, path, and regression analysis with a range of criteria measures, assessed via self-report, biographical data, and peer-report, we hope to obtain a clearer understanding of the aging of the factors circumscribing the domain of EI.

Affective computing.   Improved understanding of academic intelligence has generally been enriched by developments in both cognitive psychology and artificial intelligence (see, e.g., Carroll, 1993; Roberts et al., 2005). Significantly, leaders in the cognitive revolution, among them Simon, Norman, and Neisser, always envisaged better representation of affect in their models, a point that for many years seems to have passed relatively unnoticed (Picard et al., 2004). Over the past decade, however, there appears to have been a significant shift towards redressing this imbalance, giving rise to the field of affective computing. Picard (1997), a pioneer of this field, defines affective computing as "computing that relates to, arises from, or deliberately influences emotions ... (and includes) giving a computer the ability to recognize and express emotions, developing its ability to recognize and express emotions, and enabling it to regulate and utilize its emotions" (p. 3).

Despite being a relatively new field, affective computing boasts an impressive array of applications in the research and/or development phase. These include technologies for mirroring affect, devices for assisting those with autism and those without effective speech communication; principles for improving correspondence over the internet; technologies for improving consumer feedback; and a range of interventions aimed at improving student learning, including those based on intelligent tutors that impact (e.g., through the use of avatars) or otherwise adapt (e.g., through monitoring interest level) to the learner and her/his environment (see, e.g., Picard, 1997; Picard et al., 2004; Trappl, Petta, & Payr, 2002). Research at the MIT Media Lab also appears directed towards a variety of new measures of affective state. For example, Picard et al. (2004) report promising correlates of teacher's ratings of student affect from measures of chair pressure patterns (assessed with a device that records how postures shift during learning), upper facial features (captured using a sophisticated video camera and analyzed with a proprietary algorithm), and a skin-conductivity sensing glove that communicates wirelessly with the computer.

15.5   CONCLUSIONS

Our concluding commentary has suggested that there are many research issues requiring attention in order to advance a coherent scientific approach to the study of EI. We contend that the following are especially relevant:

1. Currently, there appear at least four different theoretical meanings attached to the concept of EI (as well as frequent conceptual confusions with other classes of construct). These different meanings carry with them various suggestions for further concept development, assessment, and real world applications. We have provided a working model that links several of these concepts, though clearly there is an urgent need to build on this model and explore its various implications both for research and practice. Related to this issue, there appears a need to develop fully formed developmental accounts, evolutionary hypotheses, genetic, biological, and cognitive models, and a scientifically grounded taxonomy. Advances in each of these domains will depend on valid measurement and carefully designed experimental, multivariate, and longitudinal studies that make use of advanced statistical procedures (e.g., polytomous IRT, Bayesian nets).

2. Across all disciplines of human endeavor, measurement is often considered that which separates science from pseudoscience. In the interests of advancing the field, we contend that a moratorium is needed on the development of still further measures assessing the more temperamental aspects of EI. Considerable resources are nonetheless required to develop and research information processing and emotional knowledge measures, in particular. Techniques should not be limited simply to existing approaches that borrow on self-assessment, consensual scoring techniques, and/or paper-and-pencil methodologies. Rather, attempts should be made to develop tests that are based in multimedia, with alternative scoring rubrics and a range of parameters, perhaps buttressed by the methods and technologies suggested from emerging advances in affective computing.

3. Applications of EI are already being touted in business, health and clinical psychology, human factors, education, and even educational policy. Conservatively, one might imagine that the science underlying the domain needs to be further advanced before its effectiveness is fully realized. At the same time, history suggests that a symbiosis between science

and practice is commonplace; the lessons learned from attempts to institute available research on EI into practice will feed into scientific models.
Disciplines covered in the section on applications, as well as those we
have added (i.e., gerontology and computer science), have previously
impacted on the development of psychology from a fledgling discipline
towards a more mature science. Prediction, implementation, intervention, and relevance to policy will ultimately stand as tests of the veracity
of the field.

We contend that each of the aforementioned issues will require a number of
scientists and practitioners to invest considerable resources of time, effort, and
intellectual capital; perhaps the current reader pursuing an academic or professional career will be among those who direct their energy towards addressing
some of these core concerns. Tantamount to such efforts will be demonstration that EI predicts important outcome variables (over and above personality
and intelligence) and buy-in from various professional bodies, testing corporations, businesses, and/or governmental agencies. Given the history of intelligence testing per se and some of the ill-conceived research programs it has
led to, it is hoped this will be done with due diligence.

Author Note

The ideas expressed in this manuscript are those of the authors and not necessarily of ETS. While both
of the first two authors are currently at ETS, they would like to acknowledge the support of both Sydney
University and the Westfälische Wilhelms-Universität Münster where they first conceptualized the idea
of this volume (and ensuing chapters), and remain affiliated. We would also like to thank the following
colleagues who have shaped ideas, contributed to technical aspects of this chapter, or are collaborating
with us in some of the studies mentioned throughout this commentary: Cristina Aicher, Paul Cruz,
Walter Emmerich, Shlomo Hareli, Kathy Howell, Rob Jagers, Larry James, Kathrin Jonkmann, Carolyn
MacCann, Jennifer Minsky, Franzis Preckel, and Katherine White.

REFERENCES

Ackerman, P. L. (1996). A theory of adult intellectual development: Process, personal-
ity, interests, and knowledge. *Intelligence, 22*, 227–257.
Aicher, C., Storladen, M., Schulze, R., Zeidner, M., Matthews, G., & Roberts, R. D.
(2005). *A multivariate investigation of emotional intelligence and social support.* Man-
uscript in preparation.
Anastasi, A., & Urbina, S. (1997). *Psychological testing* (7th ed.). Princeton, NJ: Prentice
Hall.
Bandura, A. (1999). Self-efficacy: Toward a unifying theory of behavioral change. In
R. F. Baumeister (Ed.), *The self in social psychology* (pp. 285–298). Philadelphia:
Psychology Press.
Bar-On, R. (1997). *The Emotional Intelligence Inventory (EQ–i): Technical manual.* Toronto:
Multi-Health Systems.

Bar-On, R., & Parker, J. D. A. (Eds.). (2000). *Handbook of emotional intelligence: Theory, development, assessment, and application at home, school, and in the workplace*. San Francisco: Jossey-Bass.

Baum, K. M., & Nowicki, S. (1998). Perception of emotion: Measuring decoding accuracy of adult prosodic cues varying in intensity. *Journal of Nonverbal Behavior, 22*, 89–107.

Baumeister, R. F., Campbell, J. D., Krueger, J. I., & Vohs, K. D. (2003). Does high self-esteem cause better performance, interpersonal success, happiness, or healthier lifestyles? *Psychological Science in the Public Interest, 4*, 1–44.

Baumeister, R. F., Smart, L., & Boden, J. M. (1996). Relation of threatened egotism to violence and aggression: The dark side of high self-esteem. *Psychological Review, 103*, 5–33.

Bellack, J. P., Morjikian, R., & Barger, S. (2001). Developing BSN leaders for the future: The Fuld Leadership Initiative for Nursing Education (LINE). *Journal of Professional Nursing, 17*, 23–32.

Cacioppo, J. T., Petty, R. E., Feinstein, J., & Jarvis, B. (1996). Dispositional differences in cognitive motivation: The life and times of individuals varying in need for cognition. *Psychological Bulletin, 119*, 197–253.

Campbell, J. P., & Knapp, D. J. (Eds.). (2001). *Exploring the limits in personnel selection and classification*. Mahwah, NJ: Lawrence Erlbaum.

Carroll, J. B. (1993). *Human cognitive abilities: A survey of factor-analytic studies*. New York: Cambridge University Press.

Carstensen, L. L., Pasupathi, M., Mayr, U., & Nesselroade, J. R. (2000). Emotional experience in everyday life across the adult life span. *Journal of Personality and Social Psychology, 79*, 644–655.

Charles, S. T., Mather, M., & Carstensen, L. L. (2003). Aging and emotional memory: The forgettable nature of negative images for older adults. *Journal of Experimental Psychology: General, 132*, 310–324.

Ciarrochi, J., Forgas, J. P., & Mayer, J. D. (Eds.). (2001). *Emotional intelligence in everyday life: A scientific inquiry*. New York: Psychology Press.

Cronbach, L. J. (1957). The two disciplines of scientific psychology. *American Psychologist, 12*, 671–684.

Deary, I. J., & Derr, G. (2005). Reaction time explains IQ's association with death. *Psychological Science, 16*, 64–69.

Donaldson-Feilder, E. J., & Bond, F. W. (2004). The relative importance of psychological acceptance and emotional intelligence to workplace well-being. *British Journal of Guidance & Counseling, 32*, 187–203.

Epstein, S. (1998). *Constructive thinking: The key to emotional intelligence*. New York: Praeger.

Feyerherm, A. E., & Rice, C. L. (2002). Emotional intelligence and team performance: The good, the bad and the ugly. *International Journal of Organizational Analysis, 10*, 343–362.

Gardner, H. (1993). *Frames of mind: The theory of multiple intelligences* (2nd ed.). New York: Basic Books.

Goldberg, L. R. (in press). The comparative validity of adult personality inventories: Applications of a consumer-testing framework. In S. R. Briggs, J. M. Cheek,

& E. M. Donahue (Eds.), *Handbook of adult personality inventories*. New York: Plenum.

Goleman, D. (1995). *Emotional intelligence: Why it can matter more than IQ*. New York: Bantam Books.

Goleman, D. (1998). *Working with emotional intelligence*. New York: Bantam.

Greenberg, M. T., Weissberg, R. P., O'Brien, M. U., Zins, J. E., Fredericks, L., Resnik, H., et al. (2003). Enhancing school-based prevention and youth development through coordinated social, emotional, and academic learning. *American Psychologist, 58*, 466–474.

Guttman, L., & Levy, S. (1991). Two structural laws for intelligence tests. *Intelligence, 15*, 79–103.

Hemmati, T., Mills, J. F., & Kroner, D. G. (2004). The validity of the Bar-On emotional intelligence quotient in an offender population. *Personality and Individual Differences, 37*, 695–706.

Herrnstein, R. J., & Murray, C. (1994). *The bell curve: Intelligence and class structure in American life*. New York: Free Press.

Horn, J. L., & Noll, J. (1997). Human cognitive capabilities: Gf-Gc theory. In P. Flanagan, J. L. Genshaft, & P. L. Harrison (Eds.), *Contemporary intellectual assessment: Theories, tests, and issues* (pp. 53–91). New York: Guilford.

Isaacowitz, D. M., Charles, S. T., & Carstensen, L. L. (2000). Emotion and cognition. In F. I. M. Craik & T. A. Salthouse (Eds.), *The handbook of aging and cognition* (pp. 593–631). Mahwah, NJ: Lawrence Erlbaum.

James, L. R. (1998). Measurement of personality via conditional reasoning. *Organizational Research Methods, 1*, 131–163.

James, L. R., McIntyre, M. D., Glisson, C. A., Bowler, J., & Mitchell, T. R. (in press). The conditional reasoning measurement system for aggression: An overview. *Human Performance*.

James, L. R., McIntyre, M. D., Glisson, C. A., Green, P. D., Patton, T. W., LeBreton, J. M., et al. (2005). A conditional reasoning measure for aggression. *Organizational Research Methods, 8*, 69–99.

Kyllonen, P. C., & Lee, S. (2005). Assessing problem solving in context. In O. Wilhelm & R. W. Engle (Eds.), *Understanding and measuring intelligence* (pp. 11–26). Thousand Oaks, CA: Sage.

Landy, F. (in press). Social intelligence: An historical perspective. In K. R. Murphy (Ed.), *The EI bandwagon: The struggle between science and marketing for the soul of emotional intelligence*. Mahwah, NJ: Lawrence Erlbaum.

Lane, R., Quinlan, D., Schwartz, G. E., Walker, P., & Zeitlin, S. (1990). The levels of emotional awareness scale: A cognitive–developmental measure of emotion. *Journal of Personality Assessment, 55*, 124–134.

Lazarus, R. S. (1999). *Stress and emotion: A new synthesis*. New York: Springer.

Legree, P. J. (1995). Evidence for an oblique social intelligence factor established with a Likert based testing procedure. *Intelligence, 21*, 247–266.

Leible, T. L., & Snell, W. E., Jr. (2004). Borderline personality and multiple aspects of emotional intelligence. *Personality and Individual Differences, 37*, 393–404.

Lopes, P. N., Salovey, P., & Strauss, R. (2003). Emotional intelligence, personality, and the perceived quality of social relationships. *Personality and Individual Differences, 35*, 641–658.

MacCann, C., Matthews, G., Zeidner, M., & Roberts, R. D. (2004). The assessment of emotional intelligence: On frameworks, fissures, and the future. In G. Geher (Ed.), *Measuring emotional intelligence: Common ground and controversy* (pp. 21–52). Hauppauge, NY: Nova Science.

MacCann, C., Roberts, R. D., Matthews, G., & Zeidner, M. (2004). Consensus scoring and empirical option weighting of performance-based emotional intelligence (EI) tests. *Personality and Individual Differences, 36*, 645–662.

Marshall, C. (2001). Make the most of your emotional intelligence. *Chemical Engineering Progress, 97*, 92–95.

Matsumoto, D., LeRoux, J., Wilson-Cohn, C., Raroque, J., Kooken, K., Ekman, P., et al. (2000). A new test to measure emotion recognition ability: Matsumoto and Ekman's Japanese and Caucasian Brief Affect Recognition Test (JACBART). *Journal of Nonverbal Behavior, 24*, 179–209.

Matthews, G., Emo, A., Funke, G., Zeidner, M., & Roberts, R. D. (2003). *Emotional intelligence: Implications for human factors.* In Proceedings of the Human Factors and Ergonomics Society 47th Annual Meeting (1053–1057). Santa Monica, CA: Human Factors and Ergonomics Society.

Matthews, G., Emo, A., Zeidner, M., & Roberts, R. D. (in press). What is thing called "emotional intelligence"? In K. R. Murphy (Ed.), *The EI bandwagon: The struggle between science and marketing for the soul of emotional intelligence.* Mahwah, NJ: Lawrence Erlbaum.

Matthews, G., Roberts, R. D., & Zeidner, M. (2004). Seven myths about emotional intelligence. *Psychological Inquiry, 15*, 179–196.

Matthews, G., & Wells, A. (1999). The cognitive science of attention and emotion. In T. Dalgleish & M. Power (Eds.), *Handbook of cognition and emotion* (pp. 171–192). New York: John Wiley.

Matthews, G., Zeidner, M., & Roberts, R. D. (2002). *Emotional intelligence: Science and myth.* Cambridge, MA: MIT Press.

Matthews, G., Zeidner, M., & Roberts, R. D. (2005). Emotional intelligence: An elusive ability. In O. Wilhelm & R. W. Engle (Eds.), *Understanding and measuring intelligence* (pp. 79–99). Thousand Oaks, CA: Sage.

Matthews, G., Zeidner, M., & Roberts, R. D. (in press-a). Measuring emotional intelligence: Promises, pitfalls, solutions? In A. D. Ong & M. Van Dulmen (Eds.), *Handbook of methods in positive psychology.* Oxford, UK: Oxford University Press.

Matthews, G., Zeidner, M., & Roberts, R. D. (in press-b). Personality, affect, and emotional development. In P. A. Alexander & P. Winne (Eds.), *Handbook of research in educational psychology.* Mahwah, NJ: Lawrence Erlbaum.

Mayer, J. D., Salovey, P., Caruso, D. R., & Sitarenios, G. (2003). Measuring emotional intelligence with the MSCEIT V2.0. *Emotion, 3*, 97–105.

Neisser, U., Boodoo, G., Bouchard, T. J., Jr., Boykin, A. W., Brody, N., Ceci, S. J., et al. (1996). Intelligence: Knowns and unknowns. *American Psychologist, 51*, 77–101.

Nowicki, S., & Carton, J. (1993). The measurement of emotional intensity from facial expressions. *Journal of Social Psychology, 133*, 749–750.

O'Brien, K., MacCann, C., Reid, J., Schulze, R., & Roberts, R. D. (2005). *Emotional intelligence, emotional recognition ability, and intelligence.* Manuscript in preparation.

Pallier, G., Wilkinson, R., Danthiir, V., Kleitman, S., Knezevic, G., Stankov, L., et al. (2002). The role of question format and individual differences in the realism of confidence judgments. *Journal of General Psychology, 129,* 257–295.

Pennebaker, J. W. (1997). Writing about emotional experiences as a therapeutic process. *Psychological Science, 8,* 162–166.

Petrides, K. V., Frederickson, N., & Furnham, A. (2004). The role of trait emotional intelligence in academic performance and deviant behavior at school. *Personality and Individual Differences, 36,* 277–293.

Picard, R. W. (1997). *Affective computing.* Cambridge, MA: MIT Press.

Picard, R. W., Papert, S., Bender, W., Blumberg, B., Breazel, C., Cavallo, D., et al. (2004). Affective learning: A manifesto. *BT Technology Journal, 22,* 253–269.

Roberts, R. D., Markham, P. M., Zeidner, M., & Matthews, G. (2005). Assessing intelligence: Past, present, and future. In O. Wilhelm & R. W. Engle (Eds.), *Understanding and measuring intelligence* (pp. 333–360). Thousand Oaks, CA: Sage.

Roberts, R. D., & Stankov, L. (1999). Individual differences in speed of mental processing and human cognitive abilities: Towards a taxonomic model. *Learning and Individual Differences, 11,* 1–120.

Rothbart, M. K., & Bates, J. E. (1998). Temperament. In W. Damon & N. Eisenberg (Eds.), *Handbook of child psychology: Vol. 3. Social, emotional, and personality development* (5th ed., pp. 105–176). New York: John Wiley.

Rusting, C. L., & Larsen, R. (1998). Personality and cognitive processing of affective information. *Personality and Social Psychology Bulletin, 24,* 200–213.

Sackett, P. R., Schmitt, N., Ellingson, J. E., & Kabin, M. B. (2001). High stakes testing in employment, credentialing, and higher education: Prospects in a post-affirmative action world. *American Psychologist, 56,* 302–318.

Salovey, P., Bedell, B. T., Detweiler, J. B., & Mayer, J. D. (1999). Coping intelligently: Emotional intelligence and the coping process. In C. R. Snyder (Ed.), *Coping: The psychology of what works* (pp. 141–164). New York: Oxford University Press.

Salovey, P., Mayer, J. D., & Caruso, D. R. (2002). The positive psychology of emotional intelligence. In C. R. Snyder & S. J. Lopez (Eds.), *Handbook of positive psychology* (pp. 159–171). London: Oxford University Press.

Scherer, K. R. (2001). Appraisal considered as a process of multilevel sequential checking. In K. R. Scherer, A. Schorr, & T. Johnstone (Eds.), *Appraisal processes in emotion: Theory, methods, research* (pp. 92–120). London: Oxford University Press.

Scherer, K. R., Banse, R., & Wallbott, H. (2001). Emotion inferences from vocal expression correlate across languages and cultures. *Journal of Cross-Cultural Psychology, 32,* 76–92.

Schmidt, F. L., & Hunter, J. E. (1998). The validity and utility of selection methods in personnel psychology: Practical and theoretical implications of 85 years of research findings. *Psychological Bulletin, 124,* 262–274.

Schulze, R. (2004). *Meta-analysis: A comparison of approaches.* Seattle, WA: Hogrefe & Huber.

Shimazu, A., & Kosugi, S. (2003). Job stressors, coping, and psychological distress among Japanese employees: Interplay between active and non-active coping. *Work and Stress, 17,* 38–51.

Shimokawa, A., Yatomi, N., Anamizu, S., Ashikari, I., Kohno, M., Maki, Y., et al. (2000). Comprehension of emotions: Comparison between Alzheimer type and vascular type dementias. *Dementia and Geriatric Cognitive Disorders, 11,* 268–274.

Silver, M. A. (1999). Emotional intelligence and legal education. *Psychological Public Policy, 5,* 1173–1203.

Slaski, M., & Cartwright, S. (2002). Health, performance and emotional intelligence: An exploratory study of retail managers. *Stress and Health, 18,* 63–68.

Spearman, C. (1927). *The abilities of man: Their nature and measurement.* London: Macmillan.

Sternberg, R. J. (1985). *Beyond IQ: A triarchic theory of human intelligence.* New York: Cambridge University Press.

Thorndike, E. L. (1920). Intelligence and its use. *Harper's Magazine, 140,* 227–235.

Trappl, R., Petta, P., & Payr, S. (Eds.). (2002). *Emotions in humans and artifacts.* Cambridge, MA: MIT Press.

Van Rooy, D. L., & Viswesvaran, C. (2004). Emotional intelligence: A meta-analytic investigation of predictive validity and nomological net. *Journal of Vocational Behavior, 65,* 71–95.

Wells, A., & Matthews, G. (Eds.). (1994). *Attention and emotion: A clinical perspective.* Hove, UK: Lawrence Erlbaum.

Wilhelm, O., Schulze, R., Schmiedek, F., & Süß, H.-M. (2003). Interindividuelle Unterschiede im typischen intellektuellen Engagement [Individual differences in typical intellectual engagement]. *Diagnostica, 49,* 49–60.

Zeidner, M., Matthews, G., & Roberts, R. D. (2001). Slow down, you move too fast: Emotional intelligence remains an "elusive" intelligence. *Emotion, 1,* 265–275.

Zeidner, M., Matthews, G., & Roberts, R. D. (2002). Can emotional intelligence be schooled? A critical review. *Educational Psychologist, 37,* 215–231.

Zeidner, M., Matthews, G., & Roberts, R. D. (2004). Emotional intelligence in the workplace: A critical review. *Applied Psychology: An International Review, 53,* 371–399.

Zeidner, M., Matthews, G., & Roberts, R. D. (in press). Emotional intelligence, adaptation, and coping. In J. Ciarrochi, J. P. Forgas, & J. D. Mayer (Eds.), *Emotional intelligence in everyday life: A scientific inquiry* (2nd ed.). Philadelphia: Psychology Press.

Zeidner, M., Matthews, G., Roberts, R. D., & MacCann, C. (2003). Development of emotional intelligence: Towards a multi-level investment model. *Human Development, 46,* 69–96.

Zeidner, M., Roberts, R. D., & Matthews, G. (2002). Can emotional intelligence be schooled? A critical review. *Educational Psychologist, 37,* 215–231.

Zins, J. E., Weissberg, R. P., Wang, M. C., & Walberg, H. J. (Eds.). (2004). *Building school success through social and emotional learning: Implications for practice and research.* New York: Teachers College Press.

Author Index

Subject Index